THE GRAYING OF AMERICA

The
GRAYING
of
AMERICA

· ·

AN ENCYCLOPEDIA OF
AGING, HEALTH, MIND,
AND BEHAVIOR

· ·

Donald H. Kausler and
Barry C. Kausler

University of Illinois Press
URBANA AND CHICAGO

© 1996 by Donald H. Kausler and Barry C. Kausler
Manufactured in the United States of America
C 5 4 3 2 1

This book is printed on acid-free paper.

Library of Congress Cataloging-in-Publication Data

Kausler, Donald H.
    The graying of America: an encyclopedia of aging, health, mind,
and behavior / Donald H. Kausler and Barry C. Kausler.
        p.   cm.
    Includes indexes.
    ISBN 0-252-02159-2 (cloth: acid-free paper)
    1. Aged—United States—Encyclopedias.   2. Aging—United States—
Encyclopedias.   3. Old age—United States—Encyclopedias.
4. Gerontology—United States—Encyclopedias.   I. Kausler, Barry
C., 1961– . II. Title.
HQ1064.U5K39   1996
305.26'03—dc20   95-8810
                                                                 CIP

Contents

. . . .

91/79

Introduction

· ·

In 1870 the first census of people in the United States who were 65 years of age or older was conducted. It was estimated that about 1.2 million people (3%) of the total population of 40 million were "old." The years since 1870 have seen a remarkable phenomenon—the graying of America. The years between 1960 and 1980 were especially dramatic ones in their contribution to the graying phenomenon. From 1960 to 1980 the total population of the United States increased about 19%, but the population of people age 65 and older increased by about 35%. In 1980 there were about 25 million people age 65 and older. The phenomenon has not diminished since 1980. Today it is estimated that there are about 31 million people who are age 65 or older (about 12% of the total population), and that by the year 2030 the number of "old" people may reach 66 million. Moreover, the expansion of the elderly population has been especially pronounced for the "old" old, those individuals age 85 and older. The proportion of the "old" old in our total population has seen dramatic increases in recent years. As viewers of the *Today* television program know, it is no longer unusual to encounter people who have aged normally beyond 100 years.

The graying of America has brought with it an ever-increasing need to understand what happens as we age. Organisms *do* age, and the human organism is no exception. In fact, aging begins at birth and continues throughout life. We have come to realize that aging is as inevitable as death and taxes. What makes human aging unique among organisms is that human beings alone are aware of their own aging and may anticipate its consequences. Fortunately, the rapid increase in the number of older people in our population has been accompanied by a comparable expansion in research on aging. The past 20 years have been especially productive ones for research on the biology, psychology, and sociology of aging. This research has provided an enhanced understanding of how aging, both normal and abnormal, affects our health, our mental abilities, and our personal and social behaviors. The outcome has been to replace many myths about aging with knowledge derived from research. The objective of this book is to relate in nontechnical language the results of this research about health, mental functioning, and social functioning.

The format of this book is encyclopedic. That is, the more than 300 entries covering many topics about aging are arranged in alphabetical order. These entries are listed in the first index, along with many subtopics that are discussed within the contents of the entries and with many cross-references to entries where additional information may be found. For example, arthritis is listed with reference to the entry on diseases, and bereavement with reference to the entry on widowhood and widowerhood. Many of the entries themselves also include cross-references to other entries relevant to their topics. To facilitate finding information about topics of particular interest to any reader, a second index follows the first. It identifies broad areas of aging (e.g., adjustment in aging, stress, and coping with stress; mental capabilities and functions; and physical and mental health), and individual entries relevant to each area are listed accordingly.

Many of the entries deal with mental functions and how they are affected by aging. These include such topics as intelligence, learning, memory, problem solving, and reasoning. Myths abound about our mental functioning as we grow old; many of these myths have been dispelled by scientific evidence. For example, contrary to popular belief, senility is *not* inevitable with aging, nor are all components of memory greatly affected by aging. Our intent is to relate, in nontechnical language, the current knowledge of each of these mental functions as they are affected by both normal aging and abnormal aging (e.g., Alzheimer's disease). Our behavior is certainly affected as we age by changes in the senses of hearing, vision, smell, taste, touch, and pain. The entries on the senses summarize what is presently known about age-related changes in sensory functioning.

Knowing what happens to both physical and mental health with aging is of great importance to understanding aging. Relevant entries in this area deal with such topics as exercise and health, diseases associated with late adulthood, the aging brain, alcohol consumption, drug abuse, anxiety, depression, psychosis, neurosis, stress and coping with stress, suicide, and senility caused by Alzheimer's disease and other diseases that affect the brain, such as multi-infarct dementia (stroke). Also included are entries on the tests and procedures commonly used to diagnose depression, to diagnose Alzheimer's disease, to treat mental health problems, and to evaluate personality and intelligence. Other entries discuss the concerns and the means of alleviating the burdens of the caregivers for mentally or physically impaired older adults.

The human organism plays many social roles, and older adults are no exception. Several entries deal with the various ways that aging affects these roles. Thus there are entries on friendships, sibling relationships, parenthood, grandparenting, widowhood and widowerhood, retirement, religion, sexuality, and death and dying, as well as many other entries.

Finally, there are a number of entries that provide general information about aging and the individuals and organizations involved in aging research. These entries are intended to inform you of the ways in which aging may be defined, the demography of aging, the current theories of why we age, the major long-term aging studies currently being conducted, and the national organizations that are relevant to aging and our elderly population.

A cautionary note must be sounded. Aging research is usually characterized by the reporting of *averages* for different age groups, with an indication of the variability around those averages. In some cases, research reveals that *on the average* elderly adults perform at a level below that of younger adults. For example, this finding may be true for some forms of memory and memory functions. However, it is important to realize that many elderly adults perform at a level that exceeds that of the average younger adults, even though the average performance for elderly adults may be below that for younger adults.

The information reported in our entries is derived from numerous sources. Much of the information was taken directly from research reports in major journals dealing with human aging, such as *The Gerontologist, The Journals of Gerontology, Psychology and Aging, Experimental Aging Research, Developmental Psychology, Human Development, Educational Gerontologist,* and *International Journal on Aging and Human Development.* Other information came from recent textbooks on human aging and from more advanced technical books. Both the journals and the books are likely to be found in a university library, and they should be available to you for further reading on the various topics covered in this book. A listing of the books is given below.

Textbooks

Cavanaugh, J. C. (1993). *Adult development and aging* (2nd ed.). Belmont, CA: Wadsworth Publishing Company.

Hayslip, B., Jr., & Panek, P. E. (1993). *Adult development and aging* (2nd ed.). New York: Harper Collins.

Huyck, M. H., & Hoyer, W. J. (1982). *Adult development and aging.* Belmont, CA: Wadsworth Publishing Company.

Kimmel, D. C. (1990). *Adulthood and aging* (3rd ed.). New York: John Wiley & Sons.

Rebok, G. W. (1987). *Life-span cognitive development.* New York: Holt, Rinehart, & Winston.

Schaie, K. W., & Willis, S. L. (1991). *Adult development and aging* (3rd ed.). New York: Harper Collins.

Schulz, R., & Ewen, R. B. (1988). *Adult development and aging: Myths and emerging realities.* New York: Macmillan.

Woodruff-Pak, D. (1988). *Psychology and aging.* Englewood Cliffs, NJ: Prentice Hall.

Advanced Technical Books

Binstock, R. H., & George, L. K. (Eds.). (1990). *Handbook of aging and the social sciences* (3rd ed.). San Diego: Academic Press.

Birren, J. E., & Schaie, K. W. (Eds.). (1990). *Handbook of the psychology of aging* (3rd ed.). San Diego: Academic Press.

Kart, C. S., Metress, E. K., & Metress, S. P. (Eds.). (1988). *Aging, health and society.* Boston: Jones and Bartlett Publishers.

Kausler, D. H. (1991). *Experimental psychology, cognition, and human aging.* New York: Springer-Verlag.

Kausler, D. H. (1994). *Learning and memory in normal aging.* San Diego: Academic Press.

Lewis, C. B. (Ed.). (1994). *Aging: The health care challenge.* Philadelphia: FA Davis Company.

Maddox, G. L., Atchley, R. C., Poon, L. W., Roth, G. S., Siegler, I. C., & Steinberg, R. M. (Eds.). (1987). *The encyclopedia of aging.* New York: Springer-Verlag.

THE GRAYING OF AMERICA

Abilities (Physical and Mental) and Activity

Running, jumping, throwing a baseball. These are all physical abilities nearly all of us possess—but in levels of skill that vary from low to very high. Few people are truly competitive in a marathon race, and few of us could even complete one. Virtually none of us could challenge Carl Lewis in jumping or Nolan Ryan in the speed of throwing a baseball. These are all examples of physical abilities. Individual differences clearly exist at all age levels. The average levels of such physical abilities do change with normal aging. In general, they tend to decline, but the extent of the decline depends on many other factors besides aging itself. Certainly health and regular exercise are critical factors. There is considerable evidence to indicate that physical abilities remain at a much higher level for those elderly adults who are in good health, are physically active, and who have been long-time regular exercisers (see Exercise and Physical/Mental Performance). Although it is highly unlikely that an elderly adult will win the Boston Marathon, it is true that many elderly adults do complete a marathon race. Muscle strength in elderly people can be increased, especially by following a training program that requires the appropriate exercise.

A number of physical abilities are specific to those individuals who acquired them through learning and practice early in life. Typing and playing the piano are examples. There is also evidence revealing that such skills are retained at a relatively constant level well into late adulthood, provided good health is retained and the skills have been practiced regularly and intensively over the years. This is the case for professional typists (see EXPERTISE) and for professional pianists (see MOTOR SKILL LEARNING).

Most of us also possess a number of mental abilities, such as reasoning ability, spatial ability, and verbal ability. There are large individual differences in the amount of ability at all age levels. Average levels of most mental abilities change with normal aging. Some decline modestly with aging, whereas others remain relatively constant, and still others may even increase by late adulthood. Those abilities that decline are components of what psychologists call fluid intelligence (see INTELLIGENCE). Spatial ability is an example. However, we know that elderly adults who had a high level of spatial ability as young adults continue to have a high level as elderly adults, relative to other elderly adults and even to most young adults (see SPATIAL ABILITY). Reading ability is another example of an ability that shows modest declines with normal aging. Elderly adults do read, on the average, more slowly than younger adults, and they also demonstrate less comprehension of what they read, but only when the material contains complex phrasing (see READING SKILLS). We also know that at least some of the declines in late adulthood can be reversed by appropriate interventions, such as training and practice (see MEMORY TRAINING; PLASTICITY THEORY; TRANSFER OF LEARNING/TRAINING). Whether "mental exercise" of various kinds (e.g., playing chess, bridge, or other challenging mental games) aids in retaining mental skills is still an unresolved issue (see ACTIVITY AND MENTAL PERFORMANCE). Also largely unresolved is the role that might be played by lifelong physical exercise in maintaining these abilities at the levels achieved earlier in adulthood (see EXERCISE AND PHYSICAL/MENTAL PERFORMANCE). Those abilities that remain relatively constant, and often increase in amounts, are components of what is called crystallized intelligence (see INTELLIGENCE). An example is wisdom, an ability that clearly increases from early to late adulthood (see WISDOM). Other examples are verbal ability and general knowledge. On the average, elderly people score higher than younger adults on vocabulary tests and tests of general knowledge about the world (see INTELLIGENCE; VERBAL ABILITY; WECHSLER INTELLIGENCE TESTS).

Abnormal Aging

People who age abnormally function at levels well below those of people who age normally. Abnormal aging is used in reference either to major problems in adjustment, as found in psychosis (see PSYCHOSIS) and clinical depression (see DEPRESSION) or to major problems in mental functioning to the point of dementia (see ALZHEIMER'S DISEASE; DEMENTIA; MULTI-INFARCT DEMENTIA). Dementia is characterized primarily by memory problems that exceed those found in normal aging (see AGE-ASSOCIATED MEMORY IMPAIRMENT), problems in orientation to time and place, and attentional problems. More than 5% of the population age 65 or older has dementia. The percentage affected by dementia increases with age, becoming greater than 20% for those age 85 or over. Alzheimer's disease accounts for more than half of the cases of dementia.

Accidents (at Home)

The incidence of accidents at home is the greatest for children and elderly people. Not only is the rate of home accidents (falls, burns, accidental poisoning, and so on) greater for people age 65 and older than for younger adults, but the incidence of disability and death resulting from such accidents is also increased. The high incidence in late adulthood undoubtedly is the consequence of decreased visual ability, decreased mobility, and decreased balance, relative to earlier adulthood.

Accidents (at Work)

Older workers have a lower frequency of minor accidents and temporary injuries on the job than do younger workers. A large 1981 study of workmen's compensation records reported that the highest injury rate was for workers age 20 to 24 years and that the lowest rate was for workers age 65 and older. At the same time, time off from work as a result of these injuries is greater for older than for younger workers. Injuries resulting in death or disability are also more frequent for older workers. A major factor in the age difference in injury rates is job experience. A large proportion of job injuries occur during a worker's first year, regardless of the worker's age. In addition, less qualified people tend to be removed from jobs before they reach an advanced age. Thus most older workers are those who benefit from experience and those who have demonstrated their competence on the job.

Accidents (Automobile)

In recent years the number of automobile drivers who are 65 years old and older has been steadily increasing. Also steadily increasing has been the average number of miles driven annually by people in this age range. Unfortunately, elderly drivers also have more accidents per miles driven and more fatalities per miles driven than any other age group except the youngest drivers. Elderly adults also have the highest fatality rate for pedestrians involved in automobile accidents—about one-fourth of pedestrian fatalities involve elderly adults. They also experience more traffic violations per miles driven than any other age group. Older adults are less likely to be involved in accidents involving excessive speed, reckless driving, or intoxication than are younger drivers. Accidents involving older adults are more likely to be caused by failure to see traffic signs, failure to yield the right-of-way, making unsafe turns, stopping unnecessarily (causing rear-end collisions), and improper highway entrance and exit. Interestingly, the incidence of accidents involving pilots of private planes who are in their 60s and 70s is less than the incidence of such accidents for younger adults.

Driving an automobile is primarily a visual task. It is estimated that more than 90% of the information a driver must analyze is visual in nature. Aging is accompanied by declining proficiency in many components of vision (see VISION). Some of these declines are undoubtedly related to the greater accident-proneness experienced by elderly drivers, relative to younger drivers. Researchers at the University of Alabama at Birmingham recently provided convincing evidence that a primary factor in the high accident rate of elderly drivers is the shrinkage that occurs with aging in the useful field of vision. The useful field of vision is the extent of the visual periphery needed to perform the visual task at hand. Objects in the periphery must be detected by a driver in order for the driver to shift attention and focus on them. The researchers found that those elderly drivers with an especially large amount of shrinkage of the useful field of vision accounted for 95% of the intersection accidents surveyed in their study. Another visual function that is especially important in driving is the estimation of the velocity of an automobile being observed. Elderly adults are more likely to underestimate velocity than are younger adults. Such underestimation is surely another major contributor to the high rate of accidents for elderly adults, especially accidents involving intersection crossings and merging a car into a line of traffic. Unfortunately, tests of the useful field of vision and vehicular velocity are not included in the visual tests administered to elderly drivers when they renew their driver's licenses.

Visual impairment, however, is not the only likely contributor to the driving accidents experienced by elderly drivers. Reaction time is slower for elderly adults than it is for younger adults (see REACTION TIME). When events in a driver's pathway call for rapid braking of the car, it is likely that an elderly driver will respond more slowly than a younger driver, thus increasing the risk of an accident. Mental processes are also involved in the effective driving of an automobile. At times decisions must be made as to when it is safe to pass another vehicle, the appropriate speed for given driving conditions, and so on. Memory is not spared as a component of safe driving. Remembering that a specific road sign indicates an upcoming curve surely signals a reduction in speed. Similarly, one needs to remember especially dangerous intersections and approach them cautiously. Even mildly mentally impaired elderly adults are clearly at a greater risk than normally aging elderly drivers, given their poorer orientation and memory functioning, yet some of these individuals are still driving automobiles. A study in New Jersey indicated that one-fourth of the outpatients in a dementia diagnostic clinic were still driving. Of these drivers, more than 75% had a history during the past year of "abnormal" driving habits as indicated by such incidents as getting lost, having accidents, or receiving traffic tickets.

Researchers in Florida reported that elderly women are twice as likely as elderly men to stop driving voluntarily. For a large sample of community-dwelling, ambulatory people age 70 and older, about 17% had voluntarily stopped driving. More than 30% of the people who were no longer driving cited health concerns as the reason for not driving. Researchers at Yale University found that diminished physical activity and reduced income were also factors contributing to the cessation of driving for a sample of elderly adults in New Haven.

A very sensitive, frequently debated issue is whether drivers should receive more thorough testing for license renewal when they reach a specifically designated age. Should these drivers be required to demonstrate their competence for operating an automobile by means of tests other than a routine vision test? Such testing has been proposed by various states from time to time. Sensitivity enters the picture by the charge that selective testing is a form of age discrimination and the practice of ageism. Of course, this issue could be resolved by requiring people of *all* ages to undergo vigorous testing whenever they renew their licenses. In 1991 there were seven states (California, Connecticut, Delaware, Nevada, New Jersey, Oregon, and Pennsylvania) that required physicians to report patients with apparent serious driving impairments. There were eight other states that authorized, but did not require, physicians to make these reports. Researchers in Massachusetts have demonstrated that reliable ratings of elderly drivers by competent observers can be made when they are required to drive in traffic. These ratings were found to correlate fairly substantially with scores on a mental test—the less the mental competence and alertness of the elderly driver, the poorer the driving ability as measured by performance on the test drive.

Action Memory

"Did I turn out the lights in my car when I left it in the parking lot?" "Did I turn off the stove before leaving the kitchen?" "Was it last week Tuesday or Wednesday that I mowed the lawn?" In each of these questions, the person is testing his or her memory for actions or activities personally performed during daily living. It is not unusual to discover that our memory of our own performances is often impaired. That is, we sometimes have trouble remembering what actions we did perform or remembering when those actions were performed. The remarkable thing, however, is that we do have rather good memory of our own actions, even though we are unlikely to have the intent to remember them. We don't ordinarily say to ourselves, "I locked the door" repeatedly while making a deliberate attempt to remember to commit that action to memory. That is, our memory for actions performed is usually incidental rather than intentional.

Of interest in gerontology is the extent to which action memory diminishes in proficiency from early to late adulthood. Elderly adults report most frequently that they have trouble remembering whether they turned off the stove or left the door unlocked. Researchers have brought action memory into the laboratory by having participants of different ages perform a series of simple actions, such as clapping their hands and placing a cup on a saucer. After the series is completed, memory is then tested by either trying to recall the actions or by trying to recognize those that had just been performed from a list of actions. Several interesting findings have emerged from studies using this procedure. Participants who know their memory will be tested after the series has been completed score no higher on a recall test or a recognition test than do participants who are unaware of the subsequent memory tests. That is, incidental memory is as proficient as intentional memory. This is true regardless of the participants' age. Both elderly and young participants have virtually perfect recognition memory scores. They have no difficulty recognizing which actions had been performed and which actions in the list had not been performed. However, there is a fairly substantial age difference in the recall of actions. Young adults typically recall about 75% of those performed, and elderly adults recall only about 60%. Other researchers have found little difference for either young adult or elderly participants between the recall of unfamiliar actions (e.g., placing a straw in your ear) and familiar actions (e.g., placing a straw in a glass). The age difference in recall of actions may partially be the result of the greater difficulty experienced by elderly adults than younger adults in retrieving information that has been stored in memory. It is also likely that actions are encoded (i.e., converted into a memory trace) more thoroughly by younger than by older adults. Sufficient information about actions is probably encoded by elderly adults to permit eventual recognition of what they had been doing, but it may not be enough to permit recall of a number of those actions.

Are there any interventions that improve the recall of one's own actions? To date, this is a largely unexplored topic. No one has determined, for example, whether elderly adults who have been regular, long-term physical exercisers have better action memories than elderly adults who have lived less physically active lives (see EXERCISE AND PHYSICAL/MENTAL PERFORMANCE). However, researchers at the University of Missouri–Columbia have discovered what may be an effective mnemonic for improving recall of actions somewhat (perhaps as much as 20%) regardless of age. Young adult and elderly participants were required to recall after every few actions those that had just been performed. That is, short-term recall was required for each action in the series. Short-term recall was especially beneficial to later recall if there was a brief retention interval during which the participants performed some interfering activity, such as counting backward by three from a designated number. Short-term recall of actions seems to be beneficial to later long-term recall only if it is both somewhat effortful (as it is after an interval filled with an interfering activity) and successful. Older adults who wish to improve recall of their own actions in the everyday world should try this short-term retrieval procedure. For example, if three successive actions are turning off the lights in the living room, letting out the dog, and shutting off the garden hose, try recalling the last actions performed shortly after shutting off the hose. It should help them to recall later when they have entered the bedroom that the lights are off in the living room, that the dog is still outside, and that the hose is off.

Of further interest is the age difference in temporal memory for actions performed in the laboratory (see TEMPORAL MEMORY). Here the demand is on remembering *when* an action is performed, and not on what actions were performed. Age differences for temporal memory are tested by having participants perform a series of actions; participants then reconstruct the temporal order in which they were performed. In several studies, substantial age differences, favoring young adults, have been found in the proficiency of making these time-oriented judgments. Temporal memory, whether for actions performed in the laboratory or for words viewed sequentially in a list, appears to be a highly age-sensitive form of memory.

Activities of Daily Living

It is estimated that more than 80% of the behaviors of older people occur in the home. Moreover, about one-third of each day is spent on behaviors termed the *activities of daily living* (activities for maintaining normal home living). A survey of healthy elderly people living independently in the community revealed that, on the average, they spend daily 53 minutes on personal and health care activities, 77 minutes on eating, 68 minutes on housework and home maintenance, 69 minutes on cooking, and 22 minutes on shopping. These averages are somewhat different for impaired older people (e.g., those receiving in-home services). For example, they were found to average 71 minutes daily in personal and health care activities and only 38 minutes on housework and home maintenance. For what may be considered optional activities, the unimpaired and impaired elderly people were found to be fairly equivalent in the average daily time spent reading (59 and 52 minutes, respectively) and watching television (205 and 210 minutes, respectively). However, a major difference was found in the average time spent resting and relaxing (128 minutes for the unimpaired and 200 minutes for the impaired).

Of further interest is the difficulty experienced by elderly people in performing the activities of daily living. A national survey indicated that the percentage of elderly people who expressed difficulty in performing an activity varied greatly with the nature of the activity. For example, less than 2% expressed difficulty in eating and less than 5% in using the toilet. By contrast, nearly 10% expressed difficulty in bathing and nearly 20% in walking. However, for all of these activities the percentage of elderly people who actually received help to perform them was quite small (e.g., 6% for bathing).

Researchers at the University of Chicago recently reported that people who are age 70 and older and who have visual impairments are nearly one and a half times more likely to have difficulty in performing the activities of daily living than are people of the same ages who do not have such impairments. They also reported the absence of a relationship between hearing impairment and performance of daily activities for people in the same age range.

Elderly women with upper body disability have been found to have more difficulty in performing daily activities than elderly men with a similar disability. This is probably because dressing oneself usually requires more dexterity for women than for men. On the other hand, the reverse is true for lower body disability (i.e., elderly men have more difficulty than elderly women). This sex difference may be related to the greater willingness of women than of men to seek assistance in performing activities requiring lower body strength. Limitations in performing the daily activities produced by diseases are greatest for elderly people with cardiovascular disease or arthritis.

Activity and Mental Performance

"Use it or lose it"—a statement often heard in reference to aging and the mind. The implication is that elderly people need frequent "exercise" of their minds or they risk significant decline in their mental functioning. Do elderly adults who regularly engage in challenging mental activities, such as playing bridge, playing chess, and solving crossword puzzles, perform better on memory tasks and intelligence tests than elderly adults who are less mentally active in their everyday lives? Unfortunately, the evidence on this important issue is ambiguous.

On the one hand, several studies have revealed that older people who are currently college students perform no better on laboratory memory tasks or on intelligence tests than older people who have been away from an academic setting for many years. Taking college courses should surely qualify as a source of vigorous regular mental activity. On the other hand, there is evidence provided by Canadian researchers that older men who report frequent participation in challenging mental activities (e.g., chess) score higher on an intelligence test than less mentally active older men. Similarly, researchers in California have found that long-term skilled elderly bridge players score higher on memory tasks than do nonplaying elderly people. Researchers at the University of Victoria found that elderly people who live an active life-style score higher on tests of fluid intelligence (see INTELLIGENCE) than elderly people who have a more passive life-style. Of course, one could argue that those older people who engage in demanding mental activities were brighter throughout their lives than other older people. Current mental activity could contribute little to the better mental functioning exhibited by those who engage in it. Especially impressive evidence for the potentially positive effects of a high level of mental activity late in life comes from a study conducted at Harvard University. Physicians older than age 65 who were still working as physicians scored, on the average, much higher on a variety of mental tests than physicians of the same age who were retired.

More research is needed to determine exactly the effects of mental activity during late adulthood on reducing, or even possibly eliminating, mental decline with normal aging.

Activity (Productive)

Activity is considered to be productive when it produces goods or services, regardless of whether pay is received for it. Productive activities include housework, child care, volunteer work, and help provided for family members and friends, as well as work on salaried occupations. A common belief is that men and women become increasingly similar to one another in the kinds of productive activities they perform as they grow older. This does not appear to be true, however. Older men tend to do more paid work outside the home and more household maintenance work than do older women. Older women tend to do more housework, more child care in the home, more caregiving outside the home, and more volunteer work than do older men. Married and unmarried older men and women appear to be similar to unmarried older men and women in paid work outside the home. In general, older people who are in good health engage in more productive activity than do those older people who are less healthy. This is true for men and women and whites and blacks. There are, however, some racial differences in productive activity for older people. Blacks are less likely to retire early from paid work than are whites. In terms of work around the house, older black women and men tend to engage in equal amounts, in contrast to the pattern found for older white women and men (see also PARTICIPATION IN VOLUNTEER ORGANIZATIONS AND VOLUNTEER WORK).

Another kind of productive activity is that conducted by residents of nursing homes. It has long been known that activities of various kinds are beneficial to the welfare of the residents. In fact, in 1987 Congress passed a bill that mandated nursing homes to provide activities for their residents if they were to receive federal funds. The problem, however, is to get residents involved in activities. Residents do differ greatly in the amount of time they spend in activities. Researchers in Michigan observed residents in a number of nursing homes. They discovered that women tend to spend more time in activities than do men. They also discovered that nondepressed residents spent more time in activities than did depressed residents and that the time spent on activities decreased as the degree of mental impairment increased. Not surprisingly, they also discovered that the least time was spent by those residents who needed the greatest assistance in performing the activities of daily living (see ACTIVITIES OF DAILY LIVING).

Activity Theory

Activity theory is concerned with the conditions that promote a high level of satisfaction with life in late adulthood. It began in a rough form at the University of Chicago during the 1960s in opposition to the then-popular disengagement theory, which stressed that withdrawal from social activity is the best condition for successful aging (see DIS-ENGAGEMENT THEORY). Activity theory initially stated that optimal satisfaction occurs when elderly people continue as much as possible the activities of middle age and find substitutes for those activities that are prohibited by any declining abilities. A more systematic theory was proposed in the 1970s by gerontologists at the University of Southern California. Their theory specified three forms of activity and ordered them in terms of the magnitudes of the effects each should have on life satisfaction. The first form is *informal activity,* such as activities with friends, relatives, and neighbors. The second is *formal activity,* such as participation in voluntary organizations. The third is *solitary activity,* such as leisure pursuits and maintenance of a household. Each form was expected to increase life satisfaction as the amount of that activity increased. However, the beneficial effects of informal activity were expected to be greater than the effects of formal activity which, in turn, were expected to be greater than the effects of solitary activity.

In a test of their own theory, the gerontologists at the University of Southern California found only partial support for the theory. Only informal activity was found to be positively related to the degree of life satisfaction, and then only moderately so. A more thorough test of the theory was conducted in the 1980s by researchers at the University of Miami. They too found informal activity to be moderately and positively related to the degree of life satisfaction. However, they also found formal activity to be negatively related to life satisfaction—that is, the greater the amount of formal activity, in general, the less the degree of life satisfaction. Other research on life satisfaction in late adulthood has revealed that life satisfaction is affected by many conditions in addition to activity.

Adult Day Care

Adult day-care centers began to appear in the United States during the late 1960s, and they have increased greatly in numbers over the years. In 1974 there were only 18 centers. By the late 1980s there were 1700. Each center now provides service to an average of about 20 clients a day.

Adult day-care centers were patterned after those of Great Britain, where they have long been a part of geriatric health services. The centers in the United States provide a community care program for the frail elderly. Participants in a center's program are in residence during the day and return to their homes in the evening. The objectives of the program are to enhance the health and social functioning of the participants and to reduce the burden and stress on home caregivers by making time available for activities other than caregiving. Clients of adult day-care centers are less likely to be severely mentally impaired than are residents of a nursing home or recipients of respite care (see RESPITE CARE).

Researchers at the University of Michigan recently sampled the clientele and the services of a number of adult day-care centers. They discovered that there are two distinct types of centers (excluding specialized centers, such as those for the blind or the severely mentally ill). The first type is affiliated with a nursing home or rehabilitation hospital. This type of center usually serves a clientele composed of physically dependent older people, most of whom do not have a mental disorder. The services provided may include nursing, therapy, diet regulation, and other health and social services. Financial support usually comes from sources other than governmental (e.g., client payment). The second type is affiliated with a hospital (but unlikely to be located in the hospital) or a social service agency. The clientele is likely to have a large representation from minority populations with minimal physical disability, but frequently with some degree of mental disability. Services usually include counseling, nutrition education, and transportation to and from the center. Funding is likely to be derived from governmental sources, especially Medicaid. Results from the Michigan study also revealed that both caregivers and clients are generally pleased with the services received at such centers. In addition, the cost of day care is usually much less than either full-time care in a nursing home or respite care outside a nursing home. Not surprisingly, the number of adult day-care centers has been increasing rapidly during the past decade.

Advance Directives

An advance directive enables elderly people to maintain control over their health care if they become physically or mentally incapable of choosing medical treatment options. The two most common forms of advance directives are living wills, which state in advance one's preference regarding life-sustaining treatment, and durable powers of attorney for health care, which authorize another person to make medical decisions when a patient is unable to do so. These two directives may also be combined. The Patient Self-Determination Act of 1990 requires that patients in institutions such as hospitals, nursing homes, and hospices must be informed about advance directives and their right to accept or refuse treatment.

A recent study revealed that 90% of the patients surveyed supported the concept of an advance directive, but only 15% had actually arranged to have one. Researchers at the University of Minnesota have developed an intervention for use with elderly people that seems to work in terms of increasing the number who record an advance directive. The intervention involves interactions with a social worker who provides information and counseling about the merits of an advance directive.

Aftereffects (Visual)

An aftereffect is a sensory experience that persists after the originating physical source of that experience has ceased. A familiar aftereffect occurs when you stare for a minute or so at a piece of brightly colored paper and then turn your gaze to a piece of white paper. You will "see" on the white paper a patch of color that is the complementary color of the one at which you had been staring. Thus if the paper had been colored blue, you will "see" yellow (the complementary color of blue) as the aftereffect (or negative afterimage as it is often called). Of interest is the evidence indicating that the color aftereffect persists several seconds longer for elderly people than for younger people. Longer persistence in late adulthood is also found for other aftereffects. For example, if you stare at a rapidly rotating spiral figure for some seconds, you will "see" the spiral continue to rotate for several seconds even though the physical rotation has terminated. In such instances, the aftereffect persists longer for elderly people than for younger people. The reason for the age difference in the persistence of aftereffects is unknown. However, a popular hypothesis is that more time is required for stimulation "to clear the nervous system" in late adulthood than in earlier adulthood (see STIMULUS PERSISTENCE).

Age-Associated Memory Impairment

Diagnosis of a disorder of any kind is the all-important first step before an appropriate treatment can be applied to the disorder. The outcome of diagnosis is the classification of the client's or the patient's disorder. The currently popular classification for those normally aging individuals who have moderate memory problems, but the extent of the problem is not great enough to be considered abnormal or pathological, is age-associated memory impairment (AAMI). This classification has largely replaced the earlier one of benign senescent forgetfulness. The diagnosis of AAMI is made on the basis of the client's performance on memory tests that have had wide clinical application. One such test is the Wechsler memory test (see WECHSLER MEMORY SCALE). A client who scores well below the average typically earned by normally aging individuals (but still well above the scores earned by individuals with a pathological memory impairment) is diagnosed as having AAMI.

Diagnosis does not end with the classification of a client as having AAMI. Further information about the client is needed to determine the reason for the memory problem. Conceivably, the problem is a temporary one caused by a change in the client's physical or mental health. For example, a physical health problem may have required treatment with a medication that has moderate mental confusion as a side effect, with memory dysfunction (i.e., memory working at a level below what it should be) as the primary symptom. In this case, a different medicine may be substituted for the original one, or the client may be assured that the memory problem is likely to be eliminated when the physical problem is eliminated and the medicine is no longer needed. Alternatively, the client may be in a state of depression as a result of some recent traumatic experience. Depression can adversely affect memory functioning. Once the depression is significantly reduced by therapy or by the passage of time, the chances are good that the memory problem will also be eliminated. If these extraneous health problems are ruled out, then it may be decided that the client has a memory problem that may benefit from participation in a memory training program.

Age Change vs. Age Difference

"I'm not as fast as I used to be." If said by elderly people, this statement is probably correct. When elderly people have measurements of their reaction time, their average speed of responding is indeed slower than that of younger adults. To measure reaction time, participants listen for or watch for a cue of some kind (e.g., a tone is sounded or a light goes on) and then perform a response, such as pushing a button, as rapidly as they can. Reaction time is the time elapsed between the onset of the cue and the execution of the requested response. Our point is that the statement made by elderly people is true. They have had an age change in their speed of reacting. They were faster when they were younger, and there has been a progressive slowing of their reaction time as aging progressed. There also is an age difference in speed of responding. A group of young adults average faster responses than a group of elderly adults when individuals in both groups are given a reaction time task to perform (a cross-sectional study; see CROSS-SECTIONAL METHOD). The age *differ-ence* in this case does result because of an age *change*. An age change means that individuals are changing over the course of their adult lifespan, such that their performance on whatever task measured (speed of responding in the example given) also changes. However, it is important to realize that not all age differences are the result of an age change.

A simple example should clarify the distinction between an age difference and an age change. Suppose we were to measure the height of every man between the ages of 20 and 29 and also the height of every man between the ages of 70 and 79. Not surprisingly, we would discover that men in their 20s average several inches taller than men in their 70s. Thus there is a rather large *age difference* in height. However, very little of this age difference is the result of an *age change*. The height of elderly men is about the same as it was when they were young men. It is true that a modest age change probably did occur. Some shrinking occurs with aging, a shrinking produced largely through the thinning of the cartilage between the bones of the vertebral column. However, the amount of shrinking is not nearly pronounced enough to account for the age difference of several inches in height. Something else accounts for most of the age difference in height. Most likely, it is the difference in generations (defined by birth year) between currently young and elderly adults. Members of a later generation (such as people currently in their 20s) encountered, during their childhoods, health care and diet conditions that were more favorable to physical growth than members of an earlier generation (such as people currently in their 70s). In fact, the generational difference is part of a trend toward increasing height over the centuries. Consider, for example, the average height of young men who lived many generations ago, during the Middle Ages. People are usually shocked when they visit a museum and see for the first time a suit of armor worn by a knight of that period. Most of today's fifth-graders would find the suit to be a tight fit!

The distinction between an age difference and a true age change is an important one in understanding the effects of aging on behavior. Not all age differences in behavior are the result of people changing with age. As an example, consider the age difference in the personality trait of introversion (i.e., being shy and not very out going). Some years ago elderly people were found to have test scores for the trait of introversion that were much higher than those of young adults. Does this mean that the elderly people were much more introverted than they were when they themselves were young adults—and that they became more and more introverted as they grew older? The evidence from more recent aging research indicates that this is not the case. Introversion, like most other personality traits, tends to be stable from early to late adulthood. Today's elderly adults were probably no less introverted when they were young adults than they are today. As with the height example, the critical factor responsible for the age difference in introversion found in early studies was a difference among generations in some environmental condition (social and/or physical) present during preadulthood and not aging itself. An age difference produced by some condition other than aging may very well not be present in the future, especially if that condition stabilizes for future generations. In fact, current cross-sectional studies show little difference between younger and older individuals in their average scores on a test of introversion. By contrast, if aging is the critical factor, then an age difference in behavior may well persist for future generations, unless something has been discovered that greatly reduces or even eliminates the aging process. This is surely the fate of speed of responding. As noted above, the age difference is the result of a true age change.

Ageism

The term *ageism* was introduced in 1968 by Dr. Robert N. Butler, a prominent geriatric physician and the first director of the National Institute on Aging. Ageism refers to the then widely held (and still not completely eliminated) attitude toward elderly individuals. In effect, ageism means a negative stereotype is applied to the entire population of elderly adults, a stereotype in which they are viewed as being senile, rigid in their thinking, and having other undesirable traits and behaviors. Of course, ageism is not the only negative stereotype that has characterized large segments of our population. Others include racism and sexism. The stereotyped perception of elderly adults is, of course, false. For example, senility is rare in our elderly population, and there is no firm evidence to indicate that rigidity (i.e., inflexibility) in thinking is more prevalent among elderly people than it is among younger adults (see RIGIDITY).

The existence of ageism has been frequently demonstrated in psychological studies. For example, when college students are asked to rate a "typical" 25-year-old and a "typical" 70-year-old on a number of personality characteristics, they apply more negative characteristics to the 70-year-old individual than to the 25-year-old individual and more positive characteristics to the 25-year-old than to the 70-year-old. Most depressing is the evidence that elderly adults are nearly as likely as young adults to apply the negative stereotype in evaluating their peers. Similarly, when young adults are given a description of a fictitious person who is having a memory problem (such as forgetting a telephone number while dialing it), they are far more likely to believe that the problem is a serious one and a sign of mental difficulty if the person is described as being elderly rather than young. The fact is that people of all ages often have difficulty remembering all of the digits of a telephone number encountered for the first time. The good news is that elderly adults performing the same task are less likely than young adults to view minor memory problems as a sign of senility. A negative evaluation is also more likely to be given when participants of different ages listen to a fictitious audio interview for a supervisor's job in which the interviewee is identified as being old. However, there is some evidence to suggest that the negative stereotype is assigned more often to the "old" old (people in their 80s and beyond) than to the "young" old (especially people in their 60s). Surely forgotten by those holding this pessimistic view of the "old" old are the many great recitals by Pablo Casals, Arthur Rubinstein, Vladimir Horowitz, and others at very advanced ages.

Why does ageism exist in our society? Part of the reason is the lack of valid information that many people have about aging's effects on human behavior. The lack of information is then replaced by myths about aging, myths perpetuated by the steady diet of unflattering descriptions and portrayals of elderly people often found in folklore, literature, movies, television shows, and even the daily comics. Consider the contributions of folklore through such adages as "You can't teach an old dog new tricks" and "There's no fool like an old fool." Many jokes about elderly people emphasize mental and physical deficits. Elderly people have not fared much better in literature. Witness, for example, Shakespeare's famous description of old age in *As You Like It* as being "sans teeth, sans eyes, sans taste, sans everything." With regard to the movies and television, familiar figures are those like the elderly hospital director in *House Calls,* who was depicted as a complete idiot, and the elderly woman in *Golden Girls* who is often depicted as being foolish, tactless, and irresponsible.

There is another possible reason for ageism's presence in our society, one convincingly advanced by Dr. Butler. He argued that ageism gives many younger individuals a reason for avoiding elderly people. Since elderly people differ from themselves, there is an excuse for having little to do with them. By avoiding elderly people as much as possible, younger people are able to reduce their fears regarding their own aging. Unfortunately, many younger people do shy away as much as possible from interacting with elderly people. Medical students have been known to express a negative attitude toward their future treatment of elderly patients, so much that very few express an interest in geriatric medicine. Even members of the clergy are not completely free of what has been called the YAVIS syndrome (the preference for *y*oung, *a*ttractive, *v*erbal, *i*ntelligent, and *s*uccessful—therefore affluent—clients).

Fortunately, there is evidence to indicate that the negative view of elderly people, at least that held by many medical students, may be overcome to some degree by appropriate training. Researchers at the University of Mississippi Medical School enrolled a number of third-year medical students in four 90-minute group sessions that emphasized various aspects of aging and ways of improving communication with elderly people. Compared with other students who did not participate in the sessions, the trained students showed more positive attitudes toward elderly people, and they demonstrated more socially skilled behavior while interviewing an elderly person.

Age Simulation

An age change in some ability or characteristic results in a different performance level for elderly adults, on the average, than for younger adults on tasks that involve that ability or characteristic. It is often debatable, however, whether the observed age difference in performance actually results from a change with aging. This is especially true when the study reporting the age difference in performance used the cross-sectional method (see AGE CHANGE VS. AGE DIFFERENCE; CROSS-SECTIONAL METHOD). An alternative is to use the longitudinal method in which the same individuals perform both when they are young and when they are older. However, the longitudinal method is usually impractical and has its own biases (see LONGITUDINAL METHOD). An ideal way to determine whether aging causes an observed age difference in performance on a particular task would be to test young adults on the task and then "age" them in such a manner that the ability or characteristic required for performance on the task is believed to be like that of an average elderly adult. This procedure is called age simulation. Unfortunately, there are few abilities or characteristics that can be artificially and temporarily "aged." One that is, however, is the characteristic believed to be responsible for the greater illusory Muller-Lyer effect experienced by elderly adults than by young adults (see ILLU-SIONS). The yellowing of the lens with aging permits less light to reach the eyes' retinas. This light reduction presumably plays a major role in determining the greater illusory effect for elderly people. The age change in the amount of light reaching the retina can be simulated by having young adults perform on an illusory task while wearing goggles that diminish the amount of light reaching the retina. When this is done, the illusory experience of young adult participants approximates that of elderly participants (performing, of course, without the goggles). This correspondence strengthens the belief that the reduction in light illumination is one of the age changes responsible for the age difference observed on certain illusory tasks.

Alcoholism

Self-reports indicate that elderly people consume fewer alcoholic beverages than do younger people and that members of the present generation of elderly people drink less now than they did when they were younger. In fact, a fairly large proportion of elderly people report that they abstain completely from drinking alcoholic beverages. However, the reliability of these reports may be questioned. Many elderly people may underestimate their use of alcohol to avoid criticism. The incidence of alcoholism among elderly people is largely unknown. Estimates of the percentage of elderly people with alcohol-related problems range from 1% to 25%. The incidence of alcohol addiction appears to equal the incidence of heart attacks among elderly people. Medicare costs for treatment of alcohol-related problems exceed $200 million annually.

Elderly adults who have been alcoholics for many years (chronic alcoholics) are likely to have memory impairments that exceed those of nonalcoholic elderly adults. In fact, many chronic alcoholics are likely to have memory impairments severe enough to be considered abnormal, and they are likely to have a diagnosis of Korsakoff's disease (see KORSAKOFF'S DISEASE).

That the percentage of elderly people with alcohol-related problems may be low is suggested by the results of a large-scale survey of elderly rural residents of Arizona. The percentage may be much higher, however, for elderly people in urban areas. The same survey found little support for the popular belief that there are two kinds of elderly alcoholics, those who have been heavy drinkers for many years and those who became alcoholics late in life in response to their unwanted life-style.

Of further interest are the probable reasons that older people cite as causes for a serious drinking problem. Such problems are seemingly related to negative life events in their recent lives and/or to the presence of long-standing (chronic) sources of stress. In a recent survey in California, comparisons were made between problem drinkers and nonproblem drinkers in the same age range (participants in each age group were between the ages of 55 and 65 years of age). Important sex differences were found. Male problem drinkers were more likely than female problem drinkers to report long-term financial problems and problems with friends. By contrast, female problem drinkers reported fewer financial sources of stress but more family-related sources of stress, including their spouses, than did male problem drinkers. In addition, female problem drinkers reported receiving less support from their spouses than male problem drinkers did from their spouses. The investigators noted that women may be more likely than men to perceive nurturing someone with a drinking problem to be part of their role within a family.

There were other important findings from the California survey. Sources of stress (i.e., stressors) were found to be no more severe for older problem drinkers than for older nonproblem drinkers. Thus problem drinkers in general did not have more difficult stressors with which to cope, or manage, than nonproblem drinkers. Nevertheless, problem drinkers displayed, on the average, a different form of coping behavior than did nonproblem drinkers. The problem drinkers tended to use avoidance forms of coping with stressors in which they either avoided thoughts about a problem or resigned themselves to the belief that nothing could be done about a problem. Excessive drinking is presumably part of their failure to acknowledge and overcome their problems. By contrast, nonproblem drinkers tended to use approach-coping behaviors in which they dealt directly with a problem and tried either to resolve it or to restructure it to make it less stressful. Researchers at the University of Southern California further found that caregivers of spouses with Alzheimer's disease who detached themselves from the situation and experienced a larger burden were more likely to become heavy drinkers than caregivers who directly confronted their problems encountered in caregiving.

Alcohol (Physical and Mental Effects)

Alcohol has different effects on older people than on younger people. The intake of the same amount of alcohol raises blood alcohol levels higher in older people than in younger people. Elderly people also metabolize and excrete alcohol more slowly than do younger adults. These effects mean that alcohol abuse may produce more serious physical problems for elderly abusers than younger abusers. The physical consequences for elderly people are complicated further by the fact that the likelihood of their having a disease is greater than for younger people, and the adverse physical effects of alcohol abuse may be intensified by the presence of disease. Researchers at Harvard Medical School examined all causes of death for over 20,000 male doctors during a period of 11 years. They discovered that the risk of death was 63% higher for those doctors who had two or more drinks a day than for those who did not drink at all. The greater risk for the heavy drinkers was linked to the greater incidence of cancer, especially throat, gastric, urinary tract, and brain cancer.

There is also evidence to indicate that the mental performances of older people are more adversely affected than the mental performances of younger people when they consume the same amounts of alcohol. Memory proficiency is especially affected. Both short-term and long-term memory are less proficient after ingestion of several drinks than after abstention. A familiar scenario is the individual who, after an evening of heavy drinking, is unable to remember on the next day having said some unpleasant things to his or her boss. The reason for the age difference in the effects of alcohol on mental functioning is largely unknown. However, it is known that alcohol affects aging brain tissue differently than it affects younger brain tissue.

Not all effects of alcohol use are negative. There is evidence that residents of nursing homes benefit both psychologically and socially from the moderate use of alcoholic beverages, especially when the beverages are consumed in a group setting that relaxes the tensions of feeling institutionalized. In addition, the researchers at Harvard discovered that the doctors who had two to four drinks a week had a lower risk (22%) of death than those doctors who did not drink at all. Moderate drinking may be related to a lower incidence of heart disease.

Altruism

Altruism refers to helping others, either in the form of a donation or an intervention to aid someone in trouble. In gerontology, elderly people have commonly been viewed as the needy recipients of altruistic acts and not as the givers of these acts. Elderly people have traditionally been regarded as being less altruistic than younger people. Several possible reasons have been given for the decline in altruism in late adulthood. One is that elderly people conserve their limited resources to improve their own life. Another is that many elderly people are, in effect, repaying society for its lack of concern with their own problems.

However, there is evidence to indicate that altruism may actually increase from middle age through late adulthood. Part of that evidence comes from interviews with elderly people that revealed that most elderly people *do* have a strong interest and orientation toward altruism. More impressive evidence comes from a clever study conducted by researchers at the University of Detroit. They set up a donation booth with a canister for monetary deposits in various shopping centers and malls. Large posters in the booth indicated that the donations were for infants born with birth defects. The percentage of donors was greatest for people in the age range of 65 to 74 years, with the next greatest percentage being for people 75 and older. The percentage of donors for younger adults (e.g., 25 to 34 years) was much smaller. However, the amount of the average donation, as might be expected, was less for the oldest donors than for younger donors (the largest average amounts were for people in the age range of 45 to 64 years). The diminished economic resources of people in the post-retirement years certainly accounts for their limited monetary donation. The researchers conducted a second study in which economic status would not be a determiner in either the willingness to be a donor or the amount actually donated. The situation was much like that of the first study except that now donors were asked to pull a lever in the booth, with a poster noting that local merchants would donate five cents to the charitable fund for each pull. In terms of the percentage of donors, the outcome was the same as that of the first experiment: the percentage was highest for the oldest people. In terms of the amount of donation (now expressed in number of pulls of the lever), the outcome was quite different than that of the first experiment—the average amount was greatest for the oldest donors. There were no economic constraints placed on the oldest donors. There is good reason to believe that altruism actually *increases* rather than declines in late adulthood.

Alzheimer's Association

The Alzheimer's Association was founded in 1980 with headquarters in Chicago. Until 1989 it was known as the Alzheimer's Disease and Related Disorders Association (ADRDA). It is a privately funded, voluntary organization with over 500 support groups and more than 200 chapters for people coping with sufferers of Alzheimer's disease. The association's goals include the following: (1) supporting research into the causes, treatment, and prevention of Alzheimer's disease; (2) providing assistance to families with a relative who has Alzheimer's disease; (3) making the general public better educated and informed about Alzheimer's disease; and (4) promoting legislation at the local, state, and federal levels that responds to the needs of patients with Alzheimer's disease and their caregivers. The national office offers grants for funding new investigations into the causes, treatment, and prevention of Alzheimer's disease, and it publishes a quarterly newsletter. The association is responsible for the now national observance of Alzheimer's Disease Month (in November). There is a nationwide 24-hour telephone hotline for providing information about Alzheimer's disease (800-272-3900) and for helping families find a support group and other forms of assistance. The address of the association is 919 N. Michigan Avenue, Suite 1000, Chicago, IL 60611.

Alzheimer's Disease

The existence of both presenile dementia (in people in their 40s or 50s) and senile dementia (usually among people in their 70s or older) has been known for centuries. However, it was not until 1907 that the first neurological diagnosis of dementia as a brain disorder was made. Dr. Alois Alzheimer, a German neurologist, had a patient with presenile dementia who died at age 51. Postmortem analysis revealed massive atrophy of her brain, in particular the presence of numerous small bodies of protein (called senile plaques; see BRAIN AND AGING) composed of bits of dying or dead neurons and neurofibrillary tangles (filaments that are wrapped around one another) within the bodies and axons of neurons scattered throughout the brain. At the time it was believed that presenile dementia differed from senile dementia in terms of the brain changes responsible for each. Senile dementia was considered to be the result of "hardening of the arteries" or stroke, and presenile dementia was attributed to unknown causes. Only presenile dementia was given the name Alzheimer's disease. In the late 1960s it was discovered that the brain changes present in many cases of senile dementia are very similar to those present in presenile dementia. Consequently, senile dementia in which known causative factors (e.g., stroke) could be ruled out and for which postmortem examination revealed massive senile plaques and neurofibrillary tangles also became known as Alzheimer's disease.

It is estimated that about 5% to 10% of the population of adults age 65 or older has Alzheimer's disease. The percentage increases after age 65; perhaps more than 20% of the population age 85 or older has the disease. About two-thirds of nursing home residents are believed to have Alzheimer's disease. The presenile form of the disease (affecting people in their 40s and 50s) is much rarer. In general, patients with early Alzheimer's disease live for a number of years after the onset of the disease, whereas older victims are likely to live only a few years after its onset. Diagnosis of Alzheimer's disease presently can be made only after death when analysis of the brain confirms massive atrophy of the brain and large amounts of senile plaques and neurofibrillary tangles, especially in the cerebral cortex and hippocampus (see BRAIN AND AGING). Consequently, individuals suspected of having Alzheimer's disease have a diagnosis of senile dementia of the Alzheimer's type (SDAT), with the realization that the true disease may eventually be discovered to be something other than Alzheimer's disease.

A diagnosis of SDAT is based on results of both neurological tests and mental tests (e.g., the Blessed Mental Status Test and the Mental Status Questionnaire; see BLESSED MENTAL STATUS TEST; MENTAL STATUS QUESTIONNAIRE). There is always the danger of misdiagnosis with mental tests in that the mental problems present in the early stage of Alzheimer's disease are somewhat similar to individuals who have severe depression. Recent advancements in examining the living brain, such as computed axial tomography (CAT) scans and positron emission tomography (PET) scans have thus far not been effective in enhancing the early diagnosis of SDAT, although such tests do reveal the progressive atrophy of the brain and its functioning as the disease progresses in severity. However, there is a promising new scanning test that measures amounts of a sugar called myo-inositol and a chemical called NAA. Both substances are known to occur in larger amounts in the brains of patients with Alzheimer's disease than in the brains of normally aging individuals. Researchers at the University of California–Los Angeles recently reported that PET scans may be especially valuable in detecting early brain degeneration in individuals possessing a gene related to Alzheimer's disease. Diagnosis is complicated further by the fact that a fairly large percentage of individuals with Alzheimer's disease (perhaps as large as 20%) have dementias that are increased further by multi-infarct dementia (stroke-induced dementia). Perhaps the most promising diagnostic test is one discovered by researchers at Harvard University. They found that the drug used to dilate the pupils of the eyes during a standard eye examination (tropicamide) causes the pupils of most people who later develop the disease to dilate about four times larger than those of other people.

Early correct diagnosis would enable both eventual patients with the disease and their caregivers to prepare for the future effects of the disease. Once an effective treatment is discovered, very early diagnosis would offer a head start on that treatment.

Atrophy of the brain is especially pronounced in the cerebral cortex, the hippocampus, and other brain areas associated with memory functioning and other mental operations. A major problem is the severe decline in the amount of acetylcholine, a neurotransmitter chemical linked to memory functioning, present in the brain (see BRAIN AND AGING). This decline appears to be caused by massive destruction of neurons in a structure called the nucleus basalis of Meynert located at the base of the brain, neurons that seem to be critical in the production of acetylcholine.

The most prominent mental symptom of Alzheimer's disease is the progressive and severe decline in memory functioning. The severity of the decline is especially pronounced for the various forms of episodic memory (see EPISODIC MEMORY). Both short-term and long-term memory decline greatly in proficiency, and the decline may be seen in memory for noncontent attributes of episodic events (e.g., their frequency of occurrence and their spatial locations), as well as the contents of those events. Semantic memory is also affected, but to a lesser extent than episodic memory (see LEXICON; SEMANTIC MEMORY). Individuals with SDAT have difficulty naming pictures and objects, and their word associations differ greatly from those of normally aging people (see WORD ASSOCIATIONS), although it is uncertain whether it is the actual knowledge of words that is lost with the disease or whether it is difficulty in gaining access to words that is affected by the disease. There is some evidence to indicate that the rate of progressive decline in mental functions over time is more rapid for those with higher levels of education than for those with lower levels. Also, the rate of annual decline tends to be greater for those with an earlier onset of the disease than for those with a later onset.

Individuals with SDAT are also characterized by disorientation in terms of time and place, and various personality disorders are likely to be present, especially depression and inappropriate social behavior. Approximately 30% of patients with SDAT are believed to have severe depression in addition to their mental impairment. An even larger percentage have some form of depressive symptoms. As the disease progresses, individuals with SDAT become increasingly incapable of performing the activities of daily living (feeding themselves, personal hygiene), thus requiring considerable caregiving either at home or in a nursing home. Some patients with SDAT also have paranoia, that is, pronounced delusions or false beliefs about events in their world. Especially likely are delusions of persecution in which the patients believe they are being robbed or are being spied on. Such delusions add to the concerns and problems of the patient's caregivers. In some cases the delusions may diminish with repeated reminders by caregivers that there is no factual basis for these beliefs.

One of the most prominent physical symptoms for severely impaired individuals is agitation. Agitation consists of inappropriate verbal, vocal, or motor behavior that may be abusive toward others, such as cursing or hitting caregivers. Studies have indicated that more than half of nursing home residents scream at least once a day. The frequency of screaming has been found to be related to such factors as the ability to perform the activities of daily living and the degree of mental impairment.

Another prominent physical symptom is wandering behavior. Wandering does tend to have a positive effect for some SDAT individuals. Some evidence indicates that wandering may reduce negative aggressive behaviors when individuals are permitted to wander freely in a protected environment. The problem with wandering is that individuals may escape the so-called protected environment and enter areas that may be dangerous to their well-being. Exits from protected areas by individuals with SDAT may occur at any time during the day or night, but they are most likely to occur within a few hours after eating a meal. Researchers in Ohio discovered that nursing home residents with SDAT may best be discouraged from leaving a secured area by concealing the exit door behind a cloth panel.

The cause(s) of Alzheimer's disease remains unknown. There is the possibility of a genetic defect on a particular chromosome that encodes information about a specific brain protein. When incorrectly encoded, the result is the production of a protein fragment called amyloid beta-protein that may be responsible for the massive degeneration of the brain found in Alzheimer's disease. It appears that early Alzheimer's disease may be inheritable, although why the onset of the disease is delayed until middle age is unknown. Convincing evidence of this inheritability was obtained in 1995 by researchers at the University of Toronto. They discovered a gene that, when defective, causes a rare aggressive form of Alzheimer's disease. The disease usually appears in people much younger than 65 years, perhaps even when they are in their 30s. Inheritance may also be involved in later onset of the disease. Researchers at Duke University Medical Center recently identified a gene, called APDE-4, that appears to play a major role in causing the disease. They found that the more copies of this gene possessed by an individual, the greater the risk of having the disease—and the earlier the onset of the disease. The discovery of this genetic factor holds great promise for an eventual cure for the disease.

Also suspected of being a causative factor is a viral infection that has yet to be determined. At one time a popular theory was that aluminum toxicity was important in causing Alzheimer's disease. This theory has been largely disproved by evidence indicating no relationship between the extent of use of aluminum in daily life (e.g., cookware) and the occurrence of the disease.

A cure for the disease has yet to be found. At one time it was believed that injections of acetylcholine or its artificial equivalent would greatly reduce the memory problems of victims of the disease by replenishing the diminished supply of this critical neurotransmitter. The results of clinical trials with drugs such as lecithin, which aid in the synthesis of acetylcholine, proved disappointing. The most recent drug treatment for Alzheimer's disease, tacrine, has created a controversy regarding its effectiveness in treating the symptoms of the disease. The drug acts on the brain by inhibiting the production of an enzyme that seemingly destroys acetylcholine, thereby increasing the supply of acetylcholine in the brain of a patient with Alzheimer's disease. The results of clinical trials with the drug have yielded somewhat conflicting results. Nevertheless, in September, 1993, the federal Food and Drug Administration approved use of tacrine for patients with mild or moderate Alzheimer's disease. Currently researchers are considering the possibility that a substance known as nerve growth factor is essential for the operations of neurons that synthesize acetylcholine in the brain and that there is a major reduction of nerve growth factor in the brains of individuals with Alzheimer's disease. There is the possibility that clinical trials will be approved within the next few years for the administration of nerve growth factor to groups of patients, even though some prominent scientists believe that this may actually be more harmful than helpful.

There may be hope in the future for two new forms of treatment whose potential effectiveness was discovered largely serendipitously. One of these is estrogen replacement therapy for postmenopausal women (see MENOPAUSE). Researchers at the University of Southern California studied the health records of 9,000 women living in a retirement community. Those women who had been on estrogen replacement therapy had nearly a 40% reduction in the risk of developing Alzheimer's disease relative to those who had not had replacement therapy. The implication is that estrogen replacement therapy may help some women avoid Alzheimer's disease. Unfortunately, researchers at the University of California at San Diego failed to find a significant benefit in memory functioning for women who were undergoing estrogen replacement therapy, thus challenging somewhat the preventive value of this treatment. It should be noted that some research is presently being conducted with testosterone supplements for elderly men.

The second potentially effective form of treatment is the use of anti-inflammatory drugs (which include aspirin and aspirin-like drugs). It has been discovered that rheumatoid arthritis patients who take anti-inflammatory drugs rarely develop Alzheimer's disease. A recent theory has hypothesized that Alzheimer's disease is related to a low-grade inflammation in the brain, and it is therefore a chronic inflammatory disease, as is arthritis. The inflammation may attract certain proteins from the body's immune system that destroy healthy brain cells. Anti-inflammatory drugs may serve as a defense against these proteins. Of great interest is the outcome of a small pilot study by researchers in Arizona. They discovered that the anti-inflammatory drug indomethacin that is commonly prescribed for the treatment of arthritis appeared to slow the progression of Alzheimer's disease in a group of 14 patients over a period of 6 months.

Although the mental symptoms of Alzheimer's disease are presently immune to treatment, some of the behavioral dysfunctions (e.g., personal care, eating) may be at least partially improved by the effective use of behavioral modification procedures (see PSYCHOTHERAPY). In some cases depression may be treated by the drugs used to treat depression in normally aging adults, and some of the personality symptoms may be treated by other drugs.

Alzheimer's Disease Education and Referral Center

The Alzheimer's Disease Education and Referral (ADEAR) Center was established by the National Institute on Aging (see NATIONAL INSTITUTE ON AGING) to serve as a clearinghouse for information about Alzheimer's disease and related topics. It both collects and publishes information about the disease. The address is ADEAR, PO Box 8250, Silver Springs, MD 20907-8250 (telephone, 301-587-4352).

Alzheimer's Disease Support Center

The Alzheimer's Disease Support Center is part of a telecomputer system located at Case Western Reserve University in Cleveland that has provided a free communication network since 1986. It may be accessed 24 hours a day by a microcomputer or a terminal and a modem via a telephone. Information offered by the Center consists of five parts or modules. For example, the Alzheimer's disease information rack module lists videos and brochures that may be ordered without charge from the Cleveland chapter of the Alzheimer's Association (see ALZHEIMER'S ASSOCIATION). Another module provides useful information for caregivers to help them carry out their services.

American Association of Retired Persons

The American Association of Retired Persons (AARP) was founded in 1958 by Dr. Ethel Percy Andrus, a retired California educator. It was originally known as the National Retired Teachers Association. Its membership grew dramatically over the years, reaching about 33 million members in 1991. It is the largest organization in the United States devoted to the needs of older people (its motto is "To serve, not to be served"), and it has become what many believe to be this country's most powerful lobby. Its lobbying efforts have been especially effective for issues involving Social Security. AARP is active in many other areas of concern in gerontology. For example, its nonprofit mail-order pharmacy service is the largest in the world, and its national opinion surveys are major sources of information about social issues involving the elderly population of the United States. In addition, AARP publishes a bimonthly magazine (*Modern Maturity*) that has one of the largest circulations in the United States. Part of AARP is the Andrus Foundation, which is a major source of funding of gerontological research, especially research directed at discovering ways of improving the welfare of older people. The address of both AARP headquarters and the Andrus Foundation is 601 E Street, N.W., Washington, DC 20049.

American Geriatrics Society

The American Geriatrics Society is a professional nonprofit organization that was founded in 1942 by a small group of physicians and scientists concerned with the problem of health care for elderly people. Membership now consists of thousands of geriatric health care specialists. Throughout its history the society has been devoted to promoting research on aging and health and to expanding the training of geriatric specialists. The society publishes both a medical journal, the *Journal of the American Geriatrics Society*, and a monthly newsletter that describes recent events and developments in geriatric health care. The society's address is 770 Lexington Avenue, Suite 10021, New York, NY 10021 (telephone, 212-308-1414).

American Psychological Association

The American Psychological Association (APA) is the largest organization of psychologists in the United States, with its headquarters in Washington, D.C. It began in 1892 with a handful of members. As psychology grew as a science and profession, so did the association. In 1990 the membership exceeded 70,000. The diversity of psychology and those who practice it is evident from the fact that APA has 47 divisions, each representing a different area of psychology. For example, there are divisions on clinical psychology, consumer psychology, experimental psychology, health psychology, military psychology, and psychology of women. Of particular interest is the division on adult development and aging. It has nearly 1200 members, all of whom have an interest in gerontological psychology in terms of research on aging, teaching of courses on aging, or professional practice with elderly clients. The APA publishes a number of scientific journals, including one, *Psychology and Aging,* that is devoted exclusively to psychological research on aging. APA's address is 750 First Street, N.E., Washington, DC 20002-4242 (telephone, 202-336-5500).

American Public Health Association

The American Public Health Association (APHA) was founded in 1872. In 1992 the APHA had 31,500 members. The membership is very diverse occupationally, consisting of physicians, nurses, health educators, epidemiologists, pharmacists, mental health specialists, and so on. The objectives of APHA are to protect and promote physical, mental, and environmental health. Its many services include the promoting of health standards and the establishment of uniform health practices and medical care programs. Its primary journal is the *American Journal of Public Health* (monthly). APHA's address is 1015 15th Street, N.W., Washington, DC 20005 (telephone, 202-789-5600).

American Sociological Association

The American Sociological Association (ASA) was founded in 1905. In 1992 it had 12,300 members. ASA has 23 sections, including one on aging and another on health. It publishes eight journals. Of particular relevance to aging is the *Journal of Health and Social Behavior.* ASA's address is 1722 N Street, N.W., Washington, DC 20036 (telephone, 202-833-3410).

Amnesia

Amnesia refers to a severe loss of memory ability produced by deterioration of critical centers in the brain. One form of loss is in terms of the difficulty of acquiring new information and storing it in memory. The other form of loss is in terms of the difficulty in retrieving memories that were stored before the onset of amnesia. The former is called *anterograde amnesia* (i.e., forward in time); the latter is termed *retrograde amnesia* (i.e., backward in time).

Individuals with Korsakoff's disease (see KORSAKOFF'S DISEASE) are characterized primarily by anterograde amnesia, although retrograde amnesia also may be present to some degree (especially for more recent memories relative to the onset of the disease). Some patients with Parkinson's disease and Huntington's disease (see PARKINSON'S DISEASE; HUNTINGTON'S DISEASE) may also have both forms of amnesia but usually to a lesser extent than patients with Korsakoff's disease. Both forms of amnesia are likely to be extremely severe for patients with Alzheimer's disease and for patients with multi-infarct dementia.

Androgyny

Psychological androgyny refers to having both feminine and masculine characteristics integrated in the same individual. An androgynous person is one who has avoided being bound by rigid gender roles often associated with his or her sex. Of interest is the possibility of changes in androgyny during various periods of adulthood. A popular theory of androgyny stresses that men and women retain their traditional male and female roles, respectively, through the parenting years and then become more like each other in late adulthood. That is, elderly men and women become more like one another in terms of a blend of masculine and feminine characteristics. However, there is evidence from two studies, one conducted in the 1970s and one in the 1980s, that the trend toward androgyny is more characteristic of elderly men than it is of elderly women. The percentage of androgynous men in the samples studied was found to increase from 20% to 30% in the 41- to 60-year age range to 40% in the 61-year and older age range. By contrast, the percentage of androgynous women in the

61-year and older age range was only 10% to 30%. The percentage of men classified as being predominantly masculine in their character- istics decreased from 40% to 50% in the 41- to 60-year age range to 20% to 30% in the 61-year and older age range. The percentage of women classified as being predominantly feminine in their charac- teristics increased from about 40% in the 41- to 60-year age range to about 70% in the 61-year and older age range. The two studies were conducted nearly 10 years apart; thus the older individuals surveyed were from different generations or cohorts. The fact that the out- comes were very similar for these widely separated cohorts suggests that the change toward increasing femininity for both older men and older women may represent a true age change and not an effect at- tributable to cohort or generational differences.

Anorexia

Anorexia (or anorexia nervosa) is a disorder found in some adoles- cents and young adults, primarily female, but rarely in elderly adults. It is characterized by self-starvation and the loss of considerable body weight. There is no apparent physical reason for the eating dis- order. Various psychological causes have been proposed, such as the anorexic individual is rewarded initially by compliments of her thin- ness following dieting, and then carries the restriction of food intake to extremes. An anorexic condition may occur in late adulthood, but it is most likely the consequence of a physical disorder produced by water intoxication associated with the oversecretion of the anti- diuretic hormone.

Antioxidants

The cells of our bodies require oxygen to generate the energy our bodies need. During this process, toxic substances known as free rad- icals are produced. According to a long-standing biological theory of aging (see WHY AGING? [BIOLOGICAL THEORIES OF AGING]), free rad- icals are believed to cause many of the illnesses and biological de- clines that occur in late adulthood. That is, free radicals travel through the body and produce damage to vital cell structures. Al- though the evidence to support the free radical theory of biological aging is not strong, there has been considerable interest recently in substances called antioxidants that defend the body against oxygen's presumably harmful effects by reducing the amount of free radicals in the body. These substances are beta-carotene and vitamins C and

E. Beta-carotene is found in deeply colored orange and green fruits and vegetables, such as carrots, sweet potatoes, broccoli, spinach, oranges, apricots, and canteloupe. Vitamin C is found in citrus fruits, strawberries, peppers, broccoli, and cauliflower. The best sources of vitamin E are fatty foods, such as vegetable oils, nuts, and seeds. However, a normal diet would not include the large amounts of these foods necessary to provide sufficient vitamin E to serve as an antioxidant. Consequently, it is not unusual for physicians to recommend that elderly patients supplement their diets with vitamin E capsules.

Anxiety

Are you about to take the test to renew your driver's license? Are you feeling uneasy, nervous, tense, and dreading the future event—in other words, experiencing anxiety? Psychologists distinguish among three forms of anxiety: trait anxiety, state anxiety, and clinical anxiety (i.e., an anxiety disorder or neurosis). Both trait anxiety and state anxiety are general characteristics of normal individuals (i.e., they are not clinically abnormal). They both may affect behavior in many kinds of situations. Individuals high in trait anxiety are likely to be anxious throughout their lives in many kinds of situations, even those that are only mildly threatening to individuals with lower trait anxiety. State anxiety is more transitory and depends on situations that are threatening to one's self-esteem. When faced with an examination, some people become much more anxious than others; they have a higher degree of state anxiety. They are likely to feel very nervous and agitated and to have various physical signs of their anxiety, such as heavy perspiration and irregular breathing. There is considerable evidence to indicate that there are no adult age differences in either trait or state anxiety, at least as anxiety is measured by psychological tests. That is, the scores of elderly adults on these tests differ very little from the scores of younger adults. The absence of any pronounced increase in anxiety, in general, during late adulthood is demonstrated further by the fact that the incidence of an anxiety disorder (a clinically significant form of neurotic anxiety that is especially debilitating to the affected individual is quite low for elderly people.

A high level of state anxiety is likely to hinder performance on the task being performed while the anxiety is present. By contrast, a moderate amount of anxiety could improve performance by forcing increased concentration on the task at hand. The age differences that do exist in anxiety are seemingly too insignificant to affect age differences in performances on either laboratory tasks or everyday tasks. However, elderly people who believe they are being handicapped by excessive anxiety are as likely to benefit from training in relaxation by psychologists as are younger people.

Aphasia

Aphasia is a disorder involving either the expression of speech (expressive aphasia) or the comprehension of speech (receptive aphasia). The disorder is caused by a lesion in the brain usually resulting from a stroke or a head injury. The lesion for expressive aphasia is usually in a segment of the left frontal lobe known as Broca's area. The lesion for receptive aphasia is usually in a segment of the left temporal lobe known as Wernicke's area.

Aphasias in elderly people are more likely to be receptive than expressive. Language impairment in aphasia can often be treated effectively by speech therapy. At one time it was believed that elderly people were far less likely to benefit from therapy than younger people. However, recent studies have challenged this belief and have reported little relationship between age at the onset of an aphasia and the extent of recovery achieved by therapy.

Arithmetic Ability

Numerous studies have indicated that if there are age differences in the accuracy of simple arithmetic operations, such as addition and subtraction, they are slight. However, older adults are slower than younger adults in completing simple arithmetic problems. In terms of solving fairly simple word problems, there is also little effect of aging on accuracy, at least through the mid-70s. Our reference is to solving simple problems in which all of the elements are physically present (e.g., when participants are given 534 and 28 as addends and are asked to give the sum). It is a different matter, however, when one or both addends must be held mentally while mentally summing the two. Here there does seem to be a decided disadvantage, in general, for elderly participants. The size of the disadvantage is especially apparent when both addends must be "held in the head" while summing them. There are occasions when we may be tempted to use mental arithmetic. Consider shopping in the supermarket for two items and you have only two dollars with you. One item costs 98 cents and the other 85 cents. Do you have enough money with you to make both purchases (be sure to add the sales tax, if needed). Why rely on your mental addition? People of all ages (but especially elderly people) should carry a pocket calculator to do arithmetic when shopping, or have a small notebook and a pen so that they can do their shopping arithmetic with physically present numbers.

Army Alpha and Army Beta Intelligence Tests

The Army Alpha test was the first widely used group verbal (reading ability needed to take the test) intelligence test. Among the abilities it tested were analogies, numerical ability, and reasoning. The test was developed during World War I as a selection device for finding army officer candidates among enlisted men and for assigning soldiers to services they were deemed intellectually fit to perform. The test was administered to nearly 2 million men during the war. The results from this testing provided the first clear indication of adult age differences in scores on an intelligence test. A progressive age-related decline in scores was found from officers in their 20s to officers in their 50s. Later use of the test with civilians demonstrated further age-related declines beyond the 50s. Age-related declines were also found to vary greatly among the various subtests of the Army Alpha, suggesting that the mental abilities measured by these subtests vary greatly in the extent to which they are affected by normal aging.

The Army Alpha test requires reading ability in English. During World War I military personnel were aware that many recruits would either be illiterate or foreign-born and unable to read English. Consequently, a nonverbal (no reading ability required to take the test) group intelligence test, the Army Beta, was developed with the Army Alpha. The Army Beta test included such subtests as mazes, digit symbol, and number checking.

Arousal

When frightened, angry, or otherwise highly emotionally excited, a number of physiological changes occur in our bodies as the adrenalin (also known as epinephrine) begins to flow. Stimulation from the brain during times of excitement activates the secretion of adrenalin from the adrenal glands, which are located on top of each kidney. The physiological changes produced by the adrenalin include an increase in heart rate, an increase in breathing rate, and other changes that collectively result in a state known as physiological arousal.

Psychologists have long known that the intensity of arousal produced by a stressful or demanding situation affects one's performance in that situation. As the intensity of arousal increases, performance on a task at hand is likely to increase in proficiency. However, this is true only until some optimal level of intensity is reached. Beyond that optimal level, performance on the same task is likely to decrease in proficiency. For levels of arousal below the optimal level, people are said to be underaroused, and for levels above the optimal level, they are said to be overaroused. In either case, performance on the task confronting them is likely to be less than optimal.

For 40 years gerontological psychologists have debated whether elderly adults are characterized by underarousal or overarousal when they are requested to perform demanding and difficult tasks. Much of the difficulty in resolving the issue of underarousal or overarousal arises from the fact that there is no single measure of arousal that adequately serves to evaluate its intensity. There are a number of separate measures that have yielded different outcomes when applied in aging research. One of these measures is the amount of free fatty acids in the blood. Use of this measure has indicated that elderly people, in general, become overaroused when performing a demanding task, such as a learning task. The evidence comes from studies in which elderly participants receive either a drug known to reduce the level of free fatty acids in the blood (and therefore a decreased arousal level) or a placebo (i.e., a neutral substance) in advance of practicing a learning task. Participants receiving the drug perform at a much higher level than participants receiving the placebo, presumably because the debilitating effects on performance of overarousal present for the placebo participants are removed for the drug participants. Another measure of physiological arousal is that of the skin's electrical conductance level. Research with this measure has suggested that elderly people tend to be underaroused when confronted by demanding tasks (e.g., a learning task).

Arousal is also used in reference to the brain's activity level, particularly activity of the cortex. Cortical activity is indicated in terms of the brain's electrical output, and it is measured by means of electroencephalography. There is clear evidence of cortical underarousal on the part of elderly people in general. Most important, there is also evidence to indicate the importance of integrating cortical arousal with physiological arousal to achieve effective performances on demanding tasks. Such integration seemingly occurs to a lesser degree for elderly people than for younger people. The diminished integration of the two forms of arousal probably presents a greater problem to elderly adults than does the actual level of either physiological or cortical arousal.

Attention (Overview)
See also DIVIDED ATTENTION; SELECTIVE ATTENTION; VIGILANCE

Open up a dictionary and look up the word *attention*. You are likely to find a definition like "careful observation." This term is too vague to be useful in understanding aging. Regardless of the definition of *attention,* it is apparent that attention somehow plays an important role in our everyday lives. An indication of that importance comes from the many statements we hear or see that refer to attention in some way: "Probable cause of the accident—inattention of the driver in vehicle A." "Be on guard!" "Watch for any sign of movement by the enemy." "When is our next quiz?—I was listening to that guy talking in back of me, and I wasn't paying attention to the professor." "I heard this ad on my car radio while driving home today." These statements are also an indication that there are different forms of attention. Watching for movement by the enemy is obviously different than listening to one individual while tuning out another. Moreover, both of these forms differ from listening to the radio while driving a car. The "watching for movement" is an example of vigilance; the "tuning out of the professor's voice" is an example of selective attention; and the "listening to the ad while driving" is an example of divided attention.

Vigilance refers to monitoring a constant stream of like stimulation to detect a significant change in that stimulation. A military guard stationed near the enemy is on the alert to determine whether the steady silence of the night is interrupted by some unexpected noise. Similarly, a quality control inspector on a production line watches for the rare occurrence of a defective product. Selective attention means directing attention to one source of stimulation in the immediate environment while ignoring other sources of stimulation. We are constantly bombarded by visual and auditory stimuli, and often by stimuli from the other senses, that are present in our environment. Our interest and objective at any given moment determine which of these stimuli are selected to receive attention and therefore enter our consciousness. Those that do receive attention are called relevant stimuli (e.g., the "guy's" voice for the student), those occurring simultaneously are called irrelevant stimuli (the "professor's" voice for the student—but, if the student's interest at the time had been different, the professor's voice would surely have been the relevant stimulus). Divided attention means literally what it says. We attempt to share our attention among several sources of simultaneously present stimulation. Thus the driver listening to the car radio is sharing attention between two sources of stimuli, one visual, the other auditory. The visual stimuli from the road ahead are one source, the ad on the radio is the auditory stimulus. As long as traffic is light, the driver will not find it difficult to divide attention between the two. However, with heavy traffic the driver may begin to ignore the radio (or, alternatively, to tell a passenger to be quiet).

Psychologists believe that we possess some form of an attentional resource, one that has a limited capacity or capability for maintaining attention. That is, we can attend to only a limited amount of stimulation from our environment at any one time. Many researchers in the psychology of aging believe that this attentional capacity decreases somewhat with aging. Some forms of attention place little demand on this capacity (the attention needed to perform a simple vigilance task) and therefore are unaffected by normal aging. Other forms of attention, however, are very demanding and therefore more likely to be affected by aging (e.g., dividing attention between two tasks, each of which is difficult to perform alone). Aging's effects on each of the three basic forms of attention are discussed in other articles.

Attitudes (Political and Social)

Attitudes express our feelings and behavioral tendencies for various groups of people, organizations, and social and political issues. They are usually measured by psychologists in terms of dimensions that are anchored by opposites, such as conservative at one end of the spectrum and liberal at the other end. Some people fall at one extreme or the other while others fall in the middle. Gerontologists have most often studied age differences in attitudes toward social and political issues in which the opposites of conservative and liberal are truly applicable. These studies have typically indicated the presence of more conservative attitudes among older people than among younger people. For example, in one study, the participants, all faculty spouses at a university, were evaluated with respect to attitudes toward race, law enforcement, and patriotism. Overall, only 21% of the spouses in the 50-year and older range were classified as being liberal on the basis of their attitude test scores, in contrast to 55% of the spouses in the 20- to 29-year age range. There is good reason to believe that such age differences are more the product of memberships in different generations than the product of a true age change from liberalism to conservatism as one grows older. That is, members of earlier generations were more likely to have acquired conservative positions on many issues than were members of later generations. This may be seen, for example, in analyses of allegiance to political parties. Several years ago the proportion of elderly people who considered themselves Republicans was much greater than the proportion of young adults who considered themselves Republicans. This does not necessarily mean, however, that growing old converts Democrats into Republicans. The older Republicans were predominantly Republicans when they themselves were young adults. Other studies have revealed that age itself has little effect on attitudes toward economic and foreign policy issues.

As society and its standards change, the attitudes of many people are likely to change as well. A common belief is that elderly people are more rigid and less flexible in their ability to change their attitudes. However, this does not seem to be case. As cultural changes occur over time, they are likely to influence older people to about the same extent as they influence younger people. This seems to be true, for example, for attitudes regarding legalized abortion, businesses being open on Sundays, and so on.

Attribution

Attribution refers to the way you assign the blame when something goes wrong in your life. To determine whether there are age differences in attribution, psychologists give participants statements such as, "You give an important talk in front of a group, and the audience reacts negatively." The participants are asked to imagine that this experience happened to them, and then to rate on a scale from 1 to 7 who is to blame for the experience they had. One end of the scale is defined as "totally due to others," the other end as "totally due to me." They also rate themselves on two other 7-point scales. The first scale evaluates the stability of their attribution, and it is anchored at one end by "will never again be present" and the other by "will always be present." The other scale evaluates the global nature of their attribution (i.e., how general it is); it is anchored at one end by "influences just this particular situation" and at the other end by "influences all situations in my life." Researchers have found that elderly adults are, on the average, more likely than young adults to place responsibility for negative events on negative abilities that they possess. Elderly adults, on the average, are also more likely than young adults to perceive the situation as being stable, that is, it will continue to be present in future encounters with the same situation. However, elderly adults have also been found to be less general than young adults in their attributions. As perceived by an elderly person, the responsibility for an audience's negative reaction to his or her talk probably rests with that person (e.g., he or she had speech anxiety). Moreover, the negative audience reaction will probably occur whenever a talk is given by that person (i.e., stability), but the person's anxiety would not affect other kinds of performances. By contrast, a young adult is likely to perceive his or her poor speech as being related to something like fatigue that is only temporary, but it would affect many other kinds of performances when it is present.

Autobiographical Memory

A familiar refrain of many elderly people is that they remember well events that happened to them years ago, but they have trouble remembering what happened recently. The memory of personally experienced events is known as autobiographical memory. Is it true that the remote memories of elderly people tend to remain remarkably preserved while their recent memories fade away quickly? Memory research has indicated that this is not completely true. The standard method for testing autobiographical memory is to give participants a series of seemingly random words, with instructions to recall some personal memory in response to each word. The series may include such words as "book," "machine," "sorry," and "surprised." After all memory associations have been given, the participants are then asked to date when each recalled event occurred. Surprisingly, the most frequently recalled memories to the words by elderly participants are recent ones, dating back to the last few years or, in some cases, only to the last few months. The next most frequently recalled memories are for events that occurred in early adulthood. Mid-life events are recalled much less frequently than either recent events or events from early adulthood. Events from early childhood are rarely recalled. The unavailability of memories from early childhood also is true for younger adults. This unavailability of very early memories is known as childhood amnesia.

The decline in memory from recent events to mid-life events follows the course of normal forgetfulness. Recent events have yet to experience much interference from later events, the kind of interference that produces forgetting (see FORGETTING). By contrast, mid-life events have experienced considerable interference from years of intervening events. Why then the relatively high frequency of memories of events from early adulthood, events that surely have encountered more interfering events than those of mid-life? The probable reason for the preservation of these early adulthood memories comes from research with a different procedure than the standard one for studying autobiographical memory. With this procedure elderly participants are asked simply to identify the events that were important in their lives. The most frequently recalled important events are those of adolescence and early adulthood, with recent events having the next highest frequency. As with the individual word procedure, mid-life events have the lowest frequency of occurrence. The events of adolescence and early adulthood appear to be especially significant ones in shaping the remainder of our lives. As such, they remain highly vivid and accessible to recall. Moreover, it is these events that are likely to be recalled and therefore strengthened further to resist forgetting when people reminisce about earlier life (see REMINISCENCE).

B

· ·

Baltimore Longitudinal Study

The Baltimore Longitudinal Study is one of the major longitudinal research projects conducted in the United States. As with other longitudinal studies, the same individuals are tested and retested after a period of time. Initially the study was conducted as a collaborative effort between the National Institutes of Health and the Baltimore City Hospitals. Eventually the study became part of the operations of the National Institute on Aging. Planning for the study began in 1958; the first testing occurred in 1961. The first participants were 260 healthy men ranging in age from the 20s to age 96. They were all volunteers in the Washington, D.C./Baltimore area who agreed to return for retesting about every 2 years at the Gerontology Research Center in Baltimore. Additional male participants were included in the group over the years; by 1985, more than 1200 men had been tested once. Of these participants, nearly 600 had been retested a number of times, with retesting occurring approximately every 2 years. The study was originally restricted to men because of the limited housing facilities at the Gerontology Research Center (the complete battery of tests requires more than 2 days to complete). However, women were eventually added to the study in 1978. By 1985, more than 400 women had been tested at least once, and most were eventually retested.

Participants undergo a number of physical tests, such as heart, lungs, kidney, neuromuscular, and sensory functioning on each visit to the Center. The retesting permits an analysis of the rate at which age changes occur in vital biological functions and the determination of the course of diseases that occur with aging. A unique feature of the study has been the inclusion of a number of tests of mental functioning. Among them have been tests of learning and memory, concept acquisition, and personality. The results from these tests have been virtually the only source of information free of the problems encountered in cross-sectional studies of the same functions (see CROSS-SECTIONAL METHOD).

Biological Age

A person's biological age may be expressed in two different ways. One is in terms of how that person's health status compares with the average health status at different age levels. If his or her health and biological functioning is comparable to the average 70-year-old of the same sex, then that person's biological age would be 70 years. This would be the case whether the person's actual (chronological) age is 60 or 80 years. Stated differently, one's biological age is the number of years he or she is expected to live (see LIFE EXPECTANCY) based on his or her health status. Thus if a person's health status is comparable to the average 70-year-old of the same sex, then his or her biological age is the number of remaining years the average 70-year-old is expected to live.

Blessed Mental Status Test

The Blessed Mental Status Test is likely to be part of the battery of physical and psychological tests used in the diagnosis of senile dementia of the Alzheimer's type (i.e., a diagnosis of suspected Alzheimer's disease). It has been widely used in clinical assessment since its introduction by Dr. G. Blessed and colleagues more than 20 years ago. The validity of the test's diagnostic accuracy has received strong support from the correlation found between scores on the test and the number of senile plaques found in the cortex of the brain at autopsy (see ALZHEIMER'S DISEASE).

The test consists of two parts. For the first part, a relative or close friend of a client is asked questions about the client's competence in dealing with practical tasks in the everyday world (e.g., ability to perform common household chores). For the second part, the client is given a series of mental tasks to perform that test his or her concentration, orientation, recent memory, and remote memory. For example, the client is asked when World War II occurred and to count backward from 20.

Body Build and Body Characteristics
See also STRENGTH AND STAMINA

Height remains relatively stable until people reach their 50s. Between ages 55 and 75, men tend to lose about half an inch to an inch in height, and women lose an inch to two inches. Several factors are responsible for the decrease in height. They include compression of the spine from loss of bone strength, the thinning of the cartilage found between the bones of the vertebral column, and, alas, the effects of bad posture over the years.

From early adulthood to middle age, most people gain weight (the familiar "middle-aged spread"). The main reason is that middle-aged people tend to eat as much (or more) as they did as young adults. At the same time, many become less active physically and therefore convert less food into energy. In addition, the rate at which people convert food into energy (basal metabolic rate) slows by about 3% every 10 years. As a result, the caloric intake per day needed to maintain one's present weight decreases, on the average, about 5% to 10% every 10 years. The fact that middle-aged people are unlikely to reduce their food intake means that they do not burn up enough food. Consequently, fat accumulates throughout their bodies, and, for many middle-aged people, their weight gains by 10% to 15% of what it was in their 20s. After middle age, the body's weight usually levels off and begins a slow, progressive decrease as the body loses some bone, muscle, and fat. In late adulthood the ratio of lean body mass to fat declines, on the average, resulting in a lower basal metabolic rate because the metabolic needs of fat tissue are less than those of lean tissue. As a result, fewer calories, on the average, need to be consumed by older people even when they exercise regularly.

Light-skinned people often find their skin becoming even lighter as they age. This results from a decrease in the number of pigment cells in the skin and a decrease in the amount of pigment in the remaining cells. The skin of elderly people often contains "age spots" consisting of areas of dark pigmentation that resemble freckles. The number of moles in the skin is also likely to increase in late adulthood, and small red lines may appear in the skin as some blood vessels become dilated. Varicose veins are not common, but they do occur more often after age 65 than before that age. A 1988 survey by the U.S. Department of Health and Human Services found their incidence rate to be between 7% and 8% for people age 65 or older, about 5.6% for people in the age range of 45 to 64 years, and less than 3% for people in the 18 to 44 age range. They appear as irregular swellings in veins, especially those in the legs, and wearing of special hose may be required.

There is the tendency for older women to show sagging of the breasts. The sagging is caused by partial deterioration of the glandular tissue that produce firmness of the breasts and some stretching of the tissues connecting the breasts to their muscles. Measures may be taken earlier in life that may prevent, or at least reduce, sagging later in life. They include wearing supportive brassieres during pregnancy, breast-feeding, and exercising.

Boredom

Do you feel bored with your life and would like to add some excitement to it? On the surface, you might expect to find that elderly people experience more boredom than do younger people, especially young adults. However, recent evidence suggests that this is not the case. Age differences in boredom were investigated by researchers at the National Institute on Aging with a large sample of individuals ranging in age over the adult life span. The participants responded to such statements as "I am seldom bored" and "I am always glad to find some excuse to take me away from my work." Their responses indicated the extent to which each statement applied to them. Surprisingly, it was found that boredom tends to decrease with age, being greatest early in adulthood, after which it declines through middle age. Most surprisingly, there was no tendency for boredom to increase after middle age. That is, boredom was no greater in late adulthood than in middle age—and for both middle-aged and older adults it was found to be well below the level experienced by young adults.

Closely associated with boredom is the need to find relief from it by seeking external or internal stimulation of some kind. The need for external stimulation was tested in the boredom study by having the participants respond to such statements as "At the amusement park I like to go on the most scary rides" and "I find sitting at home a nice way to pass the time." The results were much like those found for boredom. The need for external stimulation was greatest for young adults and about the same for middle-aged and elderly adults. As the feeling of boredom decreases after young adulthood, the need for experiencing exciting events as an antidote for boredom decreases as well. The same outcome has been found by other researchers for the frequency of daydreaming, a form of internal stimulation used as an antidote for boredom. That is, elderly adults actually daydream less than young adults (see DAYDREAMING).

Brain and Aging

Several years ago, a prominent gerontologist was asked at a meeting why age-related changes occur in mental functioning. He replied, "The brain rots." This is, of course, a gross exaggeration. At the same time, it cannot be denied that changes do take place in the brain with normal aging, and even greater changes take place with abnormal aging (e.g., in Alzheimer's disease). These changes are likely to effect mental functioning, but forms of mental functioning are more affected than others. Much of our knowledge of changes in the structure of the brain is derived from autopsies in which detailed studies are made of younger and older brains. These studies reveal that, on the average, the brain decreases in weight by 5% to 10% from age 20 to age 90, with the amount of decrease varying with the presence or absence of disease. Some areas of the brain show greater decreases in size than other areas. The volume of the brain also decreases by 15% to 20%. As you look down at the brain from an open skull, you see a number of swelling-like areas known as gyri and a number of "valleys" (fissures or sulci) between the gyri. The gyri tend to become smaller in the aging brain, and the sulci become wider.

It is estimated that the human brain contains from 10 to 20 billion neurons (nerve cells) at the point of its maximum growth. How many neurons die and are not replaced as aging occurs is highly speculative. Some estimates are that 20,000 nerve cells are lost per day after age 30; other estimates have the loss rate as high as 100,000 neurons per day after age 30. Other neurons that do not die may nevertheless become less functional in late adulthood as the pigment lipofuscin accumulates in them and interferes with their functioning. Other changes in the neurons that occur with aging add to the decline in their functioning. These changes include the appearance of neurofibrillary tangles within the bodies and axons (that extension of a neuron along which neural messages are transmitted to make contact with the dendrites of other neurons) of some neurons and the presence of vacuoles (spaces) in the fluid surrounding the nucleus of some neurons. Senile plaques, consisting of hard clusters of dead or damaged neurons, are present in the aging brain; they too interfere with the normal functioning of the neurons near them. Other neurons may lose some of their dendrites (extensions that receive neural messages transmitted by axons from other neurons at points called synapses), thus diminishing the amount of neural information that may be received by those neurons.

An especially important change in the aging brain is the decrease in the amounts of neurotransmitters, both in the cerebral cortex (the gray matter you would see if you looked down on an opened skull) and in other areas. Neurotransmitters are chemicals that bridge the gap between the axon of one neuron and the dendrites of other neurons, making possible the transmission of neural information from neuron to neuron. These neurotransmitters include acetylcholine, norepinephrine, dopamine, serotonin, and gamma-aminobutyric acid. Acetylcholine is of particular importance in maintaining normal memory functioning, as is norepinephrine. Dopamine is a primary neurotransmitter in those areas of the brain controlling motor or muscular movements. Extreme declines in its production lead to Parkinson's disease. Serotonin is found in those areas of the brain controlling arousal and sleep. Declines in its presence seemingly account for many of the sleep problems encountered by a number of elderly people. Gamma-aminobutyric acid is concentrated largely in the thalamus, a bundle of neurons beneath the cerebral cortex that is involved in sensory functioning. Its reduction seemingly accounts for some of the sensory problems in elderly adults that are not explained by declining functioning of sense organs themselves.

Recent research has indicated that a protein known as nerve growth factor is important for the normal functioning of cholinergic neurons, that is, those neurons that use acetylcholine for transmission across synapses, and therefore for normal memory functioning. There seems to be a diminished supply of nerve growth factor in aging brains, a decrement that is especially pronounced for people with Alzheimer's disease.

Areas and structures of the brain are affected differentially by normal aging. One of the earliest structures adversely affected by aging is the hippocampus, a small bundle of neurons located beneath the cerebral cortex. It has long been known that the hippocampus plays a major role in transferring information from short-term storage to long-term storage. Lesions to the hippocampus often lead to major problems in registering new information in long-term memory. Neuronal loss and diminished amounts of acetylcholine in the hippocampus seemingly account for the difficulty of many elderly adults in registering new information in permanent memory. Neuronal loss or dysfunctioning with normal aging seems to be less pronounced in the prefrontal area of the cerebral cortex (the front of the brain). This area of the brain is involved in the retention of very old memories and in many higher level mental operations (e.g., reasoning). Pronounced neuronal dysfunctioning in this area, however, may result in what is called the frontal lobe deficit, characterized by difficulty in decision making, slowness of thought, and difficulty in controlling impulses. At the back of the brain are the cerebellum, medulla, and pons. The cerebellum is involved in maintaining body equilibrium and in smoothly coordinating muscular movements. Neuronal loss appears to be fairly severe in this area, sufficient in some elderly adults to result in impaired body balance (thus increasing the risk of falls) and the loss of some muscle tone that, in turn, results in greater susceptibility to muscular fatigue. Neuronal dysfunctioning in this area may also result in the tremors found in some elderly people (e.g., the shaking apparent while they try to make a deliberate movement of the hand). By contrast, normal aging seems to result in little neuronal loss or dysfunctioning in that area of the brain that controls gross body movements (the basal ganglia). The medulla controls critical biological functions, such as breathing and heartbeat.

The brain is separated into two large hemispheres, the left and right cerebral hemispheres, that have different, specialized functions. The left hemisphere controls movements for the right side of the body, and the right hemisphere controls movements for the left side of the body. Similarly, the left hemisphere determines feelings of touch from the right side of the body, the right hemisphere from the left. Moreover, for most people, verbal thought processes are controlled by the left hemisphere; spatial and imaginal thought processes are governed by the right hemisphere. Of great interest in gerontology is the possibility that the right hemisphere ages at a faster rate than does the left hemisphere. We know that verbal ability remains well preserved in late adulthood (see VERBAL ABILITY), while imaginal ability shows, on the average, fairly substantial declines with normal aging (see IMAGERY). Biological evidence in support of differential rates of cerebral aging has been conflicting, and the issue of differential hemispheric aging remains unresolved.

Most of our knowledge of aging's effects on the brain has come from postmortem examinations. In recent years two new devices and techniques have permitted examinations of the living brain. The first is called computed axial tomography (CAT) scanning. An x-ray source sends a narrow beam of x-rays through an individual's head to a detector on the other side of the head. The source and the detector are then rotated one degree for another beam to be projected through the head. This one-degree-at-a-time process continues through 180 one-degree rotations. The amount of x-ray absorbed at each point in the given slice of the brain being examined is transmitted to a computer that translates these amounts into a picture of the slice's neural structure. The individual can then be moved along the axis of rotation, and a "picture" of another slice is taken. For normally aging elderly adults, these "pictures" reveal increases in the fluid-filled spaces of the brain. However, these pictures have not been very revealing in identifying specific areas of the brain where atrophy has occurred that may then be related to specific mental and behavioral declines. CAT scans have not been very helpful in the early diagnosis of Alzheimer's disease. However, as the disease progresses in severity, CAT scans do show an atrophied brain with enlarged cortical sulci and enlarged cerebral ventricles. The second device is called positron emission tomography (PET) scanning. The procedure requires the release or emission of positively charged particles (positrons) during an individual's neural activity. The radioactive isotope is injected, which interacts with activated neurons and causes the emission of two gamma-ray photons that travel in opposite directions. These photons are delivered to a computer that constructs a "picture" of the metabolism occurring in the area where there is ongoing neural activity. Thus PET scans provide information about neural functioning rather than about neural structures. To date, PET scans have not provided any major new insights into the brain changes that occur with normal aging. Apparently, changes in brain glucose and oxygen metabolism are slight with normal aging. Moreover, measures of brain metabolism of elderly adults have not been found to correlate highly with scores on various mental tasks. However, PET scan scores do reveal pronounced reductions in the rates of glucose and oxygen metabolism in various regions of the brain for patients with severe impairments as a result of Alzheimer's disease. Research with CAT and PET scans is still in its infancy. There is great hope that future advancements in technology will lead to major discoveries about the effects of both normal and abnormal aging on the brain.

Aging of the brain occurs at different rates for different individuals. Declines in the brain's functioning with normal aging are likely to occur faster and be greater for individuals with lengthy histories of bad health practices, such as smoking and excessive drinking of alcoholic beverages. Declines are also likely to occur more slowly and to be less extensive for those individuals who have been lifelong regular exercisers.

Our focus has been on the adverse effects of aging on the brain. However, positive changes may also take place in the brain during late adulthood. Transmission across synapses may be enhanced by the increased branching of dendrites found in many old brains. The brain does show considerable plasticity or resiliency in recovering from atrophied areas of the brain. Such plasticity may be related to various factors, such as good health practices and living a mentally active and stimulating life. Much remains to be discovered about how life-styles affect the brain's structures and functions.

C

. . . .

Cardiovascular Disease and Mental Performance

The effects of aging itself on mental functioning and mental performances are complicated by the frequent presence of diseases in elderly people. Lowered mental functioning in many elderly people may be the consequence of the disease rather than the product of normal aging. The clearest evidence of the negative effects comes from studies of elderly people with cardiovascular diseases, particularly hypertension. In the early 1970s a large group of people in the 60- to 69-year age range had thorough physical examinations. On the basis of those examinations, the individuals were classified into three groups: normotensive (normal blood pressure), mildly elevated (blood pressure slightly above the normal range), and hypertensive (blood pressure significantly above the normal range). These individuals were all administered the Wechsler Adult Intelligence Scale at the beginning of the study and again after 10 years. There was no significant change in scores on those components of the test measuring crystallized intelligence (e.g., vocabulary, general information; see INTELLIGENCE) for any of the three groups. The normotensive group also showed no change in scores on the components of the test measuring fluid intelligence. By contrast, the hypertensive group, on the average, showed a significant decline in these scores. Interestingly, the group with mildly elevated blood pressure showed significant improvement in fluid intelligence test scores, suggesting to some researchers that mild increases in blood pressure may enhance intellectual functioning. Why is there a decline in fluid intelligence with more severe elevations of blood pressure? Researchers have speculated that persistent high levels of blood pressure may add to the decline in functioning of some areas of the brain brought about by normal aging, especially the hippocampus (see BRAIN AND AGING).

A more recent longitudinal study has followed groups of normotensive and hypertensive individuals who were in their 40s when the study began. Neither crystallized nor fluid intelligence test scores showed a significant decline during a 10-year period for either group, unless the hypertensive individuals had other medical complications (e.g., myocardial infarction). The adverse effects of hypertension on intellectual functioning are seemingly not manifested until the affected individuals are in their 60s.

Caregivers (Elderly Parents)

Elderly parents who function well themselves often serve as caregivers for adult children with disabilities of various kinds. Researchers at the University of Wisconsin–Madison recently surveyed several hundred mothers (average age, 65 years) of such adult children (average age, 33 years). Elderly mothers of adult children with a mental illness reported higher levels of frustration and lower levels of gratification from caregiving than did elderly mothers of mentally retarded adult children. More emotion-focused coping with stress strategy was used by mothers of adult children with mental illness than by mothers of adult children with mental retardation (see STRESS AND COPING WITH STRESS). The use of a problem-focused coping strategy was found to yield a positive sense of well-being for mothers of adult children with mental retardation but not for mothers of adult children with mental illness. There are several reasons for these differences. Social interactions are usually fewer, and families are less cohesive when mental illness is the reason for caring for an adult child than when mental retardation is the reason. In addition, leaving home during the day to work or to attend a day-care center, which allows mothers time for themselves, is more likely for adults with retardation than for adults with mental illness.

Caregivers (Family Members and Friends)

A survey conducted in 1982 revealed that there were more than 1.5 million disabled elderly people in the United States who were not residing in a nursing home or a similar facility. The average age of these people was estimated to be 78 years (more than 20% of them were age 85 and older), and it was estimated that 60% of them were women, 51% were married, and 41% were widowed. *Disability* means that the affected individuals have one or more physical or mental limitations that interfere with the activities of daily living and therefore require assistance from a caregiver to survive outside a nursing home or other institution. Many of the disabled have Alzheimer's disease. As the elderly population grows, the number of disabled older people will increase, and the need for more caregivers will increase steadily. In fact, more recent estimates suggest that the number of older individuals in the community who need assistance to live outside an institutional setting may now exceed 5 million.

The 1982 survey also revealed that 72% of caregivers were women (23% the spouse of the disabled individual, 29% a daughter, and 20% a woman who was neither a spouse nor a daughter and was usually a friend of the individual). The average age of the caregivers was 57 years; nearly half were in the 45- to 64-year age range. Adult children serving as caregivers are usually the same gender as the disabled person. Because those needing care are more likely to be mothers than fathers, the number of daughters serving as caregivers greatly exceeds the number of sons. The current estimate is that they make up nearly 40% of caregivers. The stress experienced by caregivers is less, in general, the closer they are in age to the affected individual. This accounts in part for the general success of friends as caregivers—they are closer in age to the disabled person.

Further information about caregivers was provided in a more recent national survey of nearly 500 families. In this study, 75% of caregivers were women, and the average age of the caregivers was 50 years. Of the caregivers, 65% provided services for one parent, 26% for two parents, and 9% for three parents (their own plus a partner's parent). Most important, 56% of the caregivers reported helping an elderly parent more than 12 hours a week by providing such services as cooking meals and regulating the administration of medicines. In addition, researchers at the University of California–Berkeley found that the positive effects (e.g., a sense of achievement) of outside employment for caregivers outweighed the negative effects (e.g., fatigue).

Caregiving understandably places a considerable burden on the caregiver. The consequences of this burden, and the discovery of ways to reduce the consequences, have been widely studied in recent years by gerontologists. The incidence of depression among caregivers is high (perhaps as high as 50% of the caregivers), although the extent of the depression has been found to be no greater for those caring for more impaired individuals than for those caring for less impaired individuals. Researchers at Ohio State University have found that caregivers of persons with Alzheimer's disease continue to show significant depression for at least as long as 2 years after the death of the person receiving the caregiving. In general, female caregivers appear to be more depressed than male caregivers, and wives as caregivers appear to perceive themselves as being more burdened than do husbands as caregivers. When daughters serve as caregivers, the subjective burden tends to be less if there is a stronger attachment to their mothers. In general, daughters experience the fewest negative effects of caregiving for their mothers when the mothers live separately. For two-generation households (mother and caregiving daughter, no grandchildren), daughters provide more care and experience fewer negative emotional effects than in three-generation households (grandchildren present). Adult sons usually become caregivers only if a sister is unavailable. When a sister is unavailable to serve as the caregiver, a son is likely to rely on his wife for major assistance and to provide relatively little care himself.

The frustration experienced by caregivers by the disruption of their own life plans is apparently greatest at the onset of the symptoms of the person receiving the care, and often decreases over time as the caregivers develop routines for providing care, even though the need for care increases during that period. It is not unusual to discover that caregivers have emotional symptoms other than depression, such as anxiety, guilt, and psychosomatic disorders. The personality of the caregiver also appears to have an effect on whether the caregiver will experience either mental health or physical health problems. Researchers at Syracuse University recently tested 51 spouse caregivers of persons with dementia. The caregivers who scored higher on the trait of neuroticism (see NEUROTICISM; PERSONALITY TRAITS) experienced greater depression and less of a feeling of well-being than caregivers who scored lower on neuroticism. Caregivers who scored higher in neuroticism also experienced more health problems than those with lower scores, and they were more likely to use emotion-focused coping strategies than problem-focused strategies (see STRESS AND COPING WITH STRESS). By contrast, caregivers with high scores on extroversion were more likely to cope with stress by seeking social support and less likely to depend on emotion-focused coping. Optimism was also related to the mental health of the caregivers; those who scored higher on optimism rated themselves as feeling less stress and less depression than those with lower scores. In addition, the stress of caregiving tends to be less for caregivers who have better coping skills than for caregivers with poorer coping skills.

In general, male spouses experience less distress as caregivers than do female spouses. Researchers at the University of Southern California found two likely reasons for this sex difference. First, men are less aware of their emotions than are women, and they are, therefore, less likely to realize they are feeling distress. Second, women are more likely than men to use coping styles that are ineffective for reducing distress.

Over half of the daughters who are caregivers are also married and therefore serve roles other than caregiver. Distress experienced as a caregiver is often increased by the competing demands of being a wife and perhaps a mother as well. In addition, many caregivers are employed, and they must share their job performance with caregiving. This may add to the stress of caregiving. Many offices and services are open only in the daytime and then only on weekdays, thus forcing caregivers to take time off from their jobs if they need to conduct business with these agencies. Tension at work may then be the consequence. However, there are possible positive effects of multiple roles as well. Managing more than one role successfully may enhance caregivers' feelings of self-esteem and their ability to control their own lives. Interestingly, husbands of multiple-role caregiver wives generally feel that the time and energy spent on caregiving has little negative effect on relationships with their wives and may even bring the two of them closer together.

Support groups have become a major means of trying to reduce the stress experienced by caregivers and to help them to develop the skills needed to cope with their duties. A support group consists of several caregivers who are led in their meetings by either a professional gerontologist or by one of their peers. The group usually meets for six to eight weekly sessions, with each session lasting about 2 hours. The members of the group are usually trained to use one another as a support system or network. Members of the group are encouraged to share their feelings and caregiving experiences with other group members and to maintain contact with other group members after the meetings have been completed. If the support group consists of caregivers for persons with Alzheimer's disease, then the group meetings are likely to provide information about the nature of the disease and its stages. The group members may also be trained to give their recipients exercises in memory and problem solving to help slow the decline in their abilities as much as possible. However, after analyzing the results of many studies on interventions designed to reduce stress for caregivers, researchers at the University of Southern California concluded that group interventions are less effective than individual interventions in which a caregiver is given professional counseling and other forms of psychological assistance.

Because of the stress and distress often experienced by caregivers, they should explore the services and facilities available in their communities to help them with their caregiving responsibilities. Finding and joining a support group is one possibility. Both the caregiver and the person receiving the care are likely to benefit. An alternative is to seek individual counseling and training in problem solving. Another possibility is the use of respite care services available in the community (see RESPITE CARE). Again, both the caregiver and the recipient of care are likely to benefit considerably. In a recent study, researchers at John Carroll University found that long-term male caregivers of wives with Alzheimer's disease were much more likely to use respite care than short-term caregivers. Those who used respite care used the free time effectively for their own otherwise limited enjoyment (e.g., golfing, walking). Engaging in social interactions for fun and recreation has also been found to reduce the burden of caregiving experienced by many family caregivers. A promising way of coping with the anger that may often follow the frustration of caregiving has been introduced by Dr. Dorothy Gallagher-Thompson and her associates at the Veterans Administration Medical Center in Palo Alto, California. They have developed an intervention program that teaches wives or daughters who are caregivers the skills needed to manage their frustrations without producing intense anger. The skills include learning to relax during periods of extreme stress and learning to be appropriately assertive with the recipients of their caregiving.

The American Association of Retired Persons publishes booklets that give caregivers helpful suggestions for reducing the stress they may be encountering. Write to AARP Fulfillment, 601 E Street, N.W., Washington, DC 20049.

Caregivers (Paid Workers)

Adult children, especially daughters, have traditionally been the main sources of caregivers for disabled elderly people. However, as the number of women entering the labor force has increased, the availability of daughters for caregiving has decreased. The demand for paid caregivers has consequently increased. The majority of paid caregivers have been middle-aged minority women without a high school education. As the educational level of future generations of these women increases, the number who accept low-paying jobs like caregiving will decrease. Caregiving in the home usually pays much less than nursing assistants in hospitals are paid, and the benefits are also much less for those working in homes.

There have been various attempts to fill the void in home-care workers. For example, attempts have been made to train welfare recipients as caregivers, but without much success. Men, in general, are not interested in caregiving, and young people are considered to be too immature to serve as caregivers. Given the likely future increase in the number of disabled older people and the emphasis on home care in preference to institutionalization, more innovative ways are needed to make home caregiving a more attractive occupation. Some possibilities have been explored in demonstration projects sponsored by the Ford Foundation in several cities. Overall, these projects were successful in reducing the turnover among home caregivers and in increasing on-the-job longevity. Some components of the projects were relatively inexpensive. For example, in one of the cities, both experienced and novice employees received training in home-care skills, and they received several status symbols (e.g., identification badges like those of nursing assistants in hospitals) to boost their morale. However, other components, such as providing health insurance benefits for the participants, did require a much larger expenditure. In the long term, continuation of such projects would require subsidies by either private or governmental agencies. They may well be worth the cost.

Caregivers (Positive Effects of Caregiving)

Perhaps the most common experience of family members who serve as caregivers for elderly people is stress. However, the fact that caregiving can, and often does, have positive emotional effects should not be ignored. A survey by researchers at the University of Southern California revealed that a third of the families involved in caregiving reported more positive than negative changes in their lives during the course of caregiving. The positive changes included increased closeness among the family members (e.g., among siblings). Some spouses of elderly persons with Alzheimer's disease even reported an improvement in their marital relationship.

Cautiousness

An impression held by many people is that elderly adults are more cautious in their behavior than are younger adults. A number of studies have revealed, however, that the greater cautiousness of older adults is apparent for some behaviors but not for others. There are two kinds of laboratory tasks for which elderly participants have consistently been found to be more cautious than younger participants. On learning tasks, elderly participants tend to wait until they are certain a response is correct before they give it. Until then they are likely not to respond. Thus their errors are primarily errors of omission (i.e., not responding at all). By contrast, younger participants are more willing to risk appearing foolish, and they often guess in regard to the correct response. Thus they make many more errors of commission (i.e., responding, but incorrectly) than do elderly participants. A similar age difference is found when participants are asked to decide whether a weak sensory event (e.g., a faint tone) is present or absent on each of many trials (with the tone present on half the trials and absent on the other half). Elderly participants approach this task more cautiously than do younger participants. If elderly participants suspect the event may be present, but they are not certain, they are likely to avoid appearing foolish by responding "Absent." (See also RECOGNITION MEMORY VS. RECALL MEMORY for a task in which elderly participants are likely to be less cautious than younger participants.) Age differences in cautiousness appear to be absent when the task involves a higher level of decision making. The standard procedure is to give participants a test describing lifelike situations in which they are to advise someone on the degree of risk he or she should take (e.g., leaving a secure job with low pay to take a higher-paying job with a shaky company). Participants must choose among alternatives that are more desirable in some ways but more risky in others and among alternatives that are less desirable in some ways but less risky overall. In general, studies with this kind of task indicate little age difference in the willingness to take risk. Of course, the task is only a simulation of everyday risks. Nevertheless, it does seem risky to conclude that there is some general characteristic of cautiousness—and that elderly people possess more of it than do younger people.

Classical Conditioning

You are seated in a chair with your head firmly placed in front of a glass disk. Suddenly, the disk brightens, and shortly thereafter a puff of air is shot into your eye. Of course, you blink. Blinking your eye is an example of an unconditioned response to its natural stimulus (in this case, the puff of air). An *unconditioned response* is one that is automatically evoked when its appropriate stimulus occurs. Suppose the pairing of the brightening of the disk with the puff of air continues for many trials. Eventually you will begin to blink when the disk brightens and before the puff of air is delivered. Blinking to the brightness of the disk is an example of a conditioned response. A *conditioned response* is one that has been learned in the presence of what was originally a neutral stimulus or event (in this case, the brightening of the disk). The originally neutral stimulus is called a conditioned stimulus.

The procedure described above is the most common one used to investigate age differences in classical conditioning. In classical conditioning, participants essentially learn to substitute one stimulus (the conditioned stimulus) for another stimulus (the unconditioned stimulus), such that the new stimulus takes over for the original stimulus in evoking a specific response. Classical conditioning is the simplest form of learning. It was introduced to psychology nearly a century ago by Ivan Pavlov, the famous Russian scientist, in his research with dogs and other animals. Pavlov discovered, for example, that dogs could learn to salivate to such conditioned stimuli as a bell or a flashing light when the stimuli just preceded receiving meat powder in the mouth.

There is much more to classical conditioning than simply training dogs to salivate or human beings to blink. Classical conditioning may be the simplest form of learning, but it is of great importance in shaping human behavior. Some fears and phobias appear to be acquired through classical conditioning. Consider someone who has a painful fall while trying to avoid stepping on a spider. If the pain is great enough, there is the possibility that a component of the pain (an unconditioned response to the fall) will be conditioned to the sight of the spider (a conditioned stimulus). The conditioned response to future encounters with spiders is the anticipation of pain, an anticipation we call fear. In other words, this person has acquired via classical conditioning a fear or phobia of spiders. Psychologists believe that even some prejudices may be acquired by means of classical conditioning. In addition, classical conditioning serves as a form of therapy for eliminating some kinds of unwanted behaviors (see BEHAVIOR MODIFICATION). Given the importance of classical conditioning, age differences in the rate at which it occurs are of great interest.

Numerous investigators have found that elderly adults do acquire a conditioned eye-blink response with the procedure described above. However, the rate of acquisition is much slower than it is for younger adults. In fact, the slowing of acquisition is apparent by the mid-50s. For example, researchers at Temple University gave participants in their 20s, 40s, 50s, and 60s and older more than 90 pairings of the brightening disk and the puff of air. At the end of pairings, participants in their 20s and 40s were blinking to the disk stimulus alone about 80% of the time. By contrast, the older participants were blinking only about 40% of the time. The eye-blink task may be far removed from conditioning as it occurs in the everyday world, but it does have the basic elements of classical conditioning. It is apparent that something happens with normal aging that inhibits the rate at which classical conditioning occurs. The slower rate of conditioning by older adults has both its good and bad components. The good news is that older adults are less likely than younger adults to acquire new fears and prejudices by means of classical conditioning. The bad news is that older adults are less likely than younger adults to benefit from conditioning therapy.

Why is conditioning slower among older people? There is good reason to believe that it is one of the consequences of normal biological aging. Animal research has revealed that the cerebellum (a segment of the back portion of the brain) is highly involved in acquiring a conditioned response. It is the loss of neural cells in the cerebellum that seems to result in slower conditioning by aging animals, including human beings.

Claudication

Claudication refers to a painful cramp in one or both legs that occurs while walking. It is usually caused by narrowing of the arteries in the legs that results from atherosclerosis (hardening of the arteries; see DISEASES [CHRONIC]) and subsequent peripheral vascular diseases.

Clinical Dementia Rating

Researchers at Washington University (St. Louis) have designed a widely used rating procedure to measure the course of dementia (especially Alzheimer's disease) as it progresses in severity. The rating is based on an intensive clinical interview with the patient and with others close to the patient. The rating is on a scale ranging from 0 to 3. A score of 0 indicates the absence of dementia, a score of 0.5 indicates that the presence of dementia is questionable, and scores of 1, 2, and 3 indicate that the dementia is mild, moderate, and severe, respectively. Separate scores are given for six different categories of mental functioning that are affected by dementia: memory, orientation, judgment and problem solving, involvement in community affairs, involvement at home and in hobbies, and personal care. These category scores are then combined to give a single overall score.

Clinical Psychology

Clinical psychology is the component of psychology that deals with the diagnosis and treatment of emotional, adjustment, and behavioral problems. Clinical psychologists usually have a doctor of philosophy degree, and they are certified or licensed by the state where they practice to be in private practice or to practice in hospitals or mental health clinics. They are well qualified to administer psychological tests of intelligence, memory functioning, personality, and depression, and to supervise psychotherapy for patients. By contrast, psychiatrists are medically trained therapists who have a doctor of medicine degree and are able to prescribe drugs for the treatment of depression and psychosis and to prescribe such treatments as electroconvulsive therapy.

Geriatric clinical psychologists are most likely to be involved in the diagnosis and treatment of depression and other emotional disorders in elderly people caused by stress or life crises. They may also be involved in the diagnosis and treatment of dementias, such as Alzheimer's disease. Unfortunately, clinical psychologists generally prefer to work with younger clients. Many clinical psychologists are active researchers into the causes of behavioral disorders, including those associated with aging, and in the discovery of better diagnostic tests and therapies of behavioral disorders.

Cognitive (Mental) Stages of Development

In the 1920s Jean Piaget, the late and now famous Swiss physician and psychologist, gave psychology one of its most influential theories. The theory postulated that all children go through the same progressive stages of cognitive or mental development, and in the same order. The earliest stage, the sensorimotor stage, occurs roughly from birth through age 2 years. It is characterized by the child mastering such concepts as object permanence (i.e., objects do not really disappear when they are out of sight). The second stage, the preoperational stage, occurs from about age 2 to age 7 years. It is one in which children are influenced greatly by their senses. If given two rows with equal numbers of blocks, but differences in the spacing between blocks, children in this stage of development are likely to say that the row with the greater length has more blocks in it. The third stage, the concrete operational stage, begins at about age 7 and ends at about age 11. By now the child is able to say that the rows contain an equal number of blocks. This is accomplished by the child's ability to manipulate objects mentally and observe that it is only the spaces that distinguish the two rows. The final stage, the formal operations stage, occurs during adolescence. It is characterized by the development of reasoning abilities that enable individuals to think abstractly and to solve problems with which they have had no prior experience.

Piaget's stage theory has attracted interest in gerontology from two different perspectives. The first concerns the possibility of an age regression whereby some older adults return to a preformal stage of cognitive development. That is, their thinking processes are limited to those characteristic of the concrete operational stage or even the preoperational stage. Some researchers have found that some of their elderly participants are less capable than their younger participants in solving problems that should be solvable by the thinking processes characteristic of the concrete operational stage. However, it is quite likely that many elderly participants view simple problems, such as the rows of blocks problem, as being too childish. Moreover, when the elderly participants are carefully selected to ensure the inclusion of only those in good health and who are functioning well, there is no apparent difference from younger participants in the ability to solve such simple problems.

The second interest concerns the possibility of an additional stage of cognitive development, one beyond Piaget's final stage of formal operations. This fifth, postformal stage, is one characterized by more diversified forms of thinking than found in individuals locked into the formal stage. Individuals in a postformal stage would have the capability of asking the right questions when appropriate and not just finding answers to questions. Individuals in this stage would also know that answers to questions often depend on the situations and conditions relevant to those questions. There is limited evidence to indicate that more older than younger individuals perform at this postformal level. The implication is that cognitive development may continue throughout adulthood, and does not end before early adulthood.

Cohort (Generational) Effect

People born in widely separated years necessarily come from different generations. Many conditions present during the childhood and adolescence of people born, say, in 1970 changed greatly from those present during the childhood and adolescence of people born, say, in 1920. For example, people from the 1920 cohort grew up without television and with the experience of living through a major economic depression. By contrast, people from the 1970 generation grew up with television and did not experience a major economic depression. In addition, child-rearing practices differed greatly between children born in 1920 and children born in 1970. These differences in conditions in the home and in society are likely to have produced important behavioral differences overall between people born in 1920 and those born in 1970. If people born in those years had been tested on one of those behaviors affected by variation in home and societal conditions in 1990 when they were 70 and 20 years old, they would show a pronounced age difference. The age difference, however, would not be the result of a true age change in behavior. Instead the age difference would be the result of a cohort effect. This is the case, for example, for the political and social attitudes. When tested in 1990, people who are 70 years old score, on the average, as being more conservative on attitude tests than people who are 20 years old. However, this does not mean that people become more conservative with normal aging. People now age 70 were probably just as conservative when they were 20 years old. Moreover, people now age 20 are likely to remain as liberal when they reach age 70. The present age difference in conservatism is the consequence of generational differences during the preadulthood period of development, and it therefore reflects a cohort effect rather than an age change.

In addition to political and social attitudes, there is evidence to indicate that age differences in scores on both personality tests and intelligence tests represent, at least in part, cohort effects. However, it is unlikely that age differences in performances on perceptual, learning, memory, and problem-solving tasks are greatly influenced by cohort effects. Age differences on these tasks are likely to be the consequence of normal aging.

Color Perception

Older studies on the ability of elderly people to discriminate among colors indicated that they are much less proficient in doing so than are young adults. These studies indicated that elderly adults, on the average, are about 25% less accurate in identifying the colors of objects at age 70 than are young adults, and that they are only about 50% as accurate at age 90. However, more recent evidence suggests that the color weakness of elderly people may be apparent only when finer contour discriminations are needed, discriminations of the kind needed to distinguish among the colors in a tie that contains a complex, mutable pattern of shapes and colors. Regardless of the extent of the color weakness that occurs with aging, the difficulty in identifying colors is restricted largely to colors at the short wavelengths of the spectrum (i.e., blue and violet). A major factor in producing color weakness is the yellowing of the lens of the eye that occurs with normal aging. The result is that less light reaches the retina or inner layer of the eye than in earlier adulthood.

Concept Learning

Big cars, little cars, blue cars, green cars, two-door cars, four-door cars—the list goes on and on. Despite the differences among them, they are all instances of the same category or concept, namely that of an automobile. Members of the same concept are likely to differ in a number of ways. In the case of automobiles, they differ along several irrelevant dimensions, such as size, color, and number of doors. However, members of the same concept have in common characteristics along relevant dimensions. For an automobile, the relevant dimensions are source of power and number of wheels. For the power dimension, the common characteristic (or attribute) is being engine powered as opposed to animal powered (as in a carriage or stagecoach). For the wheel dimension, the common characteristic is four wheels as opposed to two wheels (as in a motorcycle). Thus "automobile" is a concept that enables us to group together all variations of an automobile. The concept in this case is called a *conjunctive concept* in that membership within the concept demands both something *and* something else. If either is missing, the object in question is not a member of a concept. There are also *disjunctive concepts;* here, membership in the concept is defined by a rule of "something *or* something else." Consider the concept of a strike in baseball. It occurs if a batter swings and misses a pitch *or* does not swing but the umpire says he should have—*or* if the batter swings and the ball goes foul and there are fewer than two strikes. Irrelevant dimensions include the location of the ball (inside corner, outside corner, or middle of the plate) and the direction of the ball if hit foul. It is little wonder that people unfamiliar with baseball have difficulty understanding it when they see their first baseball game. Considerable concept learning must occur before they can really understand the game. Another example of a disjunctive concept is a first down in football. It may be achieved by moving 10 or more yards either in the air *or* on the ground.

Much of our concept learning takes place during childhood. We learn concepts like that of "a puppy" (a conjunctive concept—a member of the puppy concept must be both a dog *and* not fully grown), "a daddy" (a conjunctive concept—male *and* a parent), and "an automobile." Concept learning does not stop in childhood, however. In recent decades, adults have learned such new concepts as "a black hole" and "AIDS" and even variations on old concepts, such as "gas guzzler" and "compact" for "automobile."

To study age difference in concept learning, participants are given such tasks as the poisoned food task. Here, patients in a hospital are described as receiving a meal consisting of three components (e.g., rice, corn, and beef), with the patient then either dying or living after eating the meal. The task is to discover what the poisoned meals have in common and thus identify what defines the concept of "a poisoned meal." Elderly participants have greater difficulty, on the average, in learning the concept in question that do younger participants. However, as with other forms of learning, learning does take place, albeit somewhat more slowly, in general, than it does for younger adults. The implication is that normally aging elderly people are perfectly capable of learning new concepts as they occur in our world; they simply are likely to need more time to do so.

Conformity

Conformity means yielding to group pressure. Suppose you are a member of a club consisting of 10 people. You have gathered to vote on whether Mr. Smith should be admitted to your club. You have studied Mr. Smith's credentials, and you have decided he would make an excellent addition. The voting is done openly and in alphabetical order. Your name makes you last in the voting order. One by one the other members of your club vote "No" to admit Mr. Smith. Now it is your turn to vote. Would you conform to group pressure and also vote "No"—or would you stay with your original conviction and vote "Yes"?

A standard laboratory task is used to study conformity. Members of a group are shown pairs of lines differing in length, and they are asked which member of each pair is longer. One member of the group is the true participant whose conformity is being observed. The other members are all stooges of the investigator. As in the fictitious club voting situation, members of the group respond one by one with which line in a pair appears longer. The real participant is the last to respond. For some of the pairs, the stooges unanimously pick the wrong line. Surely, to the real participant, it is the other line that appears to be longer. Research with this task has revealed that a larger percentage of elderly adults than younger adults conform to group pressure in this situation. This research suggests that current elderly people, in general, may be more conforming to group pressure than are younger people. However, little is known about age differences in conformity in other situations, especially those encountered in everyday life.

There is evidence indicating that elderly people in a nursing home who are rated high in conformity to the staff's regulations are also rated higher in adjustment by the staff than are elderly people rated low in conformity. This outcome should not be surprising. Conforming residents of a nursing home are the ones who behave in a manner that pleases staff members. They therefore could be rated high in adjustment for this reason alone.

Constancies of Perception

As you are walking down the street, a stranger approaches you from the opposite direction. When first spotted, the stranger is about 50 feet from you. Eventually the stranger is within a few feet of you. Despite the changing distance that separates the two of you, the stranger does not change in your perception of his or her size. The stranger appeared to be about 6 feet tall whether 50 feet from you or 5 feet. This is true even though the image of the stranger does become larger on the retinas of your eyes as the distance separating the two of you decreases. This is an example of the important principle of size constancy in perception. Your eyes provide information that enables your brain to tell you that size is remaining constant. For example, as an object changes distance from you, so does the degree of convergence of your two eyes. That is, your eyes converge more the closer the object is to you. This helps to inform you that the distance of the object from you is changing, and therefore the size of the object's image on the retina must also be changing. This is obviously not the only source of information fed to the brain. We know that people with one eye do have size constancy. Accommodation of the lens (flattening or thickening of its shape) occurs as distance changes, thus providing additional information to the brain for size constancy. This is a monocular cue (i.e., present separately in each eye), and it is therefore present for people with only one functioning eye. We also know that size constancy is retained well with normal aging. Elderly adults are no more likely than younger adults to be deceived by changes in the size of objects on the retina when those objects are perceived at different distances.

Age changes are also likely to be slight, if any, for the other basic perceptual constancies. One of these is brightness constancy. Consider the appearance of a piece of white paper in a room you occupy. Initially, the paper appears bright in illumination. Then the lights in the room begin to dim. As they do, you perceive no change in the whiteness of the paper. Similarly, a white duck swimming in a lake on a bright sunny day continues to look white when a cloud dims the sunlight. This is because the ratio of the illumination from the object in question to the illumination from the background stays constant as the background illumination decreases. This constant ratio provides information that the brightness of the object has not changed. Another basic constancy is that of shape constancy. As you look at an opening door, the shape of the moving door projected on the retinas of your eyes keeps changing. Similarly, a coin tossed in the air continues to be perceived as circular even though the images on the retina are unlikely to be circular. These are familiar examples of shape constancy. Our past experiences with these objects provide the information needed to know that they are not changing shapes, even though what is seen by the eyes is changing.

Consumers

It is estimated that people age 50 and older spend 40% of consumer dollars. They buy about 48% of all luxury cars, and they are responsible for about 80% of luxury travel. They even buy about 25% of all toys annually (there are about 55 million grandparents age 50 years and older in the United States). Nevertheless, marketing and merchandising programs commonly treat these consumers as if they are much older. For example, there is the myth that older consumers are fixed on certain products and they are unwilling to try new alternative products. Therefore why should advertising of a new product be directed at older consumers? In fact, a recent survey of 500 people over age 50 in shopping malls revealed that about 80% of them were quite willing to try new products.

Merchants can do more to appeal to older consumers. For example, they could advertise merchandise of interest to older people at nontraditional times on television, such as during the noon news when the proportion of older adults viewing the programs is likely to be greater than the proportion of younger adults. They should also have a number of older salespeople or age-sensitive younger salespeople. Above all, they should not have rock music playing in the background when they have sales of special interest to older shoppers.

Continuity vs. Discontinuity in Adult Development

Do elderly adults behave in the same ways they did when they were younger? If they were shy as young adults, do they continue to be shy through middle age and late adulthood? Do those elderly adults who are good problem solvers as young adults continue to be so as elderly adults, at least relative to other elderly adults who were not good problem solvers earlier in life? In general, the answers to those questions is "Yes." We know that many personality traits and characteristics change little from early to late adulthood (see PERSONALITY TRAITS). Shy persons may become more or less shy as they grow older, but they are likely to remain shier than most other people their own age. Similarly, there may be some modest decline in problem-solving ability with normal aging (see PROBLEM SOLVING), but people who were proficient early in life are likely to retain their advantage later in life. These are examples of continuity in adult development. Continuity does not mean the absence of changes in behavior with aging, but it does mean that the changes are primarily quantitative in nature. That is, people may possess more or less of a behavior than they did earlier, but the basic pattern of behavior remains unaltered. In many mental processes and activities, only quantitative changes are observed with normal aging. People who are good readers early in life continue to be good readers later in life, but they read more slowly than they did earlier. Memory processes are basically unaltered, but they do occur more slowly than they did earlier in life. Older people have memory spans slightly shorter than they had as young adults, but they, nevertheless, are still able to hold considerable material in short-term memory (see MEMORY SPAN). These are all examples of quantitative changes that take place in adult development.

At the same time, there *is* some discontinuity in adult development. Some behavior and mental process changes are qualitative in nature rather than merely quantitative. In effect, elderly adults are presumed to be quite different with respect to those behaviors and processes than they were earlier in life. For example, the stresses and crises confronting elderly adults are usually quite different from the stresses and crises they faced as younger adults. The ways in which they must cope with these stresses or crises are likely to be quite different from the coping strategies they used to solve earlier crises in their lives. Some memory processes may change qualitatively from early to late adulthood. When given stories to read and remember, younger adults typically try to recall the ideas of the story. By contrast, many elderly adults will focus less on the specific content and more on the moral of the story and implications of the story's content for their own lives.

Control over Life's Events

"It's up to me to keep my mental faculties from deteriorating." "No matter what I do, if I am going to get sick, I will get sick." Responses to such statements are used to measure the personality characteristic known as locus of control. The characteristic is anchored by two extremes labeled "external" and "internal." People who score at the external end of the dimension of locus of control seemingly believe that many of the events in their lives are determined or controlled by forces external to themselves (e.g., chance, fate). Such persons are likely to respond false to the first statement, one dealing with the belief about control over one's intellectual functioning, and true to the second statement, one dealing with the belief about lack of control over one's health. A number of studies, both cross-sectional and longitudinal, have indicated that people tend to become more external in their beliefs as they age normally. They tend to lessen in their belief that they have considerable control of many of life's events. This is somewhat unfortunate since there is evidence to indicate that, with normal aging, older people who score as being internal express greater satisfaction with their current lives than do people who score as being external. The same evidence suggests that this difference in life satisfaction between "internals" and "externals" is especially pronounced for elderly women. Moreover, there is also evidence that those elderly people who appear to be "internals" in regard to their intellectual functioning score higher on intelligence tests than do those elderly people who appear to be "externals." In addition, "externals" tend to rely more heavily on assistance from other people than do "internals" when confronted by mentally demanding tasks. The reliance on others for such tasks is likely to be especially true for women and for less educated elderly people. For most older people, the decline in mental ability is likely to be so moderate (if it exists at all) that they have little reason to fear facing mentally demanding tasks. Similarly, those elderly people who appear to be "internals" in regard to their health make fewer visits per year to a physician than those who appear to be "externals."

Residents of nursing homes live in an environment where there is little opportunity to control the events in their lives. There has been research revealing that when these individuals are given an opportunity to control a major event of their lives (such as the timing and duration of visits from family members and friends), their well-being, both physically and mentally, may improve considerably.

Conversation Memory

"You did too say that!" "I did *not!*"

Such frequent conversational exchanges are testimony to the fact that our memories of past conversations with other people are often imperfect. Our interest rests in the possibility that the imperfection may increase from early to late adulthood.

As with memory for the content of television programs (see MEMORY FOR TELEVISION PROGRAMS), memory for the content of conversations in the everyday world seems to occur incidentally. That is, we neither have the intent to commit conversational content to memory nor do we even try to rehearse it in an attempt to increase its memorability. The very act of attending to and comprehending what is being said to you is sufficient to ensure the automatic registration of at least part of the content in memory, but not always accurately. Memory for conversational content is an important component of our everyday memory. Failure to remember important parts of a conversation can on occasion have serious implications. This is the case, for example, in our memory of a conversation with our physician. Inability to recall correctly parts of that conversation can result in the misapplication of a treatment for an injury or a disease. We seem to be especially vulnerable to errors in memory when the content is in terms of instructions on how to reach a specific locale or how to assemble a particular piece of equipment.

Despite the importance of conversational memory in everyday functioning, there has been little research on age differences in the proficiency of conversational memory. Researchers at the University of Missouri–Columbia did bring conversational memory into the laboratory by having young adult and elderly participants engage in a series of conversations with the investigator. Each conversation centered around a specific topic, such as the presidency of the United States. For each topic, the participants were asked several questions, and after each question they were asked to explain the reason for their answer (e.g., "Should presidents be limited to one 6-year term in office?"). They were later asked to recall the topics discussed and the specific questions asked. Interestingly, memory was almost as proficient for participants, young and elderly, who did not know in advance that their memory for the contents would be tested (i.e., incidental memory) as it was for participants who did know (i.e., intentional memory). The recall of both topics and questions was far from perfect for the young adults, and it was even more imperfect for the elderly adults (about 20% less proficient). However, when tested for the recognition of the topics discussed and the questions, both young and elderly participants had essentially perfect scores. The imperfection of conversational memory, at least for memory of recent conversations, seems to be largely in the retrieval stage (i.e., getting information out of memory storage) rather than in the encoding stage (i.e., getting information into memory storage). Elderly adults have moderately greater retrieval problems than young adults (see RECOGNITION MEMORY VS. RECALL MEMORY).

When dealing with important conversational content, such as that of the instructions of a physician or the advice of an attorney, people of all ages should not rely on their memories. The information should be written down and read back to the person delivering the message. This is especially true for elderly people.

Coping and Caring: Living with Alzheimer's Disease

This booklet contains information about Alzheimer's disease for caregivers and suggestions for better coping with the stress associated with caregiving. To obtain a free copy, write to AARP Fulfillment. Request stock no. D12441. 601 E Street, N.W., Washington, DC 20049.

Cornell Medical Index

The Cornell Medical Index (CMI) is a checklist on which people report various physical and psychological symptoms they are experiencing. The CMI includes sections for both physical and psychological symptoms. Twelve different categories of symptoms are included in the physical section (e.g., cardiovascular, respiratory) and six different categories in the psychological section (e.g., anxiety, depression).

The CMI has been widely used in studies comparing adults of different ages regarding the frequencies with which they report different symptoms, both physical and psychological. The most comprehensive of these studies are those conducted with participants in the Baltimore Longitudinal Study and participants in the Normative Aging Study. These studies revealed only a modest increase in physical symptoms with increasing age for men ranging in age from 17 to 97 years in the Baltimore Longitudinal Study and from 21 to 80 years in the Normative Aging Study, and an even smaller increase in psychological symptoms. By contrast, the personality trait of neuroticism was found to be strongly related to the number of symptoms reported quite independently of age.

Creativity

Galileo was only 20 years old when he discovered the law of the pendulum. Isaac Newton was only 23 when he began his discoveries of gravitation, and Albert Einstein only 26 when he advanced the theory of relativity. Remarkable achievements by individuals so young—sufficiently so that these individuals were labeled as "geniuses." Are youthful achievements of this magnitude limited to physicists? Certainly not. Chemistry has had its share of young superstars, such as Lavoisier who, at the age of 34, unraveled the mystery of fire as the combination of a burning substance with oxygen. Ernest Hemingway was only 27 years old when *The Sun Also Rises* was published and 30 years old when *A Farewell to Arms* was published. David Hume, the philosopher, was only 28 when his major work, *A Treatise of Human Nature*, was completed. Nor has psychology been void of its youthful masters. B. F. Skinner was in his early 30s when he discovered the principles of reinforcement and operant learning that were to make him internationally famous, as was Sigmund Freud when he published his major work on the interpretation of dreams. In each of these cases, the topic is creativity. Creativity involves originality, or the discovery of a unique solution to a problem (see ORIGINALITY). However, creativity involves much more than just originality. It also means that the solutions have significance for society, and through them important advances are made in mathematics, science, philosophy, literature, and, yes, even psychology.

Is creativity possessed only by young adults? Or, at least, are important discoveries by older individuals more the exception than the rule? Those who follow the awarding of Nobel Prizes each year may be misled to conclude that many older individuals have made great discoveries in their fields. However, in most of these cases, the discoveries were made when they were much younger. It simply took the test of time for their discoveries to be recognized. The classic analyses of the relationship between age and creativity conducted by H. C. Lehman provide partial answers to our questions. Beginning in the early 1940s and continuing through the early 1960s, Lehman reported analyses of highly creative contributions made by individuals at various age levels in several different academic disciplines. A "highly creative contribution" was one that was widely cited in introductory textbooks of a given discipline. Of interest to Lehman was the age of the contributor at the time his or her most cited contribution was produced. Overall, Lehman found that the peak age range was between 30 and 39 years. Beyond that age range there was a pronounced and progressive decline in the percentage of contributions that he ranked as being truly creative, so much so that the percentage of contributions made by individuals in their 70s was close to zero.

Lehman's classic analyses did not go unchallenged. However, the challenge rested largely on the issue of productivity and not creativity. Later researchers found that productivity in various academic and artistic endeavors shows only a modest decline after ages 30 to 39 years. At stake, however, is the quality of the products of one's creative activity. True creativity, as defined by Lehman, ends with a startling, perhaps even world-shaking, discovery that changes the course of a discipline's future. Many older scholars, researchers, inventors, and artists certainly contribute effectively to their discipline, but it does seem usually that the contributions are at the level of a modest increase to knowledge in their discipline and to their own careers. It should be noted further that a massive longitudinal study (i.e., following the same individuals over a period of years) of research psychologists indicated that researchers who were the most productive when they were young continued to hold their advantage over less productive researchers during the later stages of their careers.

There are probably many reasons why creativity appears to decline with age. One contributing factor has nothing to do with aging as a biological process. Potentially creative individuals are often "rewarded" for their earlier achievements by being made executives of an industrial company or administrators of their universities at a relatively early age. Consequently, the opportunity to further pursue their research or artistic careers is denied them. It has also been argued that creativity is adversely related to certain personality characteristics that are more pronounced in older than in younger individuals (e.g., intolerance of ambiguity). However, given the generally stable nature of personality over the adult life span (see PERSONALITY), age differences in personality seem unlikely to be a major determinant of age differences in creativity. A remaining possibility is that there is some underlying mental ability that declines with aging. We do know that there are modest age differences in originality, an ability many have suspected to be a determinant of creativity. However, the extent of these age differences does not seem to be great enough to account for the pronounced age differences in creativity reported by Lehman (see ORIGINALITY). What remains is the possibility that we have yet to discover further mental abilities that affect creativity, abilities that do decline in proficiency with aging. Considerable progress in identifying these abilities should occur in the near future because new theories of creativity and new methods of studying it have appeared at a rapid pace.

Creutzfeldt-Jakob Disease

Creutzfeldt-Jakob disease is a rare form of dementia that usually has an earlier onset than Alzheimer's disease and a very rapid progression of the severity of the dementia after its onset. Many believe that the disease is transmitted by a virus and that the transmission may occur from an animal to a human being. It is the probable viral nature of the disease that has attracted considerable attention and stimulated interest in the possibility that Alzheimer's disease may also be caused by a virus.

Crime (Victim of and Fear of)

Are you afraid to leave your home for fear of being mugged? Do you have difficulty falling asleep because you fear your home will be robbed? In some cases, of course, such fears may be realistic and serve to help an individual avoid being the victim of a crime. In other cases, however, the fear of being a victim of a crime may be irrational and interfere with normal everyday functioning. Are such fears especially prevalent among elderly adults? If so, they would provide evidence to support what is called the victimization/fear paradox. Crime statistics reveal that it is teenagers and young adults, and not elderly adults, who are most likely to be the victims of crime. For some years it was believed that fear of crime was much more prevalent among older adults than among young adults. Thus the paradox—greater incidence of fear despite the lower incidence of victimization among elderly adults. However, a recent study indicates that the paradox does not really exist. It is younger persons, and not elderly persons, who are most afraid of most types of crime. In the same study it was found that at every age women are more likely than men to fear being the victim of a crime.

Cross-Sectional Method

Are there adult age differences in the rate of solving anagrams (scrambled words), in scores on intelligence tests, in performances on various kinds of memory tasks? Do younger and older adults differ in their performances on such tasks and many other tasks? To answer this question, gerontological researchers most often use the cross-sectional method. This method requires the selection of a different group of people for each age level being compared, and comparison of the scores among the age groups for the task being evaluated. Consider the simplest kind of cross-sectional study in which young adults (e.g., 20 to 29 years of age) are to be compared with elderly adults (e.g., 65 to 74 years of age) on a learning task. A group or sample of young adults is selected along with a group of elderly adults. The two groups are then given the same learning task at approximately the same time. Suppose we discover that the young group averages 8 trials to learn the task and the elderly group averages 10 trials. Thus the cross-sectional age difference reveals an age difference in which the elderly group averaged 25% below the level of performance of the young group. What can we conclude about this age difference? Is the age difference in proficiency really the result of a decline in learning ability with normal aging? This conclusion depends on how the age groups were selected.

Suppose our participants at each age level had been selected randomly from the total populations of people in the age ranges of 20 to 29 years and 65 to 74 years. If so, then the young participants would be representative of *all* adults in the 20- to 29-year age range with respect to the proportions of men and women in the total population, proportions of different races in the total population, socioeconomic backgrounds, educational backgrounds, and so on. Similarly, the elderly participants would be representative of *all* adults in the 65- to 74-year age range. If such representation is truly satisfied, then the age difference for our two groups should be generalizable to the entire populations of millions of people in the two age ranges used in this study. We would be able to conclude that learning on this particular task occurs at a rate for all adults age 65 to 74 that is about 25% slower than the rate for all adults age 20 to 29. It is through the use of the cross-sectional method with groups that are representative of their total populations that age norms are developed (see NORMS).

Our hypothetical study with representative groups at different age levels clearly described the existence of an age difference in learning. But does it permit us to conclude that is it aging itself that caused the age difference? Not necessarily. By selecting representative groups of young and elderly adults, we had two groups that undoubtedly differed in a number of ways besides their ages. These differences arise because people of different ages who are tested at the same time must come from different cohorts or generations (see COHORT [GENERATIONAL] EFFECT). The two groups in our study probably differ on such characteristics as their years of formal education. That is, the young adults will have had, on the average, more education than the elderly adults. This creates a definite problem in concluding whether the age difference is the consequence of normal aging. We know that amount of education does correlate with learning proficiency. Consequently, it may be the difference in educational level that is responsible for our observed age difference in learning, with aging itself having little effect on the difference in scores earned by the two groups.

To determine the role of aging on the observed age difference in learning, we would have to make certain that our age groups are matched in educational level. This could be done, for example, by selecting only college graduates as participants. We may then discover that the young college graduates and older college graduates average 5 and 6 trials, respectively, to learn the task. We are now better able to view the age difference of 20% as resulting from a moderate decline in learning proficiency with normal aging. At the same time, we are likely to underestimate the magnitude of the age difference that exists in the total populations of younger and older adults. Remember that our hypothetical study with representative age groups estimated that difference to be about 25%.

The matching of age groups on such important characteristics as educational level is common practice in research with the cross-sectional method when the objective is to determine whether aging itself is the reason for an observed age difference in task performance. However, there is the risk of failing to match the age groups on some characteristics that could affect performance on a given task. For example, age groups matched only for education may differ in their degree of introversion. However, this would present a problem only if degree of introversion is known to relate to performance on the task in question. If it is, then the age groups would have to be matched on introversion as well as education. For many tasks, introversion is unlikely to be related to performance. Consequently, matching the age groups in scores on a test of introversion would not be needed. Age groups are also likely to differ in many other respects, such as their average heights, their amounts of gray hair, and so on. These are usually age differences that should not affect performances on most of the tasks used in gerontological research.

Curiosity

Curiosity is rumored to have killed the cat—but what does it do to human beings? Wouldn't life be dull if we weren't curious about the world and universe in which we live? How much of your time is spent seeking information about that world? Children are well known to be very curious individuals. But what about adults of different ages? One of the beliefs about aging is that curiosity decreases from early to late adulthood. However, there is considerable evidence to indicate that this is simply another myth of aging.

The most recent evidence was provided by researchers at the National Institute on Aging. They tested a large sample of individuals of various ages of the adult life span. The participants responded to a number of statements related to both interpersonal curiosity and impersonal-mechanical curiosity. Interpersonal curiosity refers to the desire to know more about other people. Examples of the statements for this form of curiosity were "I like to read about the personal lives of people of public prominence" and "I have little interest in the private lives of my schoolmates or fellow workers." Impersonal-mechanical curiosity refers to wanting to know more about things and science in general. Examples of the statements for this form of curiosity were "I like to read about new scientific findings" and "I do not like to visit factories and manufacturing plants." The participants' responses to these statements indicated the extent to which the statement applied to them. The researchers found the degree of curiosity to be about the same for young, middle-aged, and elderly adults. Curiosity may be considered to be a trait of personality; like other traits, it is affected little by aging (see PERSONALITY TRAITS).

D

Dark Adaptation

Most people have experienced what happens when they enter a dimly lit movie theater. It takes some time before they can see well enough to find an unoccupied seat. They are experiencing the important visual phenomenon of dark adaptation. The receptor cells in the retina are adapting to the change in illumination. This process takes a number of minutes before complete adaptation occurs. The time needed for complete adaptation may be several minutes longer for elderly adults than for younger adults, although the evidence in this area is somewhat ambiguous. However, it has been well established that the vision of elderly adults in dim illumination is impaired to a much greater degree than it is for younger adults. This is a major contributing factor to the reluctance of many elderly people to drive a car at night or at twilight.

Partial dark adaptation is a related visual phenomenon that has important implications for aging. It occurs when the eyes are exposed to intermittent changes in brightness. A familiar example occurs when driving at night and the headlights of occasional cars moving in the opposite direction are encountered. Frequent shifts from bright-light vision to dim-light vision are needed to maintain control of the car being driven. Elderly adults find these shifts more difficult to accomplish than do younger adults. This is another reason why many elderly adults, especially those age 75 years and older, should avoid driving at night as much as possible.

Daydreaming

One of the myths about aging is that elderly people daydream more than younger people. This myth probably had its origin in the belief that many older people spend much of their time reminiscing. These reminiscences are thoughts that interrupt the ongoing task in which the elderly person is engaged, whether it be listening to a lecture, raking the leaves, or washing the dishes. A daydream need not be reminiscing about the past. In fact, a daydream is any thought that intrudes while we are doing something else. For example, a college student listening to a professor's lecture may find himself or herself suddenly thinking about a party to be held that coming weekend. Daydreams are typically spontaneous. They seem to just "pop" into the mind without the individual's intent to have those intruding thoughts. In addition, daydreams need not be erotic, romantic, or bizarre. In fact, they are often routine or commonplace in content (e.g., thoughts about what in the world are we are going to serve our guests for dinner tomorrow night).

Does daydreaming actually increase from early adulthood to late adulthood? Evidence gathered by Dr. Leonard Giambra of the National Institute on Aging's Gerontology Research Center indicates that the opposite is actually true. Dr. Giambra's research has involved two different methods. The first consists simply of interviewing adults of all ages about their daydreaming and answering a questionnaire. These answers reveal that both men and women report less frequent daydreaming as aging increases. That is, the older the individual, the less frequent the daydreaming. The other method consists of studying daydreaming under controlled laboratory conditions. Adults of varying ages are given a boring laboratory task to perform for an extended period of time. They are also trained to report each time they have an intruding thought or "mindwandering." The results of this laboratory research confirm Dr. Giambra's interview data: the oldest individuals reported far fewer "mindwanderings" than the youngest individuals.

The content of the daydreams reported is of further interest. Dr. Giambra discovered that for all but the youngest adults in his studies (ages 17 to 23 years), the most frequent daydreams involved problem solving of some kind. That is, the content was concerned with some problem currently facing the individual. For the youngest adults, the most frequent daydreams were, not surprisingly, sexually oriented (but problem-solving daydreams ranked second even for them). Daydreams do seem to play an important role in our everyday lives by helping us to cope with our problems. It is as if our subconscious mind is struggling with a problem even as our conscious mind is occupied with other things, perhaps leading to a solution to that problem (e.g., "Hey, let's have stroganoff" for the guests at dinner). Even the daydreams of the most famous dreamer of all time, Walter Mitty in James Thurber's *The Secret Life of Walter Mitty*, may be viewed as a form of problem solving. Mitty frequently engaged in exotic and adventurous daydreams in which he played the heroic role. Remember that he engaged in these daydreams when he was subjected to nagging by his wife. The daydreams represented a form of coping with a problem.

Death and Dying
See also EUTHANASIA; HOSPICE CARE; SUICIDE; WIDOWHOOD AND WIDOWERHOOD

Thousands of elderly people die every year. Contrary to popular belief, most of them do not die of "old age." "Old age" is not a disease. Most elderly people who do not die as a result of an accident, murder, or suicide, die of a life-threatening disease that is more prevalent in late adulthood than in earlier adulthood (e.g., cancer, heart disease; see DISEASES, [CHRONIC]).

One of the myths about aging is that people become increasingly more fearful of death and more anxious about death as they grow older. In general, elderly people think about death more often than do younger people, but healthy, normally aging elderly adults usually express less fear and anxiety about death (at least consciously) than do younger adults. There are no apparent differences between elderly men and elderly women in their degree of fear of death. The role of religious conviction and belief in an afterlife in reducing the fear of elderly people about their impending death is ambiguous. In some cases, a strong conviction does seem to help, but in other cases, it may actually increase the intensity of fear. In general, elderly people who face old age with the feeling of integrity in their lives (their lives were worth living) have less fear of their inevitable deaths than do elderly people who are confronted by despair that their lives were not worth living.

Is there any consistent pattern to how people face death when they know they have a terminal illness and will die fairly soon? This question is of particular interest in gerontology because a large proportion of the terminally ill population consists of elderly people. In the early 1960s Elizabeth Kübler-Ross provided evidence to suggest that many terminally ill people progress through a series of emotional stages. Her stage theory was based on interviews with 200 terminally ill individuals. According to Dr. Kübler-Ross, the first stage is one of shock and disbelief in which the individual feels a diagnostic mistake must have been made and denies the reality of the diagnosis. However, most terminally ill individuals eventually accept the diagnosis and move into a stage characterized by the expression of anger and hostility directed toward healthy people. They seem to be expressing their frustration and feeling of unfairness regarding why *they*, rather than other people, are dying. This stage is followed by a bargaining stage in which they may appeal to a higher being that they will be better persons if they are allowed to live. Eventually they realize that the bargaining is ineffective, and they enter a stage in which they experience depression, guilt, and shame about their illness. Discussing these experiences with others helps them enter the final stage in which they accept the inevitability of their own deaths. Thus the five stages are disbelief and denial, anger and hostility, bargaining, depression, and acceptance. Dr. Kübler-Ross recognized that not all terminally ill people progress through all of these stages, and that even those who do, move through them at different rates.

Although the stage theory has attracted considerable attention, it has also encountered considerable criticism. Several later studies have revealed that many terminally ill people remain basically the same throughout their illness, rather than progress through stages. It was found that some terminally ill people simply continue to live their daily lives as they did before their illness had been diagnosed, whereas others withdraw from further social interactions. Most important, a number of patients were found to cling to the denial of the severity of their illness until the end, rather than accepting it fairly early after diagnosis. In addition, the presence of depression in terminally ill people may be the consequence of their medications, rather than a stage of their adjustment to their impending deaths. As the end of life nears, many terminally ill people vacillate between feelings of contentment and feelings of hopelessness, rather than being continuously depressed.

Demography of Aging

The population of elderly people in the United States has increased steadily over the years, and the rate of increase has been especially great in recent years. The trend toward an increasing population of elderly people is expected to continue through the first few decades of the next century. The United States is not alone in the population boom of older people. Similar trends have occurred in most developed countries of the world, but not in many of the underdeveloped countries where life expectancy falls well below that found for developed countries. The United Nations classifies a country as being *old* if more than 7% of its population is age 65 or older. The United States and such countries as Canada, England, Germany, Italy, Japan,

Poland, and Spain fall into this category. Countries with 4% to 7% of the population in the age 65 and older range are classified as mature countries. Included here are such countries as Brazil, Panama, South Africa, and Turkey. Countries with less than 4% of the population age 65 or older are classified as young. Among these countries are Burma, Colombia, Egypt, Ethiopia, India, Iran, and Mexico.

The 1990 U.S. census revealed that there were more than 31 million people in the United States age 65 or older (about 12% of the total population). In 1900 there were slightly more than 3 million people age 65 or older in this country and about 25 million in 1980. By the year 2030 it is estimated that the number of people 65 years and older will be 66 million. By the year 2030 the percentage of our total population age 65 or older is expected to reach 22%.

Especially striking is the increase in individuals in the more advanced age ranges. The number of people age 75 to 84 in 1990 was estimated to exceed 10 million, which is a gain of more than 30% of the number in 1980. The number of people age 85 or older in 1988 was estimated to be more than 3 million, which is 23 times larger than in 1900 and a gain of 38% over the number in 1980. With further increases in longevity, the number of the "old old" in our total population is expected to show further dramatic increases in the years ahead. The gain in the number of elderly people in our country over the years is reflected further in the dramatic increase in the median age of this country's population. In 1900 it was 22.9 years; in 1990 it was estimated to be 32.9 years.

The increase in the number of elderly people has been greater for females than for males, as might be expected given the longer life expectancy of women (see LIFE EXPECTANCY). For example, in 1980 the percentage of women age 75 and older in the total population was more than twice that of men age 75 and older.

Just as countries may be classified as "old" or "young" depending on the percentage of the population age 65 or older, so may the states of the United States. "Old" states are those in which percentage of their population of elderly people exceeds the 12% of elderly people in the total population of the United States. These states include Florida, which in 1984 already had more than 17% of its population age 65 or older. Other old states are Arkansas, Missouri, Iowa, Kansas, Nebraska, and South Dakota in the Midwest and Massachusetts and Maine in the East. "Young" states are those with less than 10% of their populations made up of people age 65 or older. Included here are Texas, New Mexico, Colorado, Utah, Wyoming, and Nevada in the

Southwest and West, Louisiana and Georgia in the South, and West Virginia in the East.

The increase in the elderly population of the United States has been accompanied by a change in their locations within states. By the late 1970s the majority of elderly people lived in metropolitan areas, rather than in small towns or in rural areas as was true for earlier periods. By the late 1980s only about one-fourth of elderly people lived in nonmetropolitan areas. Especially dense is the current population of elderly people in the suburbs of metropolitan areas, especially the older (established) suburbs. This means that suburban areas now carry the major burden of providing services and care for disadvantaged and needy elderly people, a burden once carried largely by inner cities.

Depression (Diagnostic Tests)

There are several widely used tests in which those taking the test give self-reports of the symptoms of depression. The Beck Depression Inventory is one in which the test-taker rates on a 4-point scale the intensity of various psychological and physical symptoms of depression. On the Zung Self-Rating Depression Scale, people respond to such statements as "I am more irritable than usual" and "I feel downhearted, blue, and sad." The Center for Epidemiological Studies Depression Scale (CES-D) has 20 items representing various symptoms of depression (e.g., "I felt sad") in which the respondent rates the frequency of a particular symptom during the week before the test. Various problems arise in the use of these tests with elderly people. Perhaps the greatest problem is the likelihood that they will often yield high scores indicative of severe depression, largely through the presence of physical symptoms of depression on the tests (e.g., "My sleep was restless" on the CES-D scale and similar questions on the other tests). Such physical symptoms may be indicative of depression for younger adults, but they may simply be physical problems encountered by elderly people as part of normal aging. In addition, the format of these tests in terms of forced choices or estimating frequencies of occurrence is one that discourages a number of elderly adults from completing the test. Some of the tests state some items positively and others negatively, a procedure that causes confusion for some elderly respondents. A recently published test, the Geriatric Depression Scale, was designed to avoid these problems. It has 30 true-false items dealing only with psychological symptoms. Respondents answer questions about how they felt during the past week. There is evidence to indicate that elderly adults who take the test find it easy to complete.

Depression may also be diagnosed by means of clinical interviews of patients by trained psychiatrists and psychologists. There are standard forms for the nature of the interview (e.g., the Hamilton Rating Scale for Depression).

Depression (Incidence, Symptoms, Causes)

Many adults at all age levels feel depressed at times. They feel depressed in the sense of having negative feelings (e.g., sadness or melancholy, self-disparagement), often accompanied by apathy, difficulty in concentrating, difficulty in sleeping, and some loss of appetite. The duration of their depression, however, is usually fairly brief, and they return to a more normal state in which they have positive feelings about life and themselves. Clinical depression is another matter. Intense negative feelings persist for a long time, while the physical symptoms, such as loss of appetite, intensify and effective mental functioning becomes severely reduced, as indicated by pronounced declines in memory functioning. Adaptation to the hassles of daily living become difficult, if not impossible.

A common belief is that the incidence of clinical depression is much greater for elderly adults than for younger adults. This belief received support from early studies revealing that as many as 65% of elderly adults report an excessively large number of depressive symptoms on self-report tests of depression (see DEPRESSION [DIAGNOSTIC TESTS]). The problem with these early studies is that emotional symptoms (e.g., "I feel sad") were combined with physical symptoms (e.g., I have difficulty sleeping") to yield a total symptom score. Physical symptoms such as difficulty in sleeping and loss of appetite may be symptoms of depression when present in younger adults. However, when present in elderly adults, they may simply be manifestations of normal aging. More recent studies have revealed that the incidence of elderly adults who report excessively high nonphysical symptoms of depression is far less than 65%. For example, the percentage of elderly adults in their 60s who report depressive symptoms is usually found to be only from 15% to 20% (but it is somewhat higher for people age 75 or older). High scores on self-report tests do not necessarily indicate the presence of clinical depression. More intensive evaluations with psychiatric interviews of people of various ages generally indicate that the incidence of clinical depression among elderly adults may be quite low (perhaps no more than 1%), and even lower than that found for younger adults (estimated to be about 4%).

There is the danger that the incidence of clinical dementia among elderly adults, especially those age 75 or older, may be underestimated. A diagnosis of dementia may be made in some elderly adults when their memory problems and lowered mental functioning may actually be caused by depression. The mental dysfunction may be confused with symptoms found in patients with Alzheimer's disease. An error in diagnosis could have disastrous consequences. Depression is a reversible disorder; Alzheimer's disease is not. Contemporary psychiatrists and clinical psychologists have found very effective treatments of clinical depression in late adulthood (see DEPRESSION [TREATMENT]). However, a major problem is that depression may go untreated in as many as 60% of the elderly people with depression. Much of the problem stems from the fact that Medicare pays reduced amounts for psychiatric and psychological treatment of emotional disorders, thus making this service unavailable to many depressed older people.

Melancholy and self-disparagement are the emotional symptoms commonly associated with depression. However, there is evidence indicating that these symptoms are more likely to be present in depressed younger adults than in depressed elderly adults. For elderly adults, the emotional symptoms are often those of apathy, a feeling of worthlessness, and a general sense of hopelessness with their lives.

The reasons for depression among elderly adults are many. Reduced income, for example, can be sufficiently stressful to produce depression. Elderly adults who are experiencing severe financial strain have been found to have more depressive symptoms than those elderly adults who are more financially secure. Loss of a spouse and the occurrence of a physical disability are other possible causes that are more likely to be present in late adulthood than earlier in adulthood. Depression is likely to persist longer with the occurrence of a severely restricting disability than with the death of a spouse. Another common cause of depression among elderly adults is a major change in their social support system as a result of the deaths of friends, reduced physical mobility, and so on.

Depression is also common among elderly people with dementia. Perhaps as many as 30% of patients with Alzheimer's disease have severe depression, and an even larger percentage is likely to have at least some depressive symptoms. The presence of depression limits further the ability of such individuals to function well mentally. Fortunately, some patients with mild degrees of dementia may be treated effec-

tively for their depression (see DEPRESSION [TREATMENT]; PSYCHO-
THERAPY WITH NURSING HOME RESIDENTS).

Depression (Treatment)

Mild forms of depression are usually temporary and spontaneously
disappear. By contrast, severe or clinical depression is likely to be a
long-term disorder that requires treatment to remove the symptoms.
The most effective treatment of clinical depression in young and
middle-aged patients is by the administration of antidepressant drugs,
such as heterocyclic antidepressants and Prozac. Prozac is the most
widely prescribed antidepressant drug, but there is evidence to indicate that it may be no more effective than other antidepressants. It is
also prescribed frequently for anxiety and eating disorders. However,
many elderly, clinically depressed patients are required to take other
drugs and medicines that prevent the use of antidepressant drugs. In
addition, antidepressants often have adverse side effects for many elderly people, especially when they receive improper dosages. When
antidepressants can be given to elderly patients, they have been found
to reverse the symptoms of depression in more than 70% of cases. An
alternative to antidepressant drugs is the administration of electroconvulsive (ECT) or electroshock therapy. ECT often results in some
immediate symptom relief. When it is effective with elderly patients,
it usually requires only a few administrations. ECT is no longer considered to be as risky with elderly patients as it was once thought. However, patients with severe cardiovascular problems may be advised
against its use because of the transient increase in blood pressure that
often occurs with ECT. In addition, ECT often creates some memory
problems that may add to those produced by aging. Psychotherapy,
particularly cognitive therapy, is the major alternative for those elderly patients who are at risk with either drug therapy or ECT therapy (see PSYCHOTHERAPY). In addition, cognitive therapy has also
been found to relieve depressive symptoms for some patients with
mild dementia or mental impairment as well as depression (see PSY-
CHOTHERAPY WITH NURSING HOME RESIDENTS). Psychotherapy is also
often used in conjunction with either drug or ECT therapy to accel-
erate the treatment effects. For those relatively few elderly patients
with a manic-depressive disorder (shifts from agitated to depressed
states and vice versa), the usual treatment is the administration of
lithium.

There is evidence that moderate exercise may reduce depressive symptoms. For example, in a recent Canadian study a group of

moderately depressed elderly women participated in a walking exercise program for 6 weeks. Three sessions were held each week; the duration of the early sessions was 20 minutes and the duration of later sessions was 40 minutes. After 6 weeks a significant decrease in depressive symptoms, both physical and psychological, was found, on the average, for the participants. There is also evidence indicating that combining mild exercise with listening to music and imagining pleasant things further reduces symptoms of depression in elderly adults.

There are several booklets available for further information about the symptoms and treatment of depression in elderly adults. One, titled *Depression in Later Life: Recognition and Treatment,* is published by the Oregon State University Extension Service. A copy may be obtained by writing to OSU, #PNW347, Publication Orders, Department P, Agricultural Communications, Administration Services, Room A422, Corvallis, OR 97331-2119; you must enclose a check or money order for $1.50. Another is *If You're Over 65 and Feeling Depressed.* It is published by the National Institutes of Mental Health. A free copy may be obtained by calling 800-421-4211 on a touch-tone telephone.

Depth Perception

When you look at an object you are able, usually immediately, to identify three attributes of it: its height, its width, and its depth or distance from you. What makes the perception of depth truly remarkable is the fact you are seeing a third dimension even though the image of the object on the retina (inner layer of the eye) is cast in only two dimensions. You perceive depth because of several cues provided by the eye that provide you with the necessary information to "see" a third dimension. For example, your two eyes are separated by several inches; therefore the image of an object on the retina of the left eye is slightly different than the image of the same object on the retina of the right eye. This slight difference provides important information that your brain knows how to interpret. Even people with only one functional eye have depth perception to some degree. This is because other kinds of cues from either eye alone provide further information of depth that is interpreted by the brain.

The proficiency of depth perception varies among individuals. This may be seen by measuring depth perception proficiency through the use of a device similar to the one used to test vision to obtain a driver's license. You look at three vertical bars projected on an illuminated screen and are asked to make decisions about these bars on a number of test trials. For example, is Bar X in front of or behind the other two bars? Research with this device has revealed that age differences make up a major portion of the individual differences in the proficiency of depth perception. Young adults, in general, are quite proficient. This proficiency shows little decline for people until they reach their 50s. At this age the decline is rather large. However, further decline with aging, at least through the 70s, seems to be modest. Distance perception is closely related to depth perception. Perceiving an object in depth, of course, means that you are aware that some parts of the object are at a greater distance from you than other parts. Older people are likely to have some difficulty in judging distances of objects. Certain problems in everyday living are the likely consequence. For example, parallel parking becomes more difficult because it requires judging distances between nearby cars and the car being parked. Diminished depth perception is also a likely contributor to the increased incidence of falls among older people.

Developmental Psychology

Developmental psychology is the study of behavioral changes with increasing age. Behavioral change simply means variability within an individual. An organism's behavior at an older age is likely to show differences from its behavior at an earlier age, regardless of the age levels being contrasted. The differences are likely to be in the positive direction (i.e., greater proficiency of behavior) when the contrast involves later childhood with earlier childhood, and either positive or negative (i.e., less proficiency of behavior) when the contrast involves later adulthood with earlier adulthood. In either case, these behavioral changes with changes in age are the subject matter of developmental psychology. Developmental psychologists working at any age level are concerned not only with describing these changes, but also with identifying the reasons for their occurrence. For example, what accounts for changes in memory proficiency from early to late adulthood?

Development is not confined to any one segment of the life span—it is continuous during the life span. For purposes of studying development systematically and scientifically, the life span has been separated into at least three broad age ranges: each segment yields its own specialized content area. The three age ranges are those of childhood, adolescence, and adulthood. The resulting content areas are those of child psychology, adolescent psychology, and adult development. Each age range area may be divided further into content areas that are even more limited. Thus there is the psychology of infancy as a part of child psychology; this field of psychology focuses on changes during the first 2 years after birth. Similarly, there is the study of the psychology of early or young adulthood, with the content on changes from the late teens through the late 20s. Gerontological psychology, the psychology of aging, is part of the psychology of adult development. One of the objectives of gerontological psychology is the description of and understanding of behavioral changes that may occur from early adulthood to late adulthood in, for example, learning and memory proficiency. Another objective is the study of the behavior of elderly people per se, that is, without regard to comparisons with younger adults. For example, what conditions produce differences among elderly people in their degree of life satisfaction? How do they differ in their interactions with grandchildren? How do they adjust to retirement?

DHEA Hormone

Many elderly people wish that a fountain of youth could be discovered that would reduce, or even eliminate, whatever suffering they are experiencing by slowing down the aging of their bodies. Medical researchers have been very active in their efforts to find medications that could serve as at least a partial fountain of youth. Antioxidants are one of these medications that some physicians believe might be mildly successful in slowing down aging's negative effects on the body (see ANTI-OXIDANTS). Another is a hormone secreted by the adrenal glands and known as DHEA. This hormone begins to appear in the body at about age 7, and it increases in amount until it peaks at about age 25. After age 25, the amount decreases steadily, and at age 70 it is about 10% of its peak amount. Some medical researchers believe that small doses of the hormone in elderly people will reduce physical and mental impairments occurring with aging. One experimental study did show increased mobility and decreased joint pain in its elderly participants. However, other studies have failed to find significant positive effects, and widespread use of the hormone remains very controversial.

Diary Studies of Memory Failures

Asking people of various ages to keep a daily diary in which they record each day's memory failures is one means of studying age differences in memory performances. Of interest is the extent of the probable increase in the number of everyday memory failures from early to late adulthood. Critics of laboratory studies on age differences in memory performances have argued that the memory tasks encountered in the laboratory, such as memorizing lists of words, are too artificial to indicate how memory operates in the everyday world. They believe that studies conducted with these tasks tend to overestimate the extent to which memory proficiency (especially episodic memory proficiency; see EPISODIC MEMORY) declines with normal aging. Diary studies offer an alternative to laboratory studies in determining the extent to which memory is affected by normal aging.

Several diary studies of age differences in memory have been conducted. In the most comprehensive of these studies, the participants ranged in age from 20 to 76 years. For an extended period of time participants recorded in their diaries each day's failures to remember such things as an item they forgot to purchase at the supermarket. The older participants reported themselves to be more upset about their memory failures than did the younger ones (younger adults are likely to take the imperfections of memory, which they too experience, in stride). The number of memory failures actually recorded was only moderately greater for the older than for the younger participants. This difference must be interpreted cautiously, however. Diary recordings may underestimate the magnitude of memory problems facing elderly adults. If people older than age 76 had been included in the study, the age difference may have been much greater. Moreover, older adults may forget their own memory failures more frequently than younger adults, and therefore fail to record all of them. It seems reasonable to conclude that laboratory studies do provide fairly realistic estimates of age differences in episodic memory performances. Diary studies reflect the fact that many normally aging elderly people are concerned about their memory problems, perhaps much more than necessary (see MEMORY COMPLAINTS).

Disability (Incidence)

There are two ways to define disability, both of which may be used to estimate the number of older people who have a disability. The first is based on the presence of an illness that produces long-term physical impairments. The second way is in terms of an individual's ability to perform critical activities of daily living. These activities include feeding oneself and dressing oneself (see ACTIVITIES OF DAILY LIVING). Researchers at Miami University used the latter method to estimate the percentage of elderly people affected by a disability. They further classified disability into severe disability and moderate disability. Severe disability occurs when an individual has impairments of two or more important activities of daily living, and moderate disability when only one such activity is impaired. Information from 1986 census figures enabled the researchers to estimate separately the percentages of people in the 65- to 74-year age range, people in the 75- to 84-year age range, and people age 85 and older. The percentages of people with severe disability were 4.4% in the 65- to 74-year age range, 9.9% in the 75- to 84-year age range, and 28.9% in those 85 and older. Comparable percentages for moderate disability were 5.8%, 11.0%, and 21.3%. With one exception, the percentage of women with a disability was only modestly greater than that of men. The exception was for severe disability in the 85 and older age range; the percentage was 21.7% for men and 31.7% for women.

Disability (Psychological and Social Consequences)

Disability caused by illness or an accident is a major source of stress for those elderly people who experience it. They are likely to experience considerable distress, low self-esteem, and low life satisfaction. These negative consequences of disability appear to have a longer duration than those found with other sources of stress for elderly people, such as bereavement. Researchers at Arizona State University found that depression was less pronounced for bereaved elderly people than for disabled elderly people.

Elderly women are more likely to have a functional disability than are elderly men, and they are also more likely to receive assistance from other people. Elderly women and elderly men, however, do not seem to differ in the extent to which they receive assistance from devices, such as walkers and raised toilet seats.

Adjustment to a disability typically progresses through four phases or stages. The first consists of shock, in which disabled individuals are likely to have diminished mental functioning to the point that they may even be unaware of their condition and they are likely to be dependent on others to care for them. The second phase is called defensive retreat. At this point, disabled individuals realize that they have a disability, and they are likely to be frightened greatly by it. They are also likely to begin coping with and adjusting to their disability. During this period they often deny the permanence and severity of the disability. To maintain this denial they may avoid any behavior that may call attention to their disability. This may even include avoiding social interactions with family members and friends and avoiding appearances in public places for fear of embarrassment. After a while, denial becomes ineffective in eliminating stress, and a phase called acknowledgment begins. It is during this phase that anxiety, grief, and depression are most pronounced. The final phase is called adaptation—one that will last for the remainder of the disability. Disabled individuals usually learn to cope with their disabilities and to live satisfactory lives, including renewing old friendships, finding new friends, increasing social interactions, and participating in volunteer and community services (e.g., helping other people who recently became disabled to cope with their disabilities). It is during the early period of this phase that various forms of psychotherapy are especially useful to disabled older people.

Researchers at the University of Pittsburgh have discovered that the amount of social support and social contact of disabled elderly people is strongly related to their well-being and their ability to function in the community. Depression among disabled elderly people was found to be lowest for those who were optimistic about the future and who believed that they could control important events in their lives (see CONTROL OVER LIFE'S EVENTS). Other researchers have reported that lower feelings of well-being for elderly disabled men are associated with greater reliance on others and on devices for aiding their activities. By contrast, lower feelings of well-being for elderly disabled women were found to be associated with reliance on devices but not on reliance on other people.

Self-care coping strategies tend to increase as the severity of disability increases, except for the most severely disabled. These strategies include the use of devices and appropriate risk-avoiding behaviors. Increase in the use of these strategies has also been found to be related positively to the amount of assistance received from other people.

Discourse Memory

You have just finished reading an interesting novel. The plot centers on a man living in a medium-sized town who, because of a strange genetic mutation, has become a vampire. His affliction is eventually cured by the love he feels for a small child living nearby. The child's widowed mother falls in love with the vampire, and they eventually marry. How much of the story are you likely to remember? Even some time later, you probably will recall the central theme of the story ("A vampire is cured by his love for a child"). You may even remember major subplots ("The vampire marries the child's widowed mother"). However, you probably will not remember many of the more detailed information, even after you just finished reading the story. The summary statements you have in your memory of a story are called *propositions* by memory researchers. A proposition is an abstraction of information that summarizes content. Propositions differ in *levels.* The highest-level proposition is one that summarizes the central theme of the story (e.g., "A vampire is cured by his love for a child"). Intermediate-level propositions are those that summarize more important subplots (e.g., "The vampire marries the child's widowed mother"). Low-level propositions are those that deal with more trivial information (e.g., "The action takes place in the city of Aorta, Texas"). Propositions are encoded and transmitted to your memory store by the very nature of your comprehension of what you read. This is usually accomplished incidentally. We have memory for content without the intent to remember it or to rehearse the content actively. The later retrieval of these stored propositions enables you to describe the story to someone else. Propositions are also the content in memory of informative articles we read in a newspaper, magazine, or encyclopedia. For example, after reading an article about a new treatment for arthritis, you may remember the general nature of the treatment, but have difficulty recalling a number of the details.

Memory researchers refer to the memory of stories and articles as *discourse memory.* Age differences in discourse memory are studied by having younger and older participants read an unfamiliar story or article (usually several hundred words in length) and then having them paraphrase the content. In general, the results of many studies have indicated little age difference in memory for high-level propositions, a moderate age difference favoring younger participants for intermediate propositions, and a more pronounced age difference favoring younger participants for low-level propositions. This is usually the case whether the content read is narrative (a story) or expository (an article). The inability to recall more trivial details should not concern older people. Such details are usually unimportant. One could always reread the story or article if there is a need to recover the information. In addition, older adults often go beyond the specific content of a story or article and find moral implications and lessons to be learned from what they have read that younger adults do not find (see also CONTINUITY VS. DISCONTINUITY IN ADULT DEVELOPMENT).

Diseases (Chronic)

Diseases may be classified into two broad categories, acute and chronic. *Acute diseases* are those that have a rapid onset and a short duration, usually from a few days to a few weeks. They include the common cold and acute bronchitis, as well as influenza and pneumonia (see INFLUENZA; PNEUMONIA). A myth about aging is that people age 65 or older have the highest incidence rates of acute diseases. In reality, young adults have the highest rates for most acute diseases, including the common cold. Even such conditions as sprains and muscle strains have a higher yearly incidence rate among young adults than among elderly adults.

Chronic diseases have a slower onset and a longer duration than acute diseases. They include, among many others, heart disease, diabetes, emphysema, and arthritis. Chronic diseases account for nearly all deaths that do not result from an accident, suicide, or murder. Heart and cardiovascular disease are the leading causes of death among people age 65 or older (estimated to be about 40% of yearly deaths), followed by cancer, stroke, and influenza/pneumonia. Although it is true that if all diseases were to be eliminated today that many more people would live to old age, it is also true that the average length of life would probably increase by no more than 10 to 15 years.

Although heart and cardiovascular diseases are found in younger adults, they are more prevalent in elderly adults, and more frequently in elderly men than in elderly women. The most common heart disease in late adulthood results from the muscles of the heart receiving insufficient oxygen because of obstructions in the coronary arteries. It is called ischemic heart disease (the word ischemic means deprived of blood) or coronary heart disease, and is found in about 20% of men and about 12% of women age 65 or older. The disease can lead to a myocardial infarction (heart attack). The symptoms of a heart attack are variable among elderly people. Chest pain is generally less common than when a heart attack occurs for younger people. In very old people the infarction is likely to be a "silent" heart attack in the sense of the absence of pain and discomfort.

Dysrhythmias (irregular heartbeats) are common in older people. They can be serious and may cause sudden death. There are medications that control dysrhythmias, provided they are detected and treated promptly. If the reduction of blood flow to the heart and the amount of oxygen reaching the heart are great enough, chest pains known as *angina* may occur. The pain of angina has been described by some sufferers as a burning sensation and by others as a pressure or tightness that may spread from behind the breastbone to the back and arms. Angina most often occurs after physical exertion or after an intense emotional experience, and it is usually relieved within 10 minutes. Patients with angina, regardless of age, are commonly treated by such medicines as nitroglycerin and beta-blockers (drugs that counter the effects of adrenaline [epinephrine] on the heart).

Congestive heart failure occurs when the heart is unable to sustain the needs of organs and muscles. Consequently, blood backs up in the veins and lungs. The result could be the accumulation of fluids in the legs, abdomen, and lungs that can be life-threatening. Congestive heart failure is present in more than 2 million people, and it contributes to nearly 300,000 deaths per year, largely of elderly people. Symptoms include swelling of the feet, ankles, and legs, weight gains, persistent coughing, fatigue, breathlessness, and difficulty in breathing while asleep. Unfortunately, some elderly people believe that these symptoms are simply part of growing old and are not an indication of a serious health problem. Medications may control these symptoms once diagnosed and prolong the lives of individuals with congestive heart failure. Drugs called ACE inhibitors, if given to patients within 24 hours of a heart attack and continued for 6 weeks, have been found to reduce the risk of congestive heart failure.

Disorders of the circulatory system beyond the heart include atherosclerosis and hypertension. *Atherosclerosis* is one form of a general class of cardiovascular disorders known as *arteriosclerosis* (the hardening of arteries or their loss of elasticity) that is more common in late adulthood than in earlier adulthood. Atherosclerosis is characterized by the presence of pronounced fat deposits along the inner wall of arteries and the thickening of the inner walls and the resulting interference that occurs in the flow of blood through the arteries. The walls may eventually bulge (an aneurysm) and rupture. Atherosclerosis of the coronary arteries may be so severe that a coronary bypass is needed in which an artery from another part of the body (usually the leg) is transplanted to replace the affected (clogged) coronary artery. Alternatively, a procedure known as *angioplasty* may be performed. It involves the inflation of a small balloon inserted in the affected artery to open it and increase blood flow through it. In some cases, application of a Rotor Rooter–like device may be required. In other cases, a stent (a small piece of metal) may be placed in the artery to support the inflation achieved by angioplasty. The accumulation of some fat deposits in the arteries appears to be part of normal aging. The presence of excessive deposits that may lead to artherosclerosis and eventually a heart attack is linked to such factors as smoking and elevated serum cholesterol levels that could be controlled by appropriate health habits (e.g., nonsmoking, a modified diet).

Hypertension refers to excessive arterial blood pressure (systolic pressure more than 160 mm Hg or diastolic pressure more than 95 mm Hg). Hypertension may be present in as many as 40% of people age 65 or older and 25% of people in the 45- to 64-year age range. Hypertension or high blood pressure is life-threatening because it implies reduced blood flow to vital organs and increased risk of a heart attack, stroke, or kidney failure. Medications such as diuretics are used to treat high blood pressure by ridding the body of excess fluid and sodium. Obesity, smoking, and excessive consumption of alcohol are all likely to increase the risk of hypertension in older people. There is evidence to indicate that certain pain medications (known as nonsteroidal anti-inflammatory drugs) may increase blood pressure in elderly adults if they are taken at high dosages for long periods of time.

Two recent developments offer great promise of reducing the death rate of elderly people from various forms of heart disease. The first is the discovery of new noninvasive tests for identifying with improved accuracy those elderly people likely to suffer from heart disease or stroke. The tests include special measures of blood pressure and a sonar examination that measures blockage in arteries. The second is approval by the Food and Drug Administration of the drug Zocor for use by patients with heart disease. This drug may save the lives of these patients by lowering their cholesterol to ultra-low levels. In a 5-year study of 4,000 coronary patients, use of Zocor was found to lower the death rate by 42%. The drug has only mild side effects, and it should not be used by people with liver disease.

Diabetes is another chronic and life-threatening disease that is more common in late adulthood than in earlier adulthood. Diabetes is a disease involving the metabolism of carbohydrates. It is estimated that about 10% of people age 65 or older have diabetes, compared with about 6% of people age 45 to 64 and fewer than 2% of people in their early 20s. Unfortunately, detection of type II (adult-onset) diabetes in elderly people may be difficult unless they have regular physical examinations that include tests for diabetes. Often the disease is not detected until elderly people experience conditions such as blurred vision caused by their diabetic condition. A new drug called metformin is now often used to treat type II diabetes. It controls high blood sugar levels, and, unlike other drugs used for the same purpose, it does so without harmful side effects (e.g., weight gain). Aging is often accompanied by decreased insulin sensitivity. Researchers at the University of Michigan have found the age effect to be related to increases in body mass and arterial blood pressure that often occur in late adulthood.

Chronic respiratory diseases that are especially prevalent in late adulthood include chronic bronchitis (a continuous inflammation of the bronchial tubes producing a chronic cough) and emphysema (damage to the lungs that results in diminished breathing capacity and shortness of breath). For example, the 1988 survey by the U.S. Department of Health and Human Services reported the percentage of people with emphysema to be about 4.4% and 3.3% in the 65- to 74-year and 75 or older age ranges, respectively, compared with 1.8% and less than 1% in the 45- to 64-year and 18- to 44-year age ranges, respectively. Both respiratory disorders are rarely found in nonsmokers, suggesting the critical role of smoking in the diseases of elderly people.

Gallbladder diseases, even when they are not life-threatening, present a serious problem to many older people. It is estimated that about 35% of people older than age 70, compared with less than 20% of people between 55 and 65 years of age, have gallstones. Gallstones produce pain just below the rib cage or in the right shoulder. They can result in serious damage to the pancreas or liver. Treatment for gallstones is likely to be either surgery or medical treatment consisting of weight reduction, avoidance of fatty foods, and use of antacids.

The most prevalent disease in late adulthood is arthritis, affecting nearly 50% of people age 65 or older (and about 25% of people in the 45- to 64-year age range). Overall it is estimated that 38 million people in the United States have one of the more than 100 kinds of arthritis. Each form of arthritis involves joints, but other parts of the body may be affected as well. By the year 2020 the Centers for Disease Control and Prevention predict that there will be 59 million people in the United States with some form of arthritis. Arthritis is a chronic disease that for many affected people lasts the rest of their lives. An estimated 3 million Americans have severe limitation of their activities of daily living (dressing, bathing, etc.) by arthritis. The estimated annual cost of arthritis to our economy in medical care and lost wages is estimated to be nearly 1% of the U.S. gross national product.

The two most common forms of arthritis are *rheumatoid arthritis* and *osteoarthritis*. Rheumatoid arthritis affects more than 2 million people in the United States, with women more likely to have the disease than men. It involves inflammation of joints and their capsules and ligaments. The onset of the disease usually occurs between the ages of 20 and 60; thus many elderly people already have the disease before old age. However, onset of the disease may occur after age 60, with the incidence of late onset being about the same for men and women. Stiffness and pain are commonly found in the fingers, wrists, and ankles. Rheumatoid arthritis is a progressive disease in that the symptoms often increase in intensity with the duration of the disease. However, in some patients the symptoms show a pattern of cycles of remission followed by recurrence. The reason for the disorder in the body's immunological system that causes the disease is not fully understood, and a cure has yet to be found. There are procedures for reducing the pain and increasing body movement, including drugs and some forms of exercise.

Osteoarthritis (or degenerative joint disease) is most often found in people older than age 50, and it affects nearly 16 million Americans. It is characterized by the breakdown of joint tissue and the loss of the protective cartilage of joints, usually with little inflammation of the joints. It is commonly found in the hands, hips, spine, and knees. Pain occurs with movement of the affected joints, and it may also occur during rest as the disease progresses. There is no known cure for osteoarthritis. Treatment of symptoms may include appropriate exercise, physical therapy, moist heat, and certain drugs (e.g., analgesics). Researchers in Sweden have introduced a new form of treatment that could eliminate or at least postpone the need for knee joint replacement in some cases. The procedure involves the collection of cartilage from a healthy part of the knee, growing it in laboratory test tubes, and then injecting it into the damaged joint. The procedure is likely to be most successful with damage caused by traumatic injury rather than damage related to degeneration with aging. Unfortunately, younger adults are more likely to have the healthy cartilage needed for the transplant than are elderly adults.

Gout is a rarer, but fairly well known, form of arthritis (it affects about 1 million Americans, mostly men). Gout is caused by uric acid salt deposits in joints, especially those of the feet and hands; the big toe is the most frequent site. Joints affected by these deposits are painful, swollen, and tender. Gout usually appears between the ages of 40 and 55, and the intensity of the symptoms is likely to increase with increasing age. Certain drugs are used to reduce symptoms during acute stages of the disease. Dietary restrictions are very important in reducing the frequency and duration of acute symptoms.

Research on arthritis is one of the most active areas of medical research in the United States. There are arthritis centers located in medical schools and hospitals across the country. They have the facilities for the diagnosis and treatment of arthritis and for disseminating information about arthritis. New forms of treatment, including medications, behavioral management of pain, and exercise programs that are beneficial to individuals with arthritis, appear regularly. Most recently there has been evidence indicating that the antibiotic drug minocycline improves joint swelling and tenderness for some people with mild to moderate rheumatoid arthritis. Information about advances in the understanding, diagnosis, and treatment of arthritis may be obtained from an arthritis center at a medical school or hospital, from the Arthritis Foundation, or from a regional nonmedical arthritis center. It is important that people who suspect they have arthritis arrange for a diagnosis and prescribed medical/exercise treatment. It is estimated that about 6 million Americans suspect they have the disease, but have failed to see a physician about it.

Bone loss and an increase in the porosity of their mass are part of the aging process. These processes begin in the 30s and increase in the 50s. There is some evidence to indicate that potassium bicarbonate supplements reduce the rate of bone thinning. The rate and amount of loss is greater, on the average, for women than for men. If the loss is severe enough, *osteoporosis* is the result. It is found more often in older women, especially small-boned women, than in older men, and is present in about 30% of the total population age 65 or older. Black women are less likely to have osteoporosis than are either white women or women of Asian descent. The reason for this racial difference is unknown. The most visible sign of the disease is likely to be a stooped posture resulting from a curved spine.

Osteoporosis greatly increases the risk of fractures in elderly people; hip fractures represent the greatest hazard, especially for people in their 70s and older. Researchers in Indiana produced evidence indicating that about 17% of men and about 32% of women will have suffered a hip fracture by the age of 90. Additional factors that predicted a higher risk of hip fracture were found by these researchers to be race (white greater risk than black), being hospitalized for any reason in the previous year, and a leaner body mass. Several factors have been found to predict with reasonable accuracy those elderly adults who have an early discharge from hospitalization after a hip fracture. Elderly adults under age 75 tend to have an earlier discharge than those age 75 and older. Those with greater support from caregivers tend to be discharged earlier than those with less support. Surprisingly, the presence of dementia is associated with earlier discharge than is the absence of dementia, as is the delay in having surgery after the fracture (the shorter the delay, the earlier the discharge).

It is estimated that insufficient nutrition is related to about two-thirds of the cases of osteoporosis. However, it may also result either from menopause brought about by surgical removal of the ovaries or from dysfunctioning of the ovaries as a result of chemotherapy or radiation therapy. Osteoporosis is irreversible, but there are steps that may be taken to slow its progression, including a dietary regimen and certain exercises. Consultation with one's physician is essential for elderly people to minimize the effects of bone loss as much as possible. Early detection is possible among those individuals who are especially predisposed to osteoporosis. An Australian scientist recently identified a single gene that may place some people at a high risk of the disease. The gene is involved in the utilization of vitamin D by the body, a vitamin that plays a major role in bone formation. It is estimated that bone density is determined more by hereditary factors (about 75%) than by environmental factors (about 25%). The discovery of this gene, if replicated thoroughly, offers the eventual possibility of a blood test early in life to identify high-risk individuals. Those at high risk could then increase their bone density by increasing their calcium intake, exercising regularly, and avoiding substances that increase bone loss (e.g., alcohol and cigarettes). Further precautionary measures could include vitamin D supplements and estrogen-replacement medications after menopause. The risk of osteoporosis also increases for people who take drugs called glucocorticoids (steroids). Among these drugs are cortisone and hydrocortisone.

It is estimated that half of all cancers occur in people who are older than age 65. Some kinds of cancer occur in both men and women; they include lung cancer, bladder cancer, colon cancer, stomach cancer, pancreatic cancer, and oral cancer. Lung cancer is the leading cause of death from cancer among men, and it is becoming a major cause of death in women as the number of women who smoke has increased greatly in recent years. Bladder cancer occurs most often between the ages of 50 and 70 years. The incidence of bladder cancer is four times greater in men than in women. The incidence of colon cancer increases greatly between the ages of 65 and 85 years. Interestingly, there is evidence indicating that the risk of colon cancer may be much less for women who have been on estrogen replacement therapy (see MENOPAUSE) than it is for women who have not. One possible reason for the effect of the therapy may be the reduction of bile acids it produces in the colon. Alternatively, it may simply be that women who have undergone estrogen replacement therapy are healthier overall and see their doctors more often than women who have not. About half of the cases of colon cancer are cured by surgery. Early signs of colon cancer can be detected by a test for occult blood (blood that is not visible to the eye) in the stool and then confirmed by additional tests. The blood test should be conducted regularly beginning at age 40. The incidence of stomach cancer has decreased by half over the last 25 years, probably because of better nutrition. Stomach cancer is more common in men than in women, and it usually occurs between the ages of 50 and 70. The incidence of pancreatic cancer increases greatly between the ages of 65 and 85. Oral cancer is a particular problem in late adulthood because it may be undetected for some time in those elderly people who do not visit their dentists regularly.

Cancer of the prostate gland (see PROSTATE GLAND), of course, is found only in men. It is the second leading cause of death from cancer for older men (after lung cancer). It is estimated that the disease has killed 35,000 men in the United States. Prominent older men who died recently of it include Don Ameche and Telly Savalas. Men who have a high consumption of saturated fats have a greater risk of the disease than do men with less consumption; blacks have a greater risk of the disease than do whites; and Asian Americans have less of a risk than do whites. Diagnosis of the disease is made possible in many cases by a blood test known as PSA (prostate-specific antigen). An even more effective diagnostic blood test is currently being tested and may be available for general use in the near future. However, treatment of the disease depends on whether the stage (or grade) of the tumor is low-grade or high-grade. For men with the disease in an early stage, no treatment seems to be nearly as effective as treatment by surgical removal or radiation. In a recent study in the *New England Journal of Medicine,* it was reported that men in the early stage who had no treatment, but whose disease was carefully monitored, were nearly as likely to be alive after 10 years (about 87%) as other men with treatment in the early stage (about 93%). When the cancer is in an advanced or late stage, treatment by surgery or radiation is a necessity (see also PROSTATE GLAND; SEXUAL BEHAVIOR).

The kinds of cancer occurring only in women include ovarian cancer, uterine cancer, cervical cancer, and breast cancer. There are about 22,000 new cases of ovarian cancer every year and about 13,000 deaths from this cancer every year. Ovarian cancer occurs most often in women older than age 60. Uterine cancer occurs most often in women older than age 50. Especially at risk of uterine cancer are women who have never given birth, women who are obese or diabetic, and women who have high blood pressure. In addition, women who have been taking the female hormone estrogen may be at a higher risk than women who have not been taking it. There are about 13,500 new cases of cervical cancer (the cervix is the lower part of the uterus, where it opens into the vagina) every year and about 4,000 deaths from this cancer every year. The incidence of cervical cancer is higher among black women than among white women. Nearly 100% of the deaths from cervical cancer could have been prevented if the cancer had been detected early enough. Early detection is usually possible by means of a test known as a Pap smear (the test is named after Dr. George Papanicolaou, who introduced it in the early 1950s) in which the surface of the cervix is scraped and the contents of the scraping are examined microscopically. Women age 65 and older should have a Pap smear test regularly. Medicare pays for a test every three years. For more information about ovarian, uterine, and cervical cancers write to the Society of Gynecologic Oncology, 401 N. Michigan Avenue, Chicago, IL 60611 (telephone 312-644-6610). (Oncology is that branch of medicine dealing with the diagnosis and treatment of cancer.)

Breast cancer is the leading cause of death from cancer among women. More than 40,000 women are expected to die from breast cancer in 1995. The risk of breast cancer is higher for older women than for younger women (the incidence of breast cancer increases steadily after age 40), for women who have never had children, for women who had menopause at either an early age or a late age, and for women with a higher educational level and a higher socioeconomic level. Breast cancer also occurs more often in women who have a family history of the disease and in women who have already had the disease. About 90% of breast tumors (either benign or cancerous) are discovered by self-examination. Self-examinations should be conducted frequently by women of all ages. Women of all ages, and especially women age 50 and older, should also be tested by mammography at regular intervals to determine whether lumps are present in the breasts. The cost of a mammogram is between $50 and $150 and is covered in some instances by Medicare. Unfortunately, less than 15% of older women who have no health insurance to supplement Medicare get a mammogram—they simply believe they cannot afford the cost. If a lump is found, a biopsy is then performed to determine if the tumor is cancerous. Once breast cancer is discovered, several alternative treatments are available. They all involve surgery in some form, usually followed by either chemotherapy or hormone therapy. Surgery may consist of a radical mastectomy, in which the affected breast is removed along with all of the underarm lymph nodes and the chest muscles; a modified mastectomy, in which the affected breast and the lymph nodes are removed but not the chest muscles; or a lumpectomy, in which only the tumor is removed from the affected breast. For more information about breast cancer write to the Breast Cancer Foundation, Occidental Tower, 5005 LBJ Freeway, Suite 370, Dallas, TX 75244 (telephone, 800-462-9273).

Of particular interest in gerontology is the possibility of age differences in making decisions about treatment once a diagnosis of cancer has been made. For example, are older people more or less likely than younger people to seek a second medical opinion about their diagnosis? Is there an age difference in the amount of information gathered about different treatments before a decision is made as to which treatment to have? The results of a survey conducted by researchers at Pennsylvania State University suggest that there are indeed important age differences in the decision-making process. The participants were women ranging in age from 18 to 88 years, each of whom had recent breast cancer. Younger women were more likely to seek a second medical opinion than were older women: the average age of the women who sought a second opinion was 48 years, whereas the average age of the women who did not seek a second opinion was 58 years. Younger women were also found to take longer to decide on the treatment they wanted than were the older women: the average age of the women who took weeks before deciding was 46 years, whereas the average of the women who made their treatment decisions within a day of the diagnosis was 56 years. On the other hand, age was found to be unrelated to the choice of the treatment that was selected.

Aging is also associated with an increase in the incidence of a number of other body disorders or dysfunctions that are unlikely to present great risks to life, but are unpleasant and painful. For example, the 1988 survey by the U.S. Department of Health and Human Services reported the incidence of ingrown toenails to be three times greater for people age 75 and older than for people in the 18- to 44-year age range (see also FOOT PROBLEMS). Another such disorder is shingles, a painful skin disease that has its highest incidence in late adulthood. There is one comfort for elderly people, however—the incidence of acne in late adulthood is very low.

Disengagement Theory

During the 1950s an extensive survey of elderly people living in Kansas City was conducted. One of the major products of that survey was the development of what became known as disengagement theory. The investigators found that elderly adults commonly withdraw to some degree from their earlier social roles and activities, including their involvements with other people. In effect, their increased self-preoccupation produces social "disengagement." It was theorized at the time that society *expects* elderly adults to show such individual disengagement and demonstrates this expectancy by withdrawing its interest in elderly people. Elderly adults who succeeded in conforming to the disengagement expected of them by society were viewed as being more satisfied with their lives than elderly adults who continued to strive for social engagement.

Disengagement theory is clearly contrary to the notion that keeping active is the most effective way of combating adverse effects of aging. Not surprisingly, the theory stimulated considerable research, most of which has refuted the theory. Disengagement may have been common in the 1950s when there was relatively little concern about the welfare, both financial and psychological, of elderly people. More recent years have seen dramatic changes in society's treatment of older people, most of which have been beneficial to them. Disengagement is no longer the route elderly people are encouraged by society to follow, and the conditions likely to enhance life satisfaction have changed greatly. The need for elderly adults to remain socially active is now emphasized (see ACTIVITY THEORY).

Disuse Principle

A familiar theme in gerontology is that mental skills and abilities become "rusty" if they are not used regularly, and therefore a decline in proficiency is noted. Elderly adults, in general, are commonly believed to use these skills less often than do younger adults, presumably because elderly adults are faced with fewer demands to use them than are younger adults (e.g., in job performances). Consequently, elderly adults are affected more by the negative effects of disuse than younger adults. Conceivably, the remedy for overcoming the negative effects of disuse is prolonged practice of a given task. Hopefully, with such practice, elderly adults will eventually recover their earlier skill and begin to perform as well as much younger adults. This would be true if the actual skill or ability to perform that task had not declined with aging—it had simply become "rusty" for lack of use, an impairment that could be remedied by the practice needed to restore it to its original state.

Several researchers have discovered that elderly adults do indeed greatly improve their performances of various kinds of tasks with practice. One of these tasks is the digit symbol substitution task. Participants receive rows of boxes in which different digits, such as 1 and 2, are placed in the tops of the boxes. The participants are given a code, such as 1 = * and 2 = <, and they are asked to write in the bottom of each box the symbol that codes the digit it contains. After 100 trials on this task, researchers at the University of Wisconsin–Milwaukee found that their elderly participants had increased the number of substitutions they could complete by more than 30%. However, they also found that their young adult participants also increased their number completed by more than 30%. As a result, the age difference in number of substitutions completed favoring the young participants was as great after 100 trials as it was on the first trial. It seems likely that the age difference in performance on this task is the result of a moderate decline in ability with aging, and is not simply the result of the lack of recent use of that ability by elderly adults. Researchers at the University of Missouri–Columbia reported similar outcomes for several other tasks in which the participants received hundreds of practice trials. Practice improves performance regardless of age, and no more for older adults than for younger adults. However, there is one other important result of these practice studies. At the end of a lengthy practice period, elderly participants have consistently been found to perform at a level characteristic of young adult participants at the beginning of practice. Practice may not make performance perfect, but it does have the potential for making the performances of elderly adults equivalent to those of young adults who have not had the benefit of similar amounts of practice.

Disuse has also been used in a more general sense to refer to the possibility of diminished mental activity in late adulthood and the negative effects in performance such disuse may have on a wide variety of mental tasks—that is, the "rustiness" may affect performance on virtually any demanding mental task (see ACTIVITY AND MENTAL PERFORMANCE).

Divided Attention

Many times during an ordinary day you are in situations that require you to divide your attention between two or more ongoing events. While driving, you are listening to the car radio while watching the traffic around you. When introduced to someone at a party, you may be trying to attend not only to that person's name but also to the conversation behind you. Is the ability to divide attention (or, more likely, to alternate it rapidly between simultaneous events) more difficult for elderly people than for younger people? Is there an age difference in the ability to "program" attention so that it may be divided between two events in such a way that attention to either event is not greatly diminished?

Research on age differences in divided attention began in the early 1960s with the *dichotic listening task*. Participants hear successive pairs of digits, with one member delivered to the left ear and the other member delivered at the same time to the right ear. For example, they hear 3 (left ear)/6 (right ear), followed by 7 (left ear)/4 (right ear), and then 1 (left ear)/8 (right ear). Note that as each pair is presented, the participants must divide their attention between the left ear and the right ear. After the last pair is presented, the participants attempt to recall the digits, one ear at a time. For some sequences of pairs they may be asked to recall first what was heard in the left ear, and then recall what was heard in the right ear. For other sequences, the order of reporting is reversed (i.e., right ear first). In general, digits delivered to the right ear tend to be recalled better than digits delivered to the left ear. This is an example of what is called the *right ear advantage*, an advantage found for adults of all ages. The right ear advantage results from the fact that messages delivered to the right ear are transmitted directly to the left cerebral hemisphere of the brain where language centers are located for most people. By contrast, messages delivered to the left ear are transmitted directly to the right cerebral hemisphere and must then be relayed to the language centers in the left hemisphere. Elderly adults perform more poorly on the dichotic listening task than do younger adults. However, their poorer performance is found mainly for the left ear, with little age difference in memory for what was heard in the right ear. This complicates any conclusion that can be reached about a declining ability in dividing attention with normal aging. The age difference in performance on this task could be the result of greater degeneration of the right hemisphere than the left hemisphere with normal aging (see BRAIN AND AGING). In addition, the age difference in dichotic listening performance could be largely the result of memory deficits that accompany aging rather than divided attention deficits.

Not surprisingly, more recent research has turned to other kinds of tasks to determine whether there are indeed age differences in the ability to divide attention. For example, in a recent study participants were given a visual and an auditory task to perform. Two different versions of the tasks were constructed, one easy, the other difficult. On some trials one task was performed alone—sometimes the easy visual task, other times the difficult visual task, or the easy or the difficult auditory task. Two tasks had to be performed on other trials. Sometimes the two tasks consisted of the easy visual task and the easy auditory task. At other times the easy visual task was performed along with the difficult auditory task (or the easy auditory with the difficult visual task). Finally, on some trials the two difficult tasks were performed together. Evidence from this study and other recent studies using related procedures indicates that elderly participants, like young participants, experience little difficulty when two easy tasks are performed together. Both tasks are performed nearly as well when combined as when they are performed alone. However, the more difficult the combined tasks are, the greater the advantage favoring young adults. Thus performance on the two difficult tasks when performed together, relative to their performances singly, is especially difficult for older participants. Provided the two tasks are relatively easy, little decline in the ability to perform them together would be expected with aging. This would be the case, for example, in dividing attention between the car radio and watching the traffic flow when traffic is very light. As one or both tasks become more difficult, elderly adults, on the average, would be expected to have greater difficulty than younger adults in dividing attention between the two. This would be the case when the traffic flow is heavy. At this point it would probably be a greater advantage for the older driver than for the younger driver to turn off the radio (or tell a passenger to be quiet) and concentrate on the traffic alone.

Divorce

Divorce occurs most frequently for people in the age range of 30 to 45 years. The incidence of divorce is higher for those people who marry before the age of 20 than those who marry after age 20. Although divorce is less common for elderly adults than for younger adults, its incidence is, nevertheless, fairly high. It is estimated that more than half a million people age 65 or older are divorced, and that about an additional 10,000 elderly people join the ranks of the divorced annually.

Divorce is usually a stressful even for elderly people—more so, on the average, than it is for younger people. Divorce is less a normative (or expected) event in late adulthood than in earlier adulthood. In general, divorce is likely to be more stressful to elderly people than is widowhood or widowerhood (which is a normative event in late adulthood). Surveys of divorced people of various ages indicate that, immediately after separation, older people tend to show greater negative emotions and unhappiness and fewer positive emotional experiences than younger people do. In general, people age 50 and older show the most maladaptive behavior after separation. People in their 40s more closely approximate the functioning level of young adults after separation. Elderly men tend to show greater unhappiness after divorce and greater change in their perceived health status than do elderly women. However, older women tend to have more psychological symptoms and appear to be more disorganized after divorce than do elderly men. Elderly women also tend to express greater dissatisfaction with their lives for more years before the divorce than do elderly men. In general, elderly women tend to show improvement in physical health status after divorce, seemingly reflecting their release from what they may perceive to have been confining lives. However, there is also evidence that, over the long term, elderly women may experience more problems in their daily lives than do elderly men. Part of the difficulty facing many elderly divorced women is their poor financial status. A 1989 survey revealed that more than a fourth of divorcées age 62 and older had incomes below the official poverty level. Only 4% of elderly divorcées received any alimony payments, and only 23% had an income from both Social Security and an employer pension plan.

Divorce is usually a crisis situation for elderly people. Both spouses would profit greatly from psychological counseling at least as much as, if not more than, younger divorced people. Of course, divorce is an alternative to what is usually an unhappy marriage. Researchers in California have found that there is a relationship between marital satisfaction and health, one that is stronger for women than for men. In unhappy marriages, elderly wives tend to report more mental health and physical health problems than do their husbands.

There is another aspect of divorce that has important implications for elderly people. Of concern is the effect of divorce in early adulthood on relationships years later with their now adult children. In general, these adult children have less contact with both elderly parents, and their relationships with both parents are more negative, than is the case for adult children whose parents stayed together while they were growing up. Negative relationships are likely to be more pronounced with fathers than with mothers. In addition, adult children are likely to feel less loved by divorced fathers than by divorced mothers.

Drug Abuse

Researchers of drug abuse generally agree that, relative to younger people, the use of illegal drugs (e.g., marijuana) by older people is rare. The main problem for community-dwelling elderly people is the misuse of legal drugs, both those prescribed by physicians and those bought over the counter. However, the problem is more likely to be the underuse of prescribed drugs than the overuse. By contrast, elderly people in nursing homes are often the victims of overuse as a result of physicians' instructions to "administer as needed" and by errors in the administration of the drugs.

Researchers at the University of California–Berkeley have compared normally aging misusers and nonmisuers on a number of psychological characteristics. In general, misusers did not differ from nonmisuers on most characteristics, including the number of "hassles" or stresses they had experienced. However, misusers reported that they experienced their hassles more intensely than nonmisuers, and they also reported greater dissatisfaction with their ability to cope with stressors than did nonmisusers.

Drug Tests (Clinical Trials)

New drugs that may aid patients in combating a physical or a mental disorder are constantly being discovered. Before these drugs are made available to the general public by the U.S. Food and Drug Administration, they must pass a series of rigorous clinical tests to determine whether they are actually beneficial and whether they may have harmful side effects. Testing usually starts with animals. If these tests are successful, the next step is likely to be tests with healthy volunteers who are free of the disorder for which the drug is intended. If no harmful side effects are found, the next step is usually the testing of a small group of volunteer patients with the disorder. If these patients show both some improvement in their clinical condition and the absence of serious side effects, then the final step is extensive clinical trials with larger numbers of volunteer patients at many locations across the country. These tests are carefully controlled and include treating other patients with a placebo (a neutral substance) in place of the new drug. Neither the patient nor the physician knows whether the patient is receiving the drug or the placebo. A careful evaluation is then made of the drug's effect on the disorder before it is available for physicians to prescribe to their patients.

This is the procedure used to determine the effectiveness of a new drug in treating, for example, the memory problems encountered by patients with Alzheimer's disease. A number of drugs have been so tested in recent years, and clinical trials are presently planned for still other drugs (see ALZHEIMER'S DISEASE).

Duke Longitudinal Studies

The Duke Longitudinal Studies consist of three separate longitudinal studies (see LONGITUDINAL METHOD), each conducted at Duke University Medical Center. The first study began in 1955 with several hundred healthy participants aged 60 to 90. They received medical and psychological examinations every few years through 1976 when the study ended. The second study began in 1968 with several hundred participants aged 46 to 70. These participants also received medical and psychological examinations every few years through 1976 when this study also ended. The third study has been concerned only with the "old" old. It began in 1980 with several hundred participants, all age 75 years or older. As with the first two studies, this study is a longitudinal one in which the initial participants are retested several times (in this case annually).

The results of the Duke studies have revealed that normal aging is typically accompanied by declining health and physical functioning. For example, cardiovascular diseases increase in frequency, vision and hearing proficiency decline, and sexual activity decreases. However, the studies have also revealed that there is a substantial minority of aging individuals who are exceptions to the typical pattern of decline. These individuals demonstrate that physical decline is not an inevitable consequence of aging. The Duke studies have also revealed that, in general, mental health and life satisfaction show little decline with normal aging.

Dysarthria

Dysarthria consists of a group of speech impairments caused by neurological disorders that are fairly common among elderly adults. The speech impairments range from mild to severe. With mild impairment, speech is likely to be intelligible, but it sounds as if it is being spoken by a drunken individual. For this reason the impairment is often a source of embarrassment to the affected individual. With severe impairment, speech is likely to be unintelligible. There are five different forms of dysarthria that vary in terms of the location of the neurological disorder and their specific speech symptoms. Speech therapists recommend that affected individuals be encouraged to speak slowly and to use shorter utterances when speaking, as well as other steps to make communication more understandable.

E

. . . .

Ecological Validity

Ecological validity in aging research refers to the generalizability to the everyday world of the results obtained in a laboratory study on age differences for some mental task. For example, substantial age differences favoring younger adults may be found in the acquisition of face-name pairs studied in the laboratory with a number of such pairs. Are elderly adults likely to be this different than younger adults in acquiring names to pair with faces in their everyday encounters with new people? That is, to what extent does the laboratory age difference in acquisition apply to real-life acquisition? The less the result can be generalized, the lower the ecological validity of the study from which the generalization could be made. The nature of the laboratory task may be such that the results exaggerate the extent of the age difference outside the laboratory (see EVERYDAY MEMORY). Nevertheless, the study may have some degree of ecological validity in terms of the determination that there is a likely difference of some kind between younger and older adults in performance on the task investigated in the laboratory. Researchers must then determine the reason for that age difference.

Educational Level

For some years elderly adults have averaged fewer years of formal education than have younger adults. The age difference in educational level in the 1950s may be readily seen from the nature of the large sample used by David Wechsler in the standardization of his revised intelligence test. At each age level a major, and largely successful, attempt was made to make the tested sample representative of the total population in the United States at that age level. More than 43% of the sample in the age range of 25 to 34 years had attended college for 1 or more years. By contrast, only 16% of the sample in the age range of 70 to 74 years had attended college for 1 or more years. In 1960 it was estimated that fewer than 20% of the elderly population of the United States had graduated from high school. Even in the 1980s a substantial "educational gap" separated elderly and younger adults. In the mid-1980s it was estimated that nearly 72% of those adults age 25 and older had completed high school, but only 34% of those adults age 75 and older. Nevertheless, there has been a definite trend toward a better-educated elderly population. Between 1970 and 1985 the median number of years of formal education for elderly people increased from 8.7 to 11.7, with about 50% of elderly white persons completing high school. Unfortunately, the educational level of older members of minority groups has lagged well behind that of elderly white people. In the mid-1980s fewer than 20% of elderly minority group members had completed high school. In the near future it is estimated that two-thirds of the elderly population will have at least graduated from high school. However, to increase this trend even more for future generations as they age, it is clear that greater educational opportunity must be given to members of minority groups.

The age difference in educational level is important in evaluating the effects of aging on mental functioning. At all ages educational level is known to correlate positively and moderately with scores achieved on an intelligence test. When younger and older participants are carefully equated in educational level, much of the age difference in scores disappears. In most cross-sectional aging studies on learning, memory, problem solving, reasoning, and so on, the investigators are very careful to ensure that their younger and older age groups are equal in terms of educational level. An age difference in performance that persists with this condition is likely to be related to aging itself rather than to a generational difference in education.

Interestingly, the number of years of formal education also correlates positively with longevity. Of course, this does not mean that more education causes people to live longer. It suggests that people with higher levels of education find better-paying occupations. With better pay they can afford better nutrition and better health care—factors that do affect longevity. Life expectancy tables estimate how much longer people are expected to live when they have attained any given age. The years a person is expected to live are increased by such factors as nonsmoking, regular exercising—and amount of education. For example, it is not unusual to see instructions telling you to add 3 years to your life expectancy if you have 4 or more years of college, 2 years if you have 1 to 3 years of college, and so on. On the other hand, some evidence suggests that the rate of mental decline in Alzheimer's disease is faster for more highly educated people than for less highly educated people with the disease (see ALZHEIMER'S DISEASE).

Elder Abuse

There is no generally acceptable definition of elder abuse. Should it include both verbal and physical abuse? Should neglect be considered a form of abuse? Must abuse be intentional to be considered abuse? State statutes regarding elder abuse are usually broad in what is to be considered abuse, but the implementation of those statutes is usually rather limited and often restricted to physical abuse.

Elder abuse has undoubtedly existed for many years. However, concern about elder abuse did not reach national attention until the 1970s. In part, society's awakening to elder abuse resulted from surveys of small samples of older people that indicated more than a million elderly people are abused annually. Such surveys received considerable attention in newspapers, and terms such as "granny bashing" became widely used. This was a period in which general concern about elderly people had been aroused, and the existence of elder abuse became a major part of that concern. How many elderly adults are the victims of abuse? As noted above, estimates in the 1970s were based on small samples of elderly people. The results of a much larger survey were published in 1988. More than, 2,000 community-dwelling elderly people in the Boston metropolitan area were surveyed. The percentage of elderly people who reported abuse in one form or another was 3.2% (32 per 1,000 elderly people). Physical abuse was the most frequent form reported (20 per 1,000 elderly people), followed by chronic verbal abuse (11 per 1,000). Projected nationally, this estimated frequency suggests that nearly 1 million elderly people are indeed the victims of abuse. This may be a conservative estimate because in many cases abuse is never reported. Moreover, various authorities are likely to have different views of what constitutes abuse. For example, police officers are likely to consider only physically aggressive acts as forms of abuse, whereas social workers are likely to consider verbally aggressive acts as being as abusive as physical acts.

In the Boston survey, elderly men and elderly women were found to be the victims of abuse with almost equal frequency. The most common abuser was the spouse of the victim. Physical abuse, however, was reported to be administered more frequently by a wife to a husband than by a husband to a wife, whereas the reverse was true for chronic verbal abuse.

Of further concern is the extent of abuse toward residents of nursing homes. In a recent survey, nearly 600 nurses and nursing aides working in nursing homes were asked how often they had observed incidents of abuse by staff members at their institutions in the past year. The most frequently observed physical abuse was the excessive use of restraints; 6% of those surveyed reported observing its occurrence 10 or more times in the past year and 79% reported never having observed it. Such acts as pushing and shoving residents were observed to occur even less frequently. Only 1% of those surveyed reported observing its occurrence 10 or more times in the past year, and 83% reported never having observed it. By contrast, verbal abuse appears to occur much more frequently in a nursing home. Of those surveyed, only 30% reported never observing residents being yelled at in anger; 15% reported observing its occurrence 10 or more times, and 11% reported residents being insulted or sworn at 10 or more times during the past year. In another survey, 10% of nursing assistants reported committing at least one act of physical abuse toward residents and 40% reported committing at least one act of psychological abuse.

Fortunately, the incidence of abuse among residents of nursing homes may be reduced greatly by providing appropriate training for nursing assistants. This has been demonstrated by the application of a training program developed by the Coalition of Advocates for the Rights of the Infirmed (CARIE). The objectives of this program are to increase staff awareness of potentially abusive situations and to teach strategies for the effective resolution of conflicts that arise with residents and lead to abusive actions (see also MEDICAL COSTS [MIS-UNDERSTANDING]).

Elderhostel

Elderhostel programs offer continuing education programs for older adults. The concept, introduced in 1975, was patterned after the youth hostels that were popular with young people traveling in Europe. The programs are given on college and university campuses both in the United States and Canada, and similar programs are now given in Europe as well. Courses are offered for 1 to 2 weeks at a low cost. Older students live in dormitories and eat with the college students. The objective is to present older adults with courses that are relevant to their everyday lives and are enjoyable. For example, one such course is on microcomputers. The students receive hands-on experience in word processing and the use of various software programs. There are no examinations and no homework. In addition, the students are given the opportunity to participate in a variety of extracurricular activities.

Emotion

Fear, anger, disgust, joy, sadness—these are all emotions experienced by adults of all ages. However, are they experienced in the same way during the course of the adult life span? A familiar theme in aging is that they are not. One of the popular beliefs has been that there is both a blunting or flattening of emotion (i.e., becoming less intense) in late adulthood and a preponderance of negative emotions (e.g., sadness) as opposed to positive emotions (e.g., joy), relative to earlier stages of adulthood. However, recent research by Dr. Carol Zender Malatesta and her associates has demonstrated that these beliefs are really among the myths about aging. The researchers extensively interviewed a large sample of adults of various ages about their emotional experiences. The results indicated that there is no reason to believe that emotions are either less intense in late adulthood than in early adulthood or more negative than in early adulthood. There is evidence to indicate that when elderly people are asked to relive a past emotional experience (e.g., sadness experienced after someone's death) that the pattern of nervous system activity is much like that found for younger adults, although the magnitude of activity is less intense than that found for younger adults.

Another important finding emerged from Dr. Malatesta's interviews. Children in our society are generally taught, as much as possible, not to display their emotions. By the time young adulthood has been reached, control of the facial muscles has largely succeeded in hiding emotional expression. By contrast, elderly adults are much less concerned with the need to conceal their inner feelings. This is especially true for elderly women. Paradoxically, elderly women seem more likely than elderly men to mask their true feelings by controlling their outer expressions of emotions. Conversely, when asked to relive a past emotional experience, older women report feeling a more intense emotion than do older men.

On many occasions we are unable to control our emotional expression. We do hear such remarks as "You look sad today" or "Something good must have happened. You sure look happy." The implication is that our nonverbal language is communicating our emotional inner feeling to other people. Especially important in this noverbal communication is our facial expression. Even with the emphasis during childhood to mask our expression of emotion, we often find it difficult to control our facial expression while experiencing an emotion. Of further interest is the extent to which our nonverbal communication becomes less reliable as an indicator of a specific emotional state for elderly people relative to younger people. Dr. Malatesta has provided some intriguing evidence with regard to this point. People of various ages were asked to recall particular experiences in their lives during which they felt sad, other experiences when they felt happy or angry, and so on. The goal of this task was to recapture to some degree the experience felt originally (a procedure known as mood induction). Participants were videotaped as they relived these experiences. The videotapes were then shown to other adults of differing ages, who were asked to evaluate each tape in terms of the intensity of emotion displayed and the specific nature of the emotion. In general, young adults were found to judge emotions most accurately when the tapes were of fellow young adults. Middle-aged and older adults were also most accurate when they judged the expressions of others their own age. Overall, the facial expressions of elderly adults were most difficult to judge accurately.

Largely unresolved is the possibility that the importance of emotions in people's lives changes from early to late adulthood. Gerontologists have debated for some years whether emotions are of greatest importance in the lives of young or elderly adults. Recent evidence provided by researchers at Stanford University suggests that salience may actually be greater for elderly adults. Participants in their study read and then recalled a story that contained both emotional and nonemotional content. The amount of emotional content recalled was found to increase progressively from the 20s through the early 80s, thus implying increasing importance of emotions from early to late adulthood.

Entitlements

An entitlement in the federal budget is a mandatory expenditure. Individuals included in some entitlement program in the federal budget are not affected by their income levels. That is, they are entitled to payments regardless of the level of their income. Social Security and Medicare are among these non–means tested entitlements (i.e., there is no test to pass in terms of a specified income level). They account for about 21% and 10%, respectively, of federal spending. Other entitlements, such as Medicaid, are means tested in the sense that only individuals who pass the test of a low income qualify to receive them.

A belief held by many younger people is that Social Security and Medicare benefits go largely to elderly people with incomes high enough that they do not need the benefits. In fact, however, less than 2% of the benefits go to those whose family income is more than $100,000, and over 67% go to those whose family income is less than $30,000.

Environmental Press

Our environment places various demands or presses on us. These demands may consist of various combinations of physical, interpersonal, and social demands. If these demands exceed our abilities, then we are likely to experience distress. Physical demands are more likely to be a problem for elderly adults than they are for younger adults. Consider, for example, an individual living in a third (or even second) floor of an apartment house without an elevator. The need to climb the stairs is surely likely to be a greater environmental press for an elderly resident than for a younger resident. The less the physical competence of the elderly resident, the greater will be the impact on him or her created by the environmental press. Distance from a shopping center is also likely to have a greater impact on an elderly individual who must walk to shop, in relation to a younger person who is more likely to drive. Fortunately, designers of residential centers and retirement communities have become increasingly aware of the need to plan physical facilities that consider the physical capabilities of their elderly residents. Similarly, manufacturers of drugs and medicines prescribed for elderly individuals are increasingly packaging them in forms that are less taxing on the memory abilities of their clientele.

Episodic Memory

Do you remember the first spill you had on a bicycle? Where did it take place? What was the name of your date at your high school prom? What did you eat for dinner last night? How many times have you seen a beer commercial on television during the past week? When was the last time you balanced your checkbook? What was it your spouse said to you when you left the house? Do you remember where you parked your car at the shopping mall?

These are all examples of what memory researchers call *episodic memory*, or memory for personally experienced events. Episodic memory and semantic memory are the main components of the human memory system. Episodic memory refers to memory for personally experienced events or episodes in your life. Such memories are stored in reference to the context in which they occurred. Context refers to the where and when of an episode, that is, the time and place that it occurred. In this respect, episodic memory differs from *semantic memory*, which contains general knowledge information that is ordinarily stored without reference to the context in which it was acquired.

When elderly people complain about their memory problems, they are usually referring to their episodic memory. The study of age differences in episodic memory, including the reasons for their occurrences, is complicated, however, by the very complexity of episodic memory. Episodic memory is both short-term and long-term in nature. Short-term episodic memory (also called primary memory) is for information briefly held in consciousness. Age-related declines in short-term memory proficiency are, in general, modest (see SHORT-TERM MEMORY). Long-term episodic memory is either for newly acquired episodic information (called secondary memory) or for information acquired some time ago (very long-term memory or tertiary memory; see AUTOBIOGRAPHICAL MEMORY; VERY LONG-TERM MEMORY).

Most laboratory research on age differences in memory has centered on secondary memory. Age-related declines in secondary memory proficiency usually range from moderate to fairly substantial, depending on the form of secondary memory involved. These deficits may occur in either the encoding of episodic information (i.e., transforming it into a memory record or trace) or the retrieval of the resulting memory traces from the long-store of episodic memory traces. The encoding of episodic information may be, in turn, either effortful or automatic.

Effortful encoding means that there is the intent to commit information to memory and mental effort is exerted to transform the information into a memory trace. Effortful secondary memory is commonly studied with familiar words as the to-be-remembered events. After studying a lengthy list of words, participants of different ages are asked either to recall the words or to recognize them among distractor or new words. Note that participants are not really "learning" the words—they are already present in the participants' semantic memories. Instead they are asked to remember which of the many words they know were encountered at a particular time and place (the where and when of episodic memory). On the average, elderly participants recall fewer words than do younger participants. Part of the problem lies in the generally less proficient encoding of the episodic events of older adults relative to younger adults. Younger adults tend to make greater use of what is called elaborative encoding than do older adults, presumably because the former have a greater capacity of what is called working memory, the place in the memory system where encoding takes place (see WORKING MEMORY).

Elaborative encoding makes the resulting memory trace more distinctive and more accessible for later recall or recognition than does simply saying a word to yourself. One form of elaboration is to form an image of a word serving as an episodic event. Another form is the use of an organizational strategy whereby a connection or relationship is found between the words in the list. For example, four different animals may be named in the list. By making use of this relatedness, you may be able to recall their names together. Memory training programs for elderly adults usually stress the use of elaboration to improve the encoding of episodic events (see MEMORY TRAINING). Part of the older adult's problem in episodic memory results from the greater difficulty in retrieving information from the episodic memory stores. This may be seen from the results of research studies in which recognition memory has been contrasted with recall of the same information (see RECOGNITION MEMORY VS. RECALL MEMORY).

Automatic encoding refers to forms of memory in which memory occurs without the intent to commit information to memory and without a conscious effort to encode that information. That is, memory occurs incidentally. This is the case for the memory people have of their own actions, the memory of conversational contents, the memory of television programs they watched, and stories they have read. In general, younger adults are more proficient in these forms of memory than are older adults, but the extent of the age difference is less pronounced than it is for effortfully encoded material.

Another important distinction in regard to episodic memory is that between retrospective memory and prospective memory. Retrospective memory, or remembrance of things past, refers to the forms of memory just discussed. That is, it consists of memory for previously encoded episodic events that have been registered in the long-term store. By contrast, prospective memory refers to memory for performing some future action, such as remembering to mail a letter or to stop at the store on the way home from work to purchase some needed item (see PROSPECTIVE MEMORY). Interestingly, recent research has indicated that prospective memory may be largely resistant to any pronounced declines in proficiency from early to late adulthood.

The complexity of retrospective episodic memory is increased further when we realize that it refers not only to memory for the content of episodic events, but also for other attributes of events. You may remember playing bridge with the Smiths, but you don't remember when. In this instance it is the temporal (time) attribute of the event and not its content that is at stake. Or you may remember how many times you played bridge during the past month. This is the frequency-of-occurrence attribute of the event and not its content that is at stake. You may remember that the last time you played bridge with the Smiths was at their house and not yours. Here it is the spatial attribute of the event and not its content that is at stake. Or you may remember that it was George Smith and not Nancy Smith who said you are a great bridge player. Here it is the source attribute of the episodic event and not its content that is at stake. Age differences in each of these attributes have been widely studied in the laboratory by the use of procedures that vary these attributes in much the same way they are varied in the everyday world (see ACTION MEMORY; FREQUENCY-OF-OCCURRENCE MEMORY; SOURCE MEMORY; SPATIAL MEMORY; TEMPORAL MEMORY). In general, this research has revealed that the extent of age differences in proficiency varies considerably among these attributes.

Euthanasia

One of the greatest ethical debates in contemporary society is in regard to the practice of euthanasia, the killing of someone with a seemingly incurable and mentally devastating disease or disorder. The debate is likely to intensify in the coming years as the elderly population increases and the number of individuals with Alzheimer's disease increases accordingly.

There are two forms of euthanasia. The first is active euthanasia in which a patient's life is deliberately cut short by some action that terminates life immediately to avoid further suffering. This form of euthanasia has received considerable attention in recent years with the advent of so-called "death machines" that, in effect, aid the person to commit suicide. The other form is passive euthanasia in which efforts are no longer made to sustain the life of the person through the use of lifesaving medical equipment. This form of euthanasia has been the center of recent court cases in which the right to withdraw lifesaving equipment has been debated. It is hoped that many of the ethical concerns about euthanasia will be reduced by the existence of advance directives, in which people make known their desire not to have their lives sustained by artificial means when there is no apparent hope for their recovery. In some states, administrators of nursing homes are required to ask about residents' wishes and to keep these documents on file. However, the extent to which these documents are legally binding and will dictate the treatment received from a medical team is debatable.

Everyday Memory

Did I mail that letter? I must remember to stop at the supermarket on my way home from work today. What is that new neighbor's name? When was it that we last played bridge together? I know the name of that movie, but I just can't think of it now.

These are examples of everyday memory experiences. One of the most frequent complaints expressed by older people is that their everyday memory is not as proficient as when they were younger. When elderly people rate their own memory proficiency, they characteristically rate it lower than do younger adults (see METAMEMORY; METAMEMORY IN ADULTHOOD QUESTIONNAIRE [MIA] AND METAMEMORY FUNCTIONING QUESTIONNAIRE [MFQ]). The implication is that the imperfections of memory found at all ages are greater in late adulthood than in earlier adulthood. How accurate are elderly people in their complaints about their memory proficiency? Ideally, it would be best to study memory as it operates in everyday life, and then compare people of different ages in its proficiency. This is difficult to accomplish. The very presence of an investigator watching you throughout the day could alter your memory performance (i.e., the Heisenberg principle—the mere act of observing an event is likely to change the nature of that event). There is the possibility that you could be your own observer by keeping a diary in which each day you record your memory failures and imperfections. There have been several diary studies of this kind. However, the procedure is not very satisfying. How can you rely on reports of memory failures from people who may have memory problems and are unable to remember their own memory failures? (see DIARY STUDIES OF MEMORY FAILURES)

Given the problems of observing memory as it functions in everyday life, memory researchers concerned about age differences in memory proficiency have turned largely to bringing everyday memory into the laboratory where it may be studied under controlled conditions. They give participants of various ages memory tasks that they believe approximate those encountered in everyday living. Thus to study age differences in learning to associate names with faces, a task elderly people commonly claim is very difficult for them, participants learn a list in which about 10 faces of strangers are paired with surnames. In general, elderly participants take much longer to learn such a list than do younger participants. What do such results reveal about the difficulty of elderly adults in learning names to go with faces in the everyday world? How often does an elderly person need to learn 10 new face-name pairings at essentially the same time? We usually meet new people one at a time or perhaps two at a time. In general, elderly people may have a bit more trouble in mastering the new names than younger people, especially when they fail to pay attention to the name(s) in the first place. The laboratory results on face-name acquisition do indicate a decline in proficiency with normal aging (see VERBAL LEARNING). However, it is likely that the extent of that decline as evidenced in everyday face-name acquisition is exaggerated (i.e., the results of the research may have limited ecological validity; see ECOLOGICAL VALIDITY). Similarly, many studies of age differences in memory for words in a lengthy series of words reveal a fairly substantial difference in the average number of words recalled between younger and older participants. Such results do suggest that older people are somewhat less proficient than younger people in both encoding and retrieving episodic information. The results seem to exaggerate the extent of the deficiency in everyday memory proficiency. How often does an elderly person attempt to memorize a lengthy series of events? The memory of older adults for a short shopping list is probably nearly as good as most younger adults. If it is a much longer shopping list, why not write the items down and take the list with you when you go shopping?

There have been important trends toward research on adult age differences for laboratory tasks that more closely approximate those of everyday memory, and therefore seem to have greater ecological validity. With verbal material, research on age differences in memory for the contents of stories, articles, conversational content, and television programs has become a popular area of aging memory research. Our everyday memory functioning surely includes encountering frequently contents of these kinds. Similarly, an important new area of laboratory research on aging memory consists of memory for actions and activities performed in the laboratory. The objective of such studies is to approximate the kinds of memories we have for our everyday actions, such as turning off the gas on a stove and locking a door. This is a component of everyday memory about which elderly people often complain.

Exercise and Physical/Mental Performance

Some elderly people have been regular physical exercisers for many years, whereas others have lived more sedentary lives. Long-term exercisers have been found to be physically healthier and to be faster in responding on a variety of tasks than nonexercisers. There is also evidence to indicate that the regular exercisers perform at higher levels on a variety of mental tasks (e.g., reasoning tasks) than the nonexercisers. Given the high proportion of currently younger adults who are regular exercisers, there is good reason to believe that future generations of elderly people will show less mental decline than current and past generations of elderly people who were less likely to be regular exercisers. This depends, of course, on current younger exercisers continuing to exercise through late adulthood.

A related question concerns what happens to those more sedentary elderly people who become exercisers late in life. Researchers at Duke University Medical Center have been active in their attempts to answer this question. In their studies, elderly participants engage in intensive aerobic exercises for several months. They are then evaluated in terms of how they compare at the end of the exercise program both with their initial findings and with other elderly people who were engaged in nonvigorous activities during the same period. The results have shown that exercise late in life does have some physical health benefits. In addition, at the end of the program the exercisers reported that they were sleeping better than at the beginning and they reported that their social life had improved. The exercisers also believed that their concentration had improved after completion of the program, as had their mental functioning. Unfortunately, laboratory performances failed to show any significant improvement in scores on either memory tests or intelligence tests. Initiating regular exercise late in life does not seem to be a cure-all for moderate mental declines that occur with normal aging. For exercise to be effective in improving mental functioning, it seemingly needs to be begin much earlier in life and to be engaged in regularly over the years.

The physical benefits of an exercise training program are not limited to community-dwelling older adults. Researchers at Tufts University have demonstrated that benefits occur for many frail residents of nursing homes as well. Many participants in their study had illnesses such as lung disease, arthritis, and high blood pressure, and many had some degree of dementia. They worked out vigorously for 45 minutes a day for 3 days a week for several weeks. The participants used exercise machines to strengthen their thighs and knees, and they lifted weights to strengthen other muscles. At the end of the program the participants averaged an increased walking speed of 12% and an increased stair climbing ability of 28%. They appeared to be less depressed than they were at the start of the program. Most important, they walked around their room on their own much more than they did before the program. This is important because many residents of nursing homes have such poor leg strength that they are confined to chairs and unable to walk to the bathroom on their own. They would benefit greatly from this kind of exercise program.

Exercise Types

One popular myth about aging is that exercise is dangerous for many elderly people. In truth, exercise in the right form and the right amount is likely to improve the health, strength, flexibility, and stamina of many older people. There are three kinds of exercise: low-intensity or anaerobic, aerobic, and resistance.

Light walking, golfing, bowling, and some calisthenics are examples of low-intensity exercises. Low-intensity exercise has little effect on improving cardiovascular and pulmonary functioning, but it does help in weight control and increasing muscle strength.

Aerobic exercise is vigorous and raises the heart rate by more than 40% from the resting rate to the maximum rate. Examples of aerobic exercising are jogging at a moderate or fast rate, walking at a brisk pace, swimming, and riding a bicycle. When used in the right form and duration, aerobic exercise should help to improve cardiovascular and pulmonary functioning for many older people. A major study of elderly male exercisers indicated that participants who exercised moderately had more than a 20% lower risk of mortality, whereas elderly men who exercised more strenuously had a 50% lower risk of mortality. Aerobic exercise is also likely to improve agility and balance. Researchers in Vermont found that even postcoronary patients (e.g., myocardial infarct) may benefit in peak oxygen consumption from aerobic exercise. Caution is important, however. An exercise regimen that is too strenuous can lead to an increased risk of mortality.

Leg presses, tricep presses, and weight lifting are examples of resistance exercise. Researchers in California recently demonstrated that resistance exercise is not just for the young. Their over-60 participants in a yearlong training program showed significant increases in muscle strength, with the increases occurring primarily during the first 3 months of training.

In addition, researchers at Tufts University found that a twice weekly weight-lifting program increased bone density of the hips and spine for their older women participants, all of whom had a prior sedentary life-style. Increases in bone density help to reduce the risk of osteoporosis (see DISEASES [CHRONIC]). In general, the participants in this training program also experienced improved balance and greater muscle strength, therefore reducing the risk of falls.

Canadian researchers found that a weight-lifting program for elderly people served to improve treadmill-walking endurance and stair-climbing ability. Experts in weight lifting recommend that trainees warm up and stretch their muscles before they begin to lift weights and that they lift weights only every other day.

Experts in exercise emphasize that a prescription for exercise is nearly as necessary as a prescription for medicines. Elderly persons planning to begin an exercise program should consult with their physicians (including a thorough physical examination) and, if possible, with an exercise expert to determine the appropriate form and duration of exercise for someone in their current health states.

Unfortunately, many elderly people ignore the benefits of exercise, either because they believe they do not need it or they have accepted the myth of exercise's dangers. Physicians and health experts need to increase their efforts of informing elderly people of the many benefits derived from regular exercise.

To find more information about exercise and other health-related topics you should consult the booklet *Healthy Aging*. To obtain a copy write to ETNET, P.O. Box 7536, Department P, Wilton, CT 06897; you must enclose a check or money order for $1.50 and a self-addressed envelope.

Experimental Psychology

Experimental psychology is the component of psychology most directly concerned with learning, memory, problem solving, and reasoning. Experimental psychologists of aging direct their research at determining both the degree of age differences and the identification of the reasons for these age differences in each of these mental activities. Many experimental psychologists of aging also are concerned with finding ways of improving the mental performances of older adults through various interventions (e.g., memory training; see MEMORY TRAINING).

Research by experimental psychologists in general is characterized by the use of the experimental method. The control of factors or conditions that may differ between the groups of participants in an experiment, other than the critical condition being varied in the experiment, is basic to this method of investigation. If the groups differ in some way other than in the condition being varied, then the reason for any difference in performance between the groups is unknown. That is, the superior performance by one of the groups could be related to the specific condition under which it performed, in contrast to the condition under which another group performed, but it could also be caused by one or more uncontrolled factors that distinguished the two groups. For example, if the critical condition (experimental variable) in a memory study is the rate at which words in a list are presented, for 2 seconds or 4 seconds, then the experimenter would make certain that the same words are presented to both groups. Word content does affect memory proficiency. If the two groups had different sets of words to memorize, then the superior memory performance for the group with the slower rate of presentation of the individual words could be because of the content of the words presented to them rather than the slower rate of presentation. Especially essential for control are the characteristics of the subjects participating in an experiment. Assigning all of the best memorizers to one of the conditions in a rate of presentation experiment and all of the poorer memorizers to the other condition would create a biased result. Is the observed difference in memory performance observed in the experiment caused by the slower rate of presentation or the presence of better memorizers, regardless of the rate condition, in the slower rate group? To avoid this problem, the ideal solution is to randomly assign participants from a pool of participants to the different conditions of an experiment. Random assignment of participants to "young" and "old" groups is, of course, impossible in aging research—age is a characteristic that cannot be controlled by random assignment (unless the experiment involves age simulation; see AGE SIMULATION). However, the researchers can ensure as much as possible that the age groups are matched as much as possible on such basic characteristics as gender and educational level (see CROSS-SECTIONAL METHOD).

Randomization affects experimental aging research in another important way. Consider an experiment comparing memory proficiency for younger and older participants under slow and fast rates of presenting the information to be remembered. Half of the older participants will receive the words at a fast rate, the other half at a slow rate, as will the younger participants. Now it is essential that at each age level, the participants be assigned randomly to the two rate conditions. This is to make the characteristics of older participants as comparable as possible between the two rate conditions, and the same for the characteristics of the younger participants.

Expertise

The United States has recently had two presidents who may be considered "old," at least in terms of their chronological ages. Numerous studies have demonstrated age-related declines on many mental abilities, including those of memory and reasoning. However, our older presidents seem to have functioned quite well in office (although one did admit to having memory problems). Older business executives have been found to perform well below the levels of younger executives on many laboratory tasks and clinical tests of mental abilities, yet the older executives were known to have performed their jobs very well, despite their apparent decline in what may be considered basic mental abilities. The same outcome has been found for university professors. Older professors who are well known for their continuing excellence in teaching and research have scored well below the levels of younger professors on tests of many basic mental abilities. Computer programmers are no exception to the continuation of expertise into later adulthood. Older, experienced programmers have been found to function at a level comparable to that of younger and equally experienced programmers. Most bridge players are likely to know elderly players who are exceptionally skilled in bridge and are regular participants in duplicate bridge tournaments. Their skill in playing the mentally challenging game of bridge seemingly defies their likely age-related declines in many basic mental abilities. In each of these cases, expertise in a particular endeavor or field is the issue. Many people who are experts in a particular endeavor, whether it be in politics, business, or a skilled game, tend to retain their high level of performance in that endeavor, despite whatever declines they may experience in various mental abilities. They apparently compensate for those declines in some way that enables them to continue their expertise.

In the cases noted above, and in most other cases, compensation is likely to be in the way of the added knowledge gained with experience in their vocation or avocation. Thus the older expert has a broader knowledge base or background for aiding in the making of decisions (e.g., what response to give to your partner's opening bid for a hand of bridge). This kind of knowledge has been well documented for older chess players. Older master chess players have the ability to scan for several seconds a chess board containing as many as 25 pieces and then reproduce the pieces in their exact locations on the board. This is true, however, only when the pieces are arranged in accordance with standard and acceptable chess moves. Less experienced players lack the knowledge of chess plays that older masters have, and they are unable to match this remarkable memory feat. The older expert's knowledge of chess enables him or her to "chunk" the information on the board so that it circumvents the ordinary limits of short-term memory (see SHORT-TERM MEMORY).

Retaining expertise in later life is also possible in some occupations by the development of a special skill that compensates in some way for a decline in other skills that are essential for a high level of job performance. This kind of compensation may be seen for older skilled typists. Rapid movement of the fingers is essential for fast typing. Such movement does slow with normal aging, thus seemingly placing the older typists at a considerable disadvantage relative to younger expert typists. However, expert older typists have been found to type at a rate that is about the same as that of younger experts. The older typists have also been able to read several characters farther ahead in the text being typed than younger typists. This skill in reading farther ahead comes with experience and seemingly compensates for the overall slowing of the finger movements of the older expert typist.

One area of mental performances in which everyone should seemingly become an expert as a result of years of experience is memory. If true, one would expect to find few age-related declines in memory performances. For several components of memory this does seem to be the case. Semantic memory involving our general knowledge of information about our world, and our knowledge of words shows relatively little decline with normal aging (see LEXICON; SEMANTIC MEMORY). Our expertise in using this knowledge seems to ensure its automatic retrieval well into late adulthood. Prospective memory (remembering to perform some future planned action; see PROSPECTIVE MEMORY) also seems to be largely immune to negative effects caused by normal aging, as is short-term episodic memory. Age-related deficits in proficiency are most likely to occur for long-term (secondary) episodic memory, which expertise with experience fails to develop (see EPISODIC MEMORY). One reason for this failure is that much of our everyday memory takes place automatically and incidentally (e.g., memory for our own actions). Consequently, there is little opportunity for people to acquire with experience compensatory strategies that may offset age-related declines. With effortful forms of long-term memory, adults are frequently unaware of the kinds of strategies that could enhance their proficiencies, thus making it unlikely that we could develop compensatory strategies to offset age-related declines in proficiency. In fact, it is the purpose of memory training programs to make elderly adults aware of such strategies and to encourage them to use them (see MEMORY TRAINING).

Eyewitness Testimony

Witnessing a criminal commit a crime usually occurs under incidental memory conditions (i.e., there is no intent to memorize) and with little opportunity to study carefully the criminal's face. Nevertheless, eyewitnesses may later be asked to identify the suspected criminal in a police lineup. Accurate identification, of course, will aid the justice system in convicting the criminal. However, a false identification could lead to the prosecution of an innocent person. Psychologists have been very active in investigating the accuracy with which people make such identifications. Of particular interest is the age of the eyewitnesses. In the laboratory setting older people have been shown to be less accurate than younger people in their memory for faces (see FACE MEMORY). Especially disturbing is the high false alarm rate (i.e., falsely identifying a new face as one previously seen) of elderly participants. This is especially true when the faces seen are those of young adults. Criminals are more likely to be young adults than older adults. The likely problems of many older people as eyewitnesses are demonstrated further by having elderly participants observe a crime that is simulated in the laboratory. In such situations they are much less accurate than younger observers and have a much higher false identification rate. However, a researcher at Mississippi State University recently found that elderly adults are as accurate as younger adults in recalling details of a crime (i.e., the actions and objects involved in a crime) simulated on a videotape.

F

. . . .

Face Memory

"I remember your face, but not your name." Such a statement implies that memory for faces is quite good. But is it, regardless of age? Face memory is tested in the laboratory by presenting a series of pictures of faces (usually from a college yearbook) to participants and then testing their memory with a list consisting of a mixture of old faces (included in the prior series) and new faces (not included in the prior series). Research with this procedure has demonstrated that even young adults have far less than perfect memory for faces. It has also been demonstrated that elderly participants are much less accurate than younger participants in recognizing old faces as being truly old. This is true even when participants are required to study each face thoroughly and to make a decision about it (e.g., how friendly does it look?). Moreover, elderly participants misidentify new faces as being old (i.e., "false alarms") considerably more often than do younger participants. Face memory does seem to decline in proficiency from early to late adulthood. This decline has implications for a probable age difference in the accuracy of eyewitness testimony (see EYEWITNESS TESTIMONY).

Facial Appearance

We are all well aware of the changes that occur in our faces from early to late adulthood. One of the first changes is the presence of lines in the forehead that usually appear by age 30. Other lines then appear in the face between the ages of 30 and 50. Many of these lines are the result of years of squinting and frowning, and these lines may be largely prevented by wearing appropriate glasses and avoiding frowning as much as possible. After age 50 more pronounced changes in the face, such as wrinkles, usually begin to appear. In addition, water inside the facial skin decreases in amount, as does collagen, a fiber that gives the skin resilience. The facial skin tends to become stiffer, leading to more pronounced lines and, in some cases, to bags under the eyes and sagging skin on the cheeks. During late adulthood, cartilage accumulates in the nose, and it may increase both the width and length of the nose. The earlobes tend to become slightly fatter and longer, and the circumference of the head increases slightly.

The rate at which these changes in the skin occur is determined in part by heredity. Slower rates of change are also possible by avoiding ultraviolet rays as much as possible. Facial cosmetic surgery is available for prolonging a more youthful skin, and cosmetics for covering up what some elderly people feel are blemishes in their skin. Changes in the face are often more noticeable in older women than in older men. This is largely because the production of skin oil declines in women after menopause.

Most people after age 40 show some graying of the hair. Thinning of the hair also occurs, especially after age 65, as the rate of growth of hair decreases and the diameters of the strands of hair decrease in size. Although many aging men retain much of their hair, some have a hereditary form of baldness known as male pattern baldness in which the top of the head eventually becomes completely bald. A substantial percentage of elderly women also experience some degree of hair thinning to the point that they may wear a wig. Facial hair of men tends to be unaffected by aging, except for turning gray. Elderly men tend to experience growth of hair in the ears, nostrils, and eyebrows, whereas many elderly women experience excessive growth of hair over the lips and on the chin.

Falls

Although elderly people fall frequently, it is estimated that only 5% to 15% of their falls result in injuries that seriously restrict their mobility. Nevertheless, there is good reason to be concerned about falls during late adulthood. Nearly two-thirds of the more than 10,000 fatal accidents each year among elderly people result from falls, making falls the most common source of fatal injury among elderly people. Elderly women fall more often than elderly men, even though there is no apparent sex difference in balance. Most falls occur in the homes of elderly people. Especially disturbing is the fact that more than one-fourth of home-related falls could be prevented by redesigning or modifying elements of their homes. Modifications include securing throw rugs from slipping, adding grab bars to bathtubs and showers, and adding railings to stairs. Floors both in the home and in other places present a particular hazard. If a floor is not level, elderly people should start walking slowly to make certain their bodies are balanced. Any slick surface should be approached cautiously. Caution should also be exerted when moving in areas where there are animals or small children whose sudden movements may produce tripping. If furniture in a familiar room has been moved, elderly people should be informed of the changes before they enter the room.

Environmental factors are not solely responsible for the high incidence of falls experienced by elderly people. Physical impairments associated with aging also play a major role. Some of these impairments occur in the inner ear where the receptors involved in the maintenance of an upright posture and balance are located. Visual impairments, including diminished acuity, diminished depth perception, poorer dark adaptation, and greater susceptibility to glare, are frequent contributors to falls, as is the frail physical condition of people at a very advanced age and their declining ability to prevent swaying while standing (see POSTURE). There is also a relationship between walking gait and the likelihood of a fall. Elderly people with a history of falls, especially nursing home residents, tend to have decreased walking speed, shorter stride lengths, and greater variability of the length of successive steps relative to elderly people without a history of falls. The staffs of nursing homes should be aware of gait abnormalities among residents and be prepared to exert precautionary measures to prevent falls.

Health experts recommend a number of steps for elderly people to help them avoid falls. For example, elderly people are advised to avoid fast changes of direction while walking and to walk with their feet turned outward to provide greater stability. They should also avoid wearing running shoes while walking. While going up or down stairs, they should always move slowly, take one step at a time, and hold onto the handrail. Elderly people need to be especially attentive when moving in an unfamiliar outdoor area. A researcher at Pepperdine University has estimated that 60% of the falls experienced by elderly people result from inattention and engagement in hazardous activities.

Some fear of falling is probably desirable for elderly people as a means of alerting them to potentially hazardous conditions in their environments. More than 40% of the community-dwelling elderly adults surveyed by Yale researchers indicated some fear of falling. Nevertheless, most of those surveyed expressed a high level of confidence in their ability to perform everyday activities without falling. The participants with the most confidence were those with a high level of physical functioning. Fear of falling is likely to increase in intensity once a fall has actually been experienced. Not surprisingly, older adults who have chronic spells of dizziness are especially likely to fear falling. There is the danger that the fear of falling will become irrational and present its own disabling consequences. Intense and irrational fears are likely to restrict the physical activities of those who possess them. A decline in mobility is the likely result of diminished physical activity. Researchers at Yale University School of Medicine have discovered various procedures that reduce irrational fears of falling. Especially important are interventions designed to improve elderly adults' self-efficacy (confidence) in controlling their own activities. Family members and friends are also cautioned to avoid excessive remarks to competent elderly people that discourage their independence (e.g., "Don't do that—you might fall").

Not surprisingly, falls are not uncommon among elderly residents with dementia living in nursing homes. Researchers in The Netherlands analyzed the incidence of such falls during a 2-year period. The residents averaged about four falls per year, with the incidence being greatest shortly after admission to the home and after transfer to a different ward in the home. The incidence also varied with the severity of the dementia and the degree of physical impairment, and was as high for men as for women. Most falls were caused either by a disruption of equilibrium or by inadequate use of available facilities. Fortunately, most falls produced relatively minor injuries, although fractures were occasionally the result.

An important objective of aging research is to identify those older people who have a high risk of falling and possibly experiencing a serious injury. A promising start in meeting this objective was offered recently by Canadian researchers. They followed a number of elderly volunteers, all of whom had received a series of postural balance tests, during a 1-year period. "Fallers" were distinguished from "nonfallers" largely in the greater amplitude of their lateral sway. Once such high-risk individuals are identified, they could benefit from the kind of balance training program developed by researchers at the University of Oregon. The program stresses greater control of balance by means of improving the use of sensory information of importance in maintaining balance.

Fatigue and Mental Performance

It is popularly believed that elderly people are more susceptible to mental fatigue from performing demanding mental tasks than are younger people. There is evidence to indicate the validity of this belief, but only when the demanding task has been performed for some time. Both younger and older participants score lower on an intelligence test when that test has been preceded by a lengthy performance of another demanding task than they do when there has been no prior task, but the negative effect on intelligence test performance is much greater for the older participants. However, when the prior task is a relatively brief one, few negative effects have been found on a subsequent task for older participants. To safeguard against the negative effects of mental fatigue, older participants in laboratory research or older patients in a clinic usually receive frequent rest breaks while performing a demanding mental task or test.

Fluid Intake

One concern about the health of elderly adults is whether they have sufficient daily intake of fluids to maintain normal biological functioning. A recent study at Georgia State University suggests that they do. Several hundred adults ranging in age from 20 to 80 years recorded in a diary every food they ate and every fluid they drank each day for a week. The diary records indicated little difference between younger and older participants in the amount of fluids consumed daily, implying that normally aging adults do regulate their intake of fluids effectively. The records did indicate, however, some qualitative differences between younger and older adults. The older adults drank fewer alcoholic beverages than the younger adults but more coffee and/or tea. On the other hand, the younger adults drank more soda, both with and without sugar.

Food and Meal Services

It is estimated that millions of elderly Americans fail to eat enough to maintain their physical health. In an effort to solve this problem, the federal government passed the Older Americans Act of 1965. The act established two free food services for anyone age 60 or older, services that were eventually administered by community Area Agencies on Aging (see UNITED STATES ADMINISTRATION ON AGING). The first provided meals at senior centers to qualified individuals and their spouses once daily for 5 or 7 days a week. Donations are likely to be asked from those who can afford to give them. Around 2.5 million meals were served in 1993. The second service is Meals on Wheels. This service is for people who have a disability that keeps them homebound. More than 800,000 people received these meals in 1993.

Unfortunately, in recent years these two services have not been able to keep up with the needs of many elderly people. The problem is that the money allotted for them has remained fairly constant over the years while the number of elderly people needing them has increased greatly.

Elderly people may also benefit from food stamps issued by the Department of Agriculture and redeemed at grocery stores. Eligibility for food stamps, and the amount of stamps received, is determined by income level, assets, and family size. In addition, food and/or meals are offered to needy elderly people by many churches and civic organizations. Elderly people who need food or meal services and are not receiving them should contact local agencies on aging, senior centers, churches, and so on to find out what services are available in their communities.

Foot Problems

It is estimated that 75% of Americans have a foot problem some time during their lives. Elderly adults are major contributors to this alarming statistic, especially elderly women. A recent issue of *Perspectives in Health and Aging* (1993, volume 8, number 2), a publication of the American Association of Retired Persons, was devoted to foot problems and their prevention or treatment. Information in this entry is derived from that publication.

Changes occur in the feet of many people as they age normally. The feet may tend to spread, they may lose some of their cushioning, and they may become discolored. The skin and nails may also become dry and brittle. Other problems may occur. One is the presence of athlete's foot, which is caused by a fungus. To avoid this condition older adults should keep their feet dry and exposed frequently to the air. Corns and calluses are caused by pressure from bony areas of the feet that rub against shoes. Their prevention requires wearing properly fitting shoes. Removal of corns and calluses should be done by a podiatrist. Some bunions are inherited, but others are caused by wearing ill-fitting shoes. Shoes that are wide at the instep and big toe may reduce discomfort from less severe bunions, as may protective pads in the shoes. For more severe and painful bunions, surgery may be required. Hammertoe, a condition in which the second toe slants toward and under the big toe, may accompany a bunion. Hammertoe may cause a problem with balance and may therefore be a contributing factor to falls. Mild cases are treated by wearing the correct shoes and stockings, but more severe cases may require surgery. Calcium growths on the heels, known as heel spurs, may be prevented by avoiding prolonged standing and by wearing well-fitted supportive shoes. Calcium growths are treated by wearing shoes with heel pads and heel cups and sometimes by drugs. Ingrown toenails consist of corners of nails that pierce the skin. They are usually the result of improper nail trimming, but they may also be caused by an injury or a fungal infection. They may be avoided by always cutting the toenails straight across.

Unfortunately, foot problems may be aggravated in many elderly adults who use walking as their form of exercise. The difficulty lies in wearing improper walking shoes and socks. A podiatrist should be consulted before purchasing walking shoes. Among the things to look for are shoes with firm heel counters to cushion the impact while walking and soles that provide a high degree of shock absorption. Equally important is the wearing of the right socks. Podiatrists often recommend wearing two pairs of socks during strenuous walking. The thin inner pair should be made of silk or wool to prevent blisters and the thicker outer pair should be made of a blend of acrylic fiber and either cotton or wool.

Forgetting

"Mommy, my forgettery is better than my memory." The little girl in the comic strip who said this was displaying a wisdom well beyond her years. She reminded us that the imperfections of memory are present at all ages, and that many of these imperfections result from forgetting information that had once been acquired. Forgetting, like memory per se, is a fact of life, and especially for episodic memory. Information in short-term memory is forgotten in a matter of seconds if it is not continuously rehearsed (see SHORT-TERM MEMORY). However, the rate of short-term forgetting appears to be no greater for older adults than for younger adults. But what about long-term episodic memory? Much of the information that has entered the long-term memory stores does seem to be forgotten. However, an important distinction must be made between the unavailability of that information and the inaccessibility of that information. Unavailability means that the once-stored information has been "lost" and is no longer available for retrieval. Inaccessibility means that at least some of the information is still present in the store, but it cannot be retrieved at a given moment. Consider a particular foreign language word that you learned in high school but you cannot recall. For example, you may be trying to recall the Spanish word for "dog," and you cannot remember it. However, on seeing it, you may immediately recognize its meaning. This surely indicates that you have not fully forgotten the word. Moreover, even if you do not recognize the word, you may still have some memory of it. This is likely to be demonstrated if you took a refresher course in Spanish. The Spanish words you seem to have forgotten are likely to be learned faster than they were learned originally. This is called a savings in learning, and it clearly demonstrates that some memory remains even though it cannot be consciously recollected (see IMPLICIT MEMORY). Most people have difficulty recalling the content of a college course after only a year has passed. However, they are likely to discover that they learn the same material much more quickly if they repeat the course. This again is a savings that indicates more memory persists than is within our conscious recollection.

We usually view forgetting in terms of our conscious recollection of information. If information can be neither recalled nor recognized, it is likely to be considered forgotten. Forgetting usually follows a normal progression, with most of it occurring shortly after information is acquired, with further forgetting occurring at a slower rate until it levels off at some residue of retained information. This is the case, for example, with the foreign language words you may have acquired in a high school language course. Most of the forgetting takes place within the first year after the course (see VERY LONG-TERM MEMORY). Why does such forgetting occur? The most important reason is the interference from other somewhat similar material acquired both before the language course and after the language course. Consider your memory of the names of television programs from 10 years ago. You probably do not recall many of their names, and you probably would not recognize many more as well. In this case, interference comes from both the names of programs you viewed more than 10 years ago and the names of programs viewed during the intervening 10 years. The interference from prior information is called proactive interference, and interference from later information is called retroactive interference. The product of the two sources of interference is the loss from the long-term store of some information and the inaccessibility of the remaining forgotten information.

Forgetting is studied in laboratory situations by having participants learn successive lists of paired words (paired-associate learning; see VERBAL LEARNING). Retention may then be determined for either the first list or the second list. The forgetting that occurs for the first list is largely the consequence of the interference produced by the second list. That is, it is the product of retroactive interference. The forgetting that occurs for the second list is the consequence of the interference

produced by the first list. That is, it is the product of proactive interference. As with real-life information, forgetting is rapid after acquisition. In this situation most of it occurs within a day after learning the
lists and then slows until a residue of still-remembered information remains. Of great importance is the general finding that the rate of forgetting is no faster for elderly participants than it is for younger
participants, provided the material has been mastered equally at each
age level. The implication is that new episodic information that has
been well registered in the long-term store should not be forgotten,
on the average, at any substantially greater rate by older adults than by
younger adults. This equality in forgetting rates is somewhat surprising in that elderly adults were once believed to be more susceptible to
the effects of interference than younger adults (see TRANSFER OF
LEARNING/TRAINING).

Form Perception

When you look at a tree, you recognize it as a tree. Similarly, a dog
is recognized as a dog, an automobile as an automobile, and so on.
These are familiar examples of form perception. We are able to "make
sense" of the "raw" visual information registered by our eyes, and perceive the forms initiating that information meaningfully. That is, we
are able to name those forms. Our visual system, including the visual
areas of the brain, automatically extracts features of the object in
question and matches that information with information stored permanently in memory. Thus the features of an automobile include
four wheels and mechanical power. When a form has features matching these and the other features we know that characterize an automobile, that form is recognized and identified as an automobile.
Extracting features and matching them with what is stored in memory is known to psychologists as pattern recognition. Consider the
form **A** that you immediately identify as the uppercase form of the
first letter of the English alphabet. The form has two distinctive features, converging slanting lines and an intersecting horizontal line.
Stored in your memory is information acquired during childhood
that these features identify the letter **A.** Whenever a new pattern is encountered that matches these features, pattern recognition occurs
rapidly and effortlessly. Even with some distortion of the features, as
in the form or pattern Pesa, there is enough commonality with the basic features to identify the novel form as an **A.**

Are elderly adults less accurate in form perception (or pattern
recognition) than young adults? Under normal circumstances, the

answer is only slightly, if at all. When young adults and older adults are compared in the accuracy of naming pictures of objects, the age differences in average accuracy is small. Normally aging older adults, like young adults, rarely make misidentifications. However, when the circumstances make pattern recognition more difficult, there is a more moderate age difference. This may be seen when segments of the pictures are deleted. In a study by researchers at the University of Missouri, young and elderly participants viewed drawings of such forms as a violin and a rabbit in which 90% of each form had been randomly deleted by means of a computer. The young participants were able to identify, on the average, about 85% of the pictures, and the elderly participants identified about 75%.

Although the effects of aging on the accuracy of form perception are modest, the effects of aging on the speed of pattern recognition are much greater (in agreement with the "slowing down" principle; see SLOWING DOWN PRINCIPLE). The age difference is demonstrated in the laboratory with simple materials in which participants receive pairs of letters and they decide whether they have the same name. Examples of such pairs are **A a, B B, H K,** and **T b.** Note that for the first two pairs the answer is yes. However, the answer will be given more quickly regardless of age for the second pair than for the first pair. This is because the letters in the second pair have completely overlapping features—and they must therefore have the same name. This is not true for the first pair where there is no overlap of features. Therefore pattern recognition takes somewhat longer while memory is searched to discover that **A** and **a** do indeed have the same name. Elderly adults are slower than young adults for both **A a** and **B B** type comparisons, but the magnitude of the age difference is greater for the **A a** type. These are simple materials of little relevance to everyday form perception. However, they do suggest that elderly adults will, on the average, be slower in identifying many forms in the everyday world. For example, is the object in the road ahead of the driver simply debris or an animal? The slower recognition by the older driver than by the younger driver could result in very different actions taken by the drivers (e.g., swerving the car or not swerving it).

Foster Grandparent Program

The Foster Grandparent Program in the United States is one of several programs established by the Domestic Service Act of 1973. The objective of this program is to encourage the participation of elderly people in activities that should improve the quality of their lives and enhance their mental health, as well as the lives of the recipients of these activities. Elderly participants are paid a small compensation for working with children in various settings, such as schools and homes for children with mental disabilities. Not only are the foster grandparents likely to benefit from their relationships with the children, but the children also are expected to receive affection that may otherwise be missing in their lives.

By the early 1980s more than 18,000 foster grandparents were employed in this program. Their average age was 69 years, and more than half were widowed. Among the reasons cited for joining the program were to make better use of their time, to help children, and to earn some badly needed money.

Frequency-of-Occurrence Memory

How many times in the past week did you see an advertisement on television for Budweiser beer? Which advertisement did you see more often in the past week, one for Budweiser beer or one for McDonald's? You are likely to be reasonably accurate in your answers to these questions (assuming you pay attention to television commercials). This is true even though you had no idea your memory for the frequency-of-occurrence of these events would be tested and you therefore acquired the frequency information without intending to do so. That is, the frequency information was acquired incidentally and without your effort to rehearse the events in question. Some memory theorists believe that the frequencies with which events occur are registered automatically in memory in the sense that they do not require the intent to register that information. Presumably, we have been programmed genetically to record frequency-of-occurrence information for the events that occur in our everyday lives. If true, then we would expect frequency-of-occurrence memory to be as proficient for normally aging elderly adults as for young adults.

To investigate these characteristics of frequency-of-occurrence memory, researchers use a laboratory task in which events occur different numbers of times. Participants are then asked to give judgments about those frequencies. The events usually are familiar words that appear in a lengthy series. Some of the words appear only once, some two times (widely separated appearances), some three times, and so on. At the end of the series participants may be asked questions such as "How many times did the word *apple* appear in the series?" Alternatively, they may be asked "Which word appeared more often, *apple* or *pencil*?" Answers to questions of these kinds are usually rather accurate. Moreover, accuracy is usually as high when the participants do not know in advance that their memory will be tested (incidental memory) as when they do know in advance exactly what kind of memory will be tested (intentional memory). This is true regardless of the age of the participants. Most important, older participants are nearly as accurate as younger participants. The magnitude of an age decline in frequency-of-occurrence memory proficiency does seem to be much less than the magnitude of the decline found in many other forms of memory (e.g., spatial memory and temporal memory). For whatever reasons, frequency-of-occurrence memory seems to be largely immune to any pronounced declines in proficiency with normal aging.

Friendships

There are two kinds of friendships: interest-related and deep. An interest-related friendship is one brought about by similar interests of the friends, such as a common hobby or playing bridge together. A deep friendship is one involving a more intimate relationship that goes beyond shared interests. There is a bond of closeness between the friends. The number of friendships, particularly interest-related ones, is likely to decline in late adulthood because of deaths, health problems, and other factors that constrain the opportunity for interactions with friends. There may be another important reason. Some gerontologists believe that many elderly people restrict their social interactions to long-time friends and avoid making new friends to conserve their physical energy and to minimize negative emotional states that might arise from social interactions with other than old and familiar friends. There is evidence to indicate that new friendships are relatively infrequent for elderly people, especially those in their 80s and older. The number of friends does decrease for those in this age range, relative to those in the 60- to 80-year age range. However, the number of close relationships for the very old remains about the same as for the younger old. Thus the proportion of close, deep attachments increases during very late adulthood.

In general, older people appear to find greater satisfaction in their relationships with friends than with family members. The apparent reason is the greater sharing of leisure activities with friends than with family members. However, there are important sex differences in the friendships of older people. Older women, in general, have more friends than older men, and they are likely to place greater value on their friendships than do older men. Older women also seem to have a greater sharing of their activities and a greater emotional involvement with their friends than do older men. For older married couples, the wife is likely to have a friend as her closest confidant, whereas the husband's closest confident is likely to be his wife.

A theory widely applied to friendships is called equity theory. According to this theory, the satisfaction gained from a friendship depends on the mutual benefit gained from a friendship. This theory has received considerable support when applied to the friendships of younger adults. However, it has received less support when applied to the friendships of older adults. A recent survey of older adults in Colorado suggests that for older adults the perception of equity or fairness in a relationship is relatively unimportant when applied to their best friends. However, perceived equity does seem to be an important factor in determining the degree of satisfaction from relationships from other "non-best" friends.

Functional Age

"I may be 70 years old, but I have the handgrip strength of a man 40 years old."

If this statement is true, then the man making the statement has a physical *functional age* that is many years younger than his chronological age, at least for the specific physical function of hand strength. If someone's level of functioning corresponds to the level of functioning of an average 40-year-old, then the person's functional age is 40 years. This would be the case whether the person is actually 30, 50, or 70 years old. Of course, that same person's functional age is likely to be different for other physical skills and functions, and may even be greater than 70 for some. For example, his lung capacity may correspond to that of the average 75-year-old man. In fact, for any given individual, there may be considerable variability in his or her various functional ages. It is this variability that makes physical functional age difficult to serve as an effective replacement for chronological age in defining the onset of old age (see OLD [DEFINING LATE ADULTHOOD]). The concept of functional age may also be applied to mental skills and abilities. Thus a 70-year-old person who has the memory proficiency of the average 40-year-old person would have a functional age of 40 in regard to memory. However, that same individual is likely to have different functional ages for other mental skills and abilities, thus making functional age on any one ability an unlikely replacement for chronological age in defining late adulthood.

There is the argument expressed by various occupational groups (e.g., airline pilots, physicians, professors) that it is functional age on job-related skills that should determine retirement and not some arbitrary fixed chronological age. Airline pilots are presently required to retire as pilots when they reach age 60. This practice seemingly conflicts with evidence indicating that the incidence of flying accidents for pilots of private airplanes is actually lower for pilots in their 60s and 70s than it is for younger pilots. Older pilots may continue to work as flight engineers. Some hospitals require physicians to retire at age 70, and professors are usually forced to retire at age 70. Pilots who are chronologically older than 60 have long argued that functionally (in terms of the skills needed to fly a large airplane) they may be much younger, and that it is their functional age and not their chronological age that should determine retirement. A similar argument has been made by many physicians, resulting in various legal cases, and most recently by a referee of the National Football League who was given duties off the field because of his age. Surely, many college professors at age 70 have a functional age for professorial skills that is well below their chronological age. Unfortunately, the difficulties in reliably and thoroughly determining functional age for any given occupation have made its substitution for chronological age in determining retirement age unacceptable. This is likely to change in the future, however, as better understanding of aging abilities and their measurements are accomplished.

G

. . . .

Gender and Sex Differences in Aging

The terms *gender* and *sex* are often confused in the everyday world. A good example is in the current issue of *gender equity* in college sports. What is really meant is *sex equity* in the form of equal funding and support for women's and men's sports. Gender actually refers to what are commonly considered to be traditional masculine and feminine characteristics and behaviors. For years, men played the role of family providers, and women played the role of child caregiver. Men were also expected to be more assertive and aggressive than women, and women were expected to be more tender and sensitive than men. Thus assertiveness and tenderness are masculine and feminine characteristics, respectively. However, there have also been gender reversals at all ages. Many men possess feminine characteristics (e.g., tenderness), and many women possess masculine characteristics (e.g., assertiveness).

One of gerontology's most interesting debates in recent years has been whether men and women become increasingly alike in their balance of masculine and feminine characteristics as they age. Do elderly men become more sensitive than they were earlier in life and elderly women more assertive? If so, they have become androgynous persons who are no longer bound to rigid gender characteristics and rigid sex-roles. There is evidence indicating that androgyny is more characteristic of elderly men than it is of elderly women (see ANDROGYNY). The trend toward androgyny is likely to increase for future generations as sex-role stereotypes become increasingly relaxed with changes in our society, and it is likely to be found in many men and women long before they reach late adulthood.

Sex differences refer to differences between men and women in physical and mental abilities and in behaviors. An obvious sex difference is in longevity, with women generally living some years longer than men (see LIFE EXPECTANCY). There are other obvious biological differences between men and women as well (e.g., in strength). There are also others that are not as obvious (e.g., in urinary incontinence; see URINARY INCONTINENCE). Declines in sensory functioning with normal aging are fairly comparable for men and women. Hearing does show a moderate sex difference. Declines in hearing proficiency with aging are greater for women than for men with low-pitched sounds, and the reverse is true for higher-pitched sounds. Elderly men and women perform at comparable levels on intelligence tests and on most tests of specific mental abilities. However, there are a few exceptions. Early in adulthood women score higher than men on tests of verbal ability, and men score higher than women on tests of spatial ability. These sex differences persist moderately through late adulthood. With one exception, memory functioning appears to be comparable for elderly men and women. The possible exception is for very long-term, or remote, memory. There is tentative evidence to suggest that elderly men may be slightly more proficient than elderly women in remembering long-past events (see VERY LONG-TERM MEMORY).

There are a number of behavioral differences between elderly men and elderly women. For example, elderly men are more likely to remarry than are elderly women. A number of these behavioral differences, along with other physical differences between elderly men and women, may be found in other entries in this book.

Generativity

Generativity is a term introduced to psychology some years ago by Dr. Erik Erikson. It refers to a person's concern about the next generation and how to help guide members of that generation through teaching, leadership, and example. Dr. Erikson assumed that generativity peaked in middle age and then declined. Researchers at Northwestern University recently challenged the suspected decline in late adulthood. They measured generativity for adults of various ages by means of a number of psychological tests (e.g., writing sentences describing personal goals). Contrary to Dr. Erikson's assumption, they found generativity to be as high in their older participants as in their middle-aged participants—and higher for both groups than for young adult participants. They also found generativity to be related positively to life satisfaction for the older participants; that is, generativity was highest for those elderly adults who were most satisfied with their current lives.

Other researchers have discovered some interesting differences between women in their 40s who are either high or low in generativity. For example, women who are high in generativity tend to have greater concern for their children's health status and to be more active politically than women low in generativity.

Geriatrics

Geriatrics is that branch of medicine concerned with the investigation of the medical problems encountered in late adulthood and with the application of knowledge about the biological and behavioral aspects of aging to the diagnosis and treatment of those problems.

Gerontological Society of America

The Gerontological Society of America (GSA) was established in 1945. From its inception, it has been the most prominent and largest organization of gerontologists, both researchers and practitioners, in the United States. Its objectives are to promote research on aging and to promote the exchange of knowledge about aging between researchers in gerontology and practitioners in various areas of gerontology. The GSA has its headquarters in Washington, D.C. Its membership (more than 6,000) represents four different areas of study; Biological Sciences; Clinical Medicine; Behavioral and Social Sciences; and Social Research, Planning, and Practice. An annual meeting is held in November with more than 1,000 presentations given across the various disciplines of gerontology. In addition, the GSA publishes two major journals in gerontology. The *Journal of Gerontology* is published bimonthly and contains basic research articles in the areas of biological sciences, medical sciences, psychological sciences, and social sciences. The *Gerontologist* is also published bimonthly; it contains largely applied research articles (e.g., research on caregivers, respite programs). The GSA has been influential in developing educational curricula in gerontology, in identifying training needs in gerontology, in advising various congressional committees, and in other important services related to the needs of the older population. It also offers annually several postdoctoral fellowships for training in various areas of gerontology. GSA's address is 1275 K Street, N.W., Washington, DC 20005-4006 (telephone, 202-842-1275).

Gerontology

Gerontology is a broad field of study concerned with every aspect of functioning in late adulthood. Thus gerontology is concerned with the many facets of aging, but especially the biological, psychological, and sociological. Research in biological gerontology is directed at the discovery of the biological mechanisms responsible for aging and at the determination of the nature of age-related changes in various biological/physiological functions. Research in psychological aging is directed at the study of what happens to various psychological processes and functions (e.g., sensory, attentional, memory) with aging and the determination of the reasons for those changes. One of the main areas of research in social gerontology deals with the demographic characteristics of elderly people. Other major areas are concerned with the family life of older people and the services available for older people.

Goals

Do you make New Year's resolutions? If so, you are setting goals or objectives you want to accomplish during the new year. Goals, of course, are not limited to such resolutions (which usually are minor ones that are soon abandoned anyway). Life goals are those that give direction to our activities and our commitments. Succeeding at one's profession or job is a common goal for younger adults, as is raising their children to a happy and healthy adulthood. But what about older people? Do they continue to set goals for themselves? If so, what kinds of goals do they have? Most important, do their goals affect their happiness and their adjustment to the demands of daily living?

Researchers at New York University have conducted studies that provide at least partial answers to these questions. They classified goals into such categories as "active improvement of one's life" (e.g., doing creative volunteer work), "maintenance of one's social values and relationships" (e.g., maintaining old friendships), "feeling safe and secure" (e.g., living in a safe neighborhood), "having an energetic life-style" (e.g., being able to do your own errands), and "disengagement" (e.g., having fewer family obligations). Not surprisingly, they found that older people vary greatly in their goals. However, they also found that certain characteristics and living conditions of elderly people are related to their goals. For example, they found that being widowed is characterized by having safety and security as a goal. They also found that retirees increasingly have the goal of an energetic life-style as the duration of their retirement increases and that healthy elderly people are more likely than less healthy ones to have an energetic life-style as a goal. Moreover, they found that satisfaction with one's present life is greater for those older people who have maintenance of social values and relationships or an energetic life-style as goals than for those elderly people who have disengagement as a goal.

Grandparenting

About three-fourths of the elderly people in the United States are grandparents. As you might expect, they show differences in their styles of interacting with their grandchildren. Twenty-five years ago, researchers at the University of Chicago identified five basic styles of grandparenting. The first is a formal style in which there is a sharp division between grandparent and grandchild. That is, the grandparent stays largely in the background with an occasional offering of a gift. The second is a fun-seeker style that is characterized by a leisurely, informal orientation, and mutual pleasure experienced by both participants in their interactions. The third is a surrogate parent style in which the grandparent substitutes for the child's parents. Not surprisingly, few grandparents select this style voluntarily. The fourth style is one in which the grandparent serves as a reservoir of family wisdom and perhaps authority. The remaining style is that of a distant figure in which the grandparent emerges from the shadows briefly at birthdays and holidays. A grandparenting style, however, may not be a fixture. A grandparent may exhibit one style with one grandchild and a different style with another grandchild. Alternatively, a grandparent may exhibit the same style to all grandchildren at one age, but may change the style as the grandparent (and the grandchildren) grow older.

Other researchers have identified the meanings found by grandparents in their roles as grandparents. For example, some perceive themselves as gaining immortality through the perpetuation of their bloodline, whereas others perceive themselves as treasured and respected elders. Typically, the role of a grandmother is broader and more intimate than that of a grandfather. In general, grandparenting is not very important in determining the degree of life satisfaction experienced by older adults. That is, life satisfaction is fairly independent of the frequency of encounters with grandchildren. However, there does seem to be a moderate tendency for grandmothers to derive more satisfaction from grandparenting than do grandfathers. Moreover, the degree of satisfaction expressed by grandmothers appears to be related positively to their responsibilities for caring and helping their grandchildren.

In general, younger grandparents have been found to feel greater responsibility for offering child-rearing advice to their children than older grandparents, regardless of the number or ages of the grand-children. Mothers, in general, have been found to take seriously the advice of grandmothers in regard to the nature of the punishments and rewards their children should receive.

There is a tendency for the contacts between grandmothers and their grandchildren to increase after the divorce of the children's parents. The frequency of the grandparents' participation in the children's recreational activities and the frequency of babysitting are also likely to increase after a divorce of the grandchildren's parents. Unfortunately, less is known about grandfathers and their grandparenting activities after the divorce of their children.

Which of a child's four grandparents is most important in that child's life? That question was asked of a number of children by researchers at Adelphi University. Maternal grandmothers were selected more than twice as often as the other three grandparents. Maternal grandmothers seem to be more involved in their grandchildren's lives than the other grandparents, probably because mothers of children visit with their own mothers more often than they do with other grandparents.

More than half a million grandparents are raising their grandchildren in a parentless home. Such caregiving is likely to place a considerable financial burden on grandparents. Their median annual income is about $18,000, which is half that of a traditional parental family. More than 90% of single grandparents who are their grandchildren's sole caregivers are women.

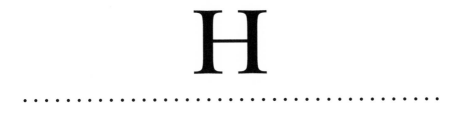

H

Health Care Costs

Health care costs for Americans have been increasing annually over the years. Statistics provided by the Health Care Financing Administration indicate that the cost increased from $250 billion in 1980 to nearly $670 billion in 1990. The costs are projected to exceed $1.5 trillion in the year 2000. A major portion of these costs is paid by Medicare. In 1990, Medicare reimbursement totaled $136 billion, and it is estimated that it will exceed $300 billion in 2000. Another large share is paid by Medicaid. In 1990, Medicaid costs exceeded $75 billion, and such costs are expected to total more than $240 billion in the year 2000.

Some reduction of these costs is offered by the increasing number of high-technology services that are available for home use. They include renal dialysis and cardiac telemetry. Dr. Leonard W. Kaye of Bryn Mawr College has prepared a consumer guidebook for those seeking such services. It includes information about the kinds of services available and how to access them.

Health Programs

Health programs are designed to provide information or experiences intended to improve the health of the participants. Such programs may include instruction and training on weight control, smoking cessation, and exercise. Older people have greater health risks than younger people, and they are therefore a group most likely to benefit from participation in health programs. Nevertheless, the percentage of elderly people who do participate is small (those who participate are more likely to be women than men). This is apparent from a study of a large sample of older people in western Washington. A number of elderly people received mailings of descriptive material for a health promotion program in which they would be visited by a nurse educator in their homes who would discuss health risks with them. In addition, they would then have the opportunity to participate in other programs, such as having a pharmacist review their medications. Only 29% of the elderly people contacted consented to be participants. Those who consented were found to be more educated, to have a higher income, and to be more involved in community organizations than those who did not give their consent. Other researchers have discovered that there are effective strategies that may increase the number of elderly participants in health programs, such as selecting program recruiters who have characteristics resembling those of the elderly adults to be recruited and good publicity of the support of the program by influential community members.

Health Status and Mental Performance
See also CARDIOVASCULAR DISEASE AND MENTAL PERFORMANCE

National statistics reveal that the health status of our elderly population is poorer than it is for younger people. A report issued in 1983 by the U.S. Special Committee on Aging indicated that about 16% of people between the ages of 65 and 74 and 20% of people age 75 or older were hospitalized during the prior year. In contrast, only 11% of people 45 to 54 years of age had been hospitalized. People 75 years or older averaged 18 days of bed disability in the previous year compared with the 8.5 day average of people in the 45- to 54-year age range. Despite these statistics of poor health in many older people, the same report indicated that about 70% of people age 65 or older described their health as being excellent or good, relative to others their own age. This percentage does not differ from the 75% of people in the 55- to 64-year age range who reported their health to be excellent or good, or from the 82% of people in the 45- to 54-year age range. Self-ratings of health are fairly valid measures of older adults' true health status. For example, mortality rates during a 3-year period have been found to be much higher for elderly adults with low self-ratings (implying poor health) than for older adults with high self-ratings (implying good health). This is true even for those elderly people with low ratings who appear to others to be healthy.

Nevertheless, a sizable percentage of people age 65 or older do perceive their health to be less than good. In most laboratory studies of normal aging and mental performances, these individuals are eliminated from participation. A standard procedure is to have potential participants rate their health status on a 5-point scale, with 1 being excellent and 2 being good. Only those participants who assign self-ratings of 1 or 2 are likely to have their scores included in age comparisons. Investigators are typically interested in how normal aging affects mental performances and not on how these effects may be complicated by disease and poor health. What happens when health status is an uncontrolled study factor? Researchers at the University of Missouri–Columbia found that it had little effect on the relationship between age and performance on a variety of learning, memory, and reasoning tasks. That is, the strong relationship between age and performance scores was about the same regardless of whether participants with low self-reported health were excluded. Conversely, researchers at both the University of Michigan and the University of Victoria found that the relationship between age and scores on tests of fluid intelligence (see INTELLIGENCE) was much less pronounced when participants who reported their health to be less than good were excluded from their analyses. The standard practice in research on the relationship between age and mental performance should be to continue to exclude participants who rate their health as poor. Of course, there is the important area of research in which the health or disease status of older people serves as the focus; that is, the interest is in how elderly people in poor health compare in their mental performances with elderly people in good health (see CARDIOVASCULAR DISEASE AND MENTAL PERFORMANCE). Except for cardiovascular disease, there is reason to believe that health status relates only moderately to performances on most mental tasks and tests.

One may question how well elderly people actually know their own health status. That is, how reliable are self-ratings of health as an indicator of true health? There is evidence to indicate that self-ratings actually relate more closely to performance on some mental tasks than do assessments of health made by physicians.

Hearing

Presbycusis is the diminished ability to hear sounds of high pitches, particularly those of 3,000 Hertz (i.e., 3,000 cycles per second of the sound waves) and higher. It is one of the most common consequences of aging. Nearly all individuals age 65 and older are affected to some degree of presbycusis. It is estimated that nearly 30% of these individuals have noticeable impairment and more than 10% have severe cases. Diminished hearing of high-frequency sounds begins for people in their 30s. By the 50s the hearing loss is already moderate, and it increases greatly during the remaining decades of life. On the other hand, the loss of hearing ability with normal aging is much less severe for sounds of lower pitch, especially those of 1,000 Hertz and lower.

There are sex differences in the rate of loss of hearing ability with aging for higher-pitched sounds. In general, the hearing loss for women is greater than that for men for sounds of 1,000 Hertz and lower, but it is somewhat greater for men for frequencies of 2,000 Hertz and above. The sex difference is probably related to differences in exposure to environmental noise rather than to sex differences in the biological components of hearing. Prolonged exposure to noise causes damage to the hair cells in the inner ear that respond to sound waves.

The importance of environmental noise in producing hearing loss is apparent from comparisons between Americans and people from other cultures who live in isolated areas that are relatively free of intense environmental noises. For example, the hearing loss for Sudanese men in their 70s has been found to be half that of American men in their 70s. Given the loud music preferred by many young people, the threat of even greater hearing loss for future generations of older people is a definite possibility.

Hearing acuity for a particular sound frequency is measured by determining an individual's absolute threshold for a pure tone at that frequency. To determine the threshold at 3,000 Hertz, the subject would receive tones of that frequency at varying levels of loudness, beginning at a very low intensity (in decibels). The intensity is increased until the level of intensity at which the subject hears the tone half of the time it is presented. The decibels at that level define the absolute threshold. For people in their 70s, the threshold value at 3,000 Hertz averages about 30 decibels greater than that of people in their 20s.

Impairment in the ability to discriminate between sounds of different pitches also accompanies normal aging. For example, can you detect the difference in pitch between tones of 3,000 Hertz and 3,330 Hertz? Between 2,000 Hertz and 2,010 Hertz? Although there are major losses with aging in the ability to discriminate between pitches, the losses are slight for tones less than 1,000 Hertz. They become much greater for higher pitches, and they are especially large for sound frequencies of 3,000 Hertz and higher. To determine pitch discrimination ability at any given sound frequency, the difference threshold is measured. If that frequency is 3,000 Hertz, a number of trials is given in which the 3,000 Hertz tone is sounded first (at about 40 decibels) and is followed by a second tone. The frequency of the second tone is gradually increased until you are able to detect the difference in pitch from the first tone half of the time. The difference in the frequencies at that point defines the difference threshold. For people in their 20s, the average difference threshold for tones in the 3,000 Hertz range is about 15 Hertz. It increases in magnitude with aging;

for people in their 60s and 70s, the difference threshold averages about 40 and 70 Hertz, respectively. Older people are obviously less sensitive to variation in pitch than are young adults.

Hearing impairment in late adulthood has obvious adverse effects on everyday living. Speech perception is affected to some degree by both declining acuity in hearing sounds and declining ability to discriminate among pitches (see SPEECH PERCEPTION). Older people are also likely to have diminished quality of the music they hear. There is also a more subtle effect of hearing impairment. Researchers have discovered that scores earned by elderly people on an intelligence test are related to some degree to the extent of their hearing impairment (see INTELLIGENCE).

Elderly people should be aware that hearing impairment may be caused by factors other than environmental noise. Ototoxic drugs (damaging to hearing receptors) may produce impairment, or they may worsen an already existing impairment. Included among these drugs are certain diuretics (furosemide and ethacrynic acid), certain antibiotics (especially streptomycin), and cisplatin (a drug used in some forms of chemotherapy). In addition, tinnitus (see TINNITUS) may be caused by high doses of aspirin. Elderly people should realize that some hearing impairments may be treatable. This is the case when the impairment is caused by excessive wax in the ear canal or by some forms of infection. Older people should be encouraged to have regular hearing tests to determine the probable cause of any new impairment.

Heat Stroke

Older adults are at a much greater risk of illness or death from heat stroke during periods of high temperatures and high humidity than are younger adults. The risk is especially high for elderly adults with respiratory or heart conditions. Symptoms of heat stroke include leg cramps, headache, nausea, and exhaustion. One reason for the greater risk is that older people perspire less than younger adults, and perspiring is a primary way for the body to cool itself. A second reason is that older adults are more likely than younger adults to be taking medications that increase the risk of heat stroke. These medications include many cold medicines, antihistamines, diuretics such as furosemide, and antidepressants.

Elderly people should avoid being outdoors during periods of extreme heat, and they should stay in air-conditioned quarters as much as possible. They should also drink plenty of cool water and splash their skin often with cool water. Unfortunately, many older adults cannot afford air conditioning in their homes. Those who do not have air conditioning should contact their local health authorities and social agencies to request help either in obtaining air conditioners or for finding temporary air-conditioned quarters. They should also contact their utility companies for budget billing.

Hiding Your Age

"You certainly don't look your age. You look great!" Many older adults would be greatly pleased to hear these words—they would be happy not to look their age. In fact, some try to look younger than they are by hiding as many signs of aging as possible. For example, they may hide the graying of their hair by dyeing it. Women are judged more often on their appearance than are men. Not surprisingly, looking old may be considered more unattractive for elderly women than for elderly men. Consequently, more older women than older men may be expected to hide their signs of aging. Evidence provided by researchers at the University of New Mexico provides strong support for this expectation. They surveyed a number of people older than 50 years of age. Only 6% of the men reported coloring their hair in contrast to 34% of the women. Similarly, only 1% of the men reported using wrinkle creams in contrast to 24% of the women.

Home Maintenance

There are about 14 million homeowners who are age 65 and older. Several surveys have shown a relationship between age and the maintenance activity of homeowners. That is, the amount of money spent annually on the upkeep of a home is less for homeowners age 65 and older than it is for younger homeowners, and the amount spent decreases progressively, on the average, with increasing age beyond age 65. For example, this is apparent in a survey of homeowners in the Houston area. The average amount spent annually for home maintenance was about $466 for homeowners younger than age 60 and only about $145 for homeowners age 75 and older. Moreover, the percentage of homeowners age 75 and older who engaged in home upkeep was about 63%, compared with the 80% of homeowners younger than age 60. The results from this survey also indicate that the major reason for this age difference is the decline in income during late adulthood. Other factors, such as the health status of the homeowner, were found to have little effect on home maintenance.

However, it was also found that elderly homeowners were just as likely as younger homeowners to maintain essential properties of their homes (e.g., roof repairs). The age difference is attributable largely to the fact that elderly homeowners spend less money than younger homeowners on what may be considered cosmetic home maintenance (e.g., painting).

Homosexuality

It is believed that the proportion of older people who are homosexual differs little from the proportion of younger people. This means that there are about 3 million elderly homosexual men and women in the United States. A myth of aging is that elderly homosexual men and women are, on the average, more lonely and more despaired than elderly heterosexual men and women. This may have been true before the onset of the gay rights movement in 1969, but it seems unlikely today. Surveys during the past 10 years have indicated that gay older men show diverse life-styles and considerable well-being. The majority do not appear to be depressed, lonely, or sexually frustrated. Many of those interviewed revealed that they are still sexually active and that their sexual relationships are very satisfactory. Virtually all of the elderly gay men interviewed indicated that they preferred their sexual contacts to be men of similar ages rather than young men. Similar surveys of older lesbians reveal that, on the average, they are comfortable with their sexual preference and that they appear to be in excellent mental health. There is some indication that lesbians may discontinue their sexual activities at an earlier age than do gay men.

It has been argued by some gerontologists that homosexuality may actually be adaptive to the usual stresses of aging caused by society's frequent devaluation of its elderly population. A homosexual preference may help the individual to become more independent early in life and to avoid being entrapped in traditional sex roles. Homosexual individuals have become familiar with the stigmatization often associated with homosexuality, and may therefore be more adaptable than heterosexual elderly people to the stigma associated with aging. However, the little evidence available fails to lend much support to this belief. A study conducted in the mid-1980s revealed that more than 80% of the older lesbians interviewed felt positively about their sexual preference, but only about 50% felt positively about aging.

A problem facing homosexual older people is the fact that senior centers, retirement communities, and nursing homes are all traditionally heterosexually oriented. Homosexual participants and residents are therefore likely to feel constrained and isolated in these facilities. Of interest are the results of a survey of older lesbians in which only 5% of those interviewed said they attended a senior center, and most of them indicated a strong preference for lesbian or gay/lesbian facilities and services. This problem is likely to be resolved in the future as the rights and needs of homosexuals, including those of elderly homosexuals, are increasingly being recognized.

Hospice Care

The term *hospice* originally meant an inn or way station for travelers. Since 1967, it has assumed another meaning, namely, a program of care for terminally ill patients, most of whom are older people dying of diseases such as cancer. The first hospice was founded that year in England by Dr. Cicely Saunders. The purpose was to provide services for the terminally ill that would allow them to be as free of pain as possible, provide emotional and social support, and fulfill as many of their desires as possible, as the end of life approached. In addition, patients were encouraged to maintain as many of their functions as they could. The concept spread to the United States in the early 1970s, and there are now thousands of hospice programs in this country. Such programs are either inpatient or outpatient. Inpatient programs may be located either within an established hospital or in a special facility designed only for hospice care. Outpatient programs are for terminally ill patients who remain in their homes while receiving care from hospice staff members. Outpatient programs are becoming increasingly popular, given their lower costs.

Patients in a hospice program are usually treated by a team consisting of a physician, a nurse, a social worker, and a counselor. The patient's dignity and self-respect are given the highest attention by such practices as maintaining physical appearance and grooming at as high a level as possible. Most patients prefer a hospice center or program to that of a regular hospital. Hospice patients tend to be more mobile and less depressed and anxious than terminally ill patients cared for in a regular hospital.

Hostility

Hostility is characterized by a negative approach to other people. It may be expressed by abusive thoughts or statements and/or abusive actions. Psychologists have known for some time that expressions of hostility decline from adolescence to mid-life, with the lowest incidence among people 30 to 60 years of age. Less certain has been the frequency of expressions of hostility after age 60. A cross-sectional study conducted several years ago found a moderate increase in the expression of hostility for people after age 60. A more recent study by researchers at Duke University reported that the older adults in their sample were generally more suspicious of other people and more cynical in their beliefs about other people than were middle-aged adults. More hostile behavior was also expressed during an interview by the elderly adults than by the middle-aged adults. The greater verbal expression of hostility was true for both older men and women. However, violent acts as expressions of hostility tend to decrease in late adulthood.

The apparent increase in hostility in elderly adults has important implications for their health. There is considerable evidence indicating that high levels of hostility have adverse effects on physical health (e.g., increased risk of heart disease) and on longevity.

Household Expenditures

Running a household requires spending money—for food, clothing, entertainment, rent or mortgage payments, and so on. Do the percentages of monthly expenditures for various household needs differ for elderly adults compared to younger adults? What little is known about possible age differences in the allotment of household expenditures comes from a study by researchers at Northwestern University. They had available the results of a consumer survey conducted by the United States Department of Labor in the mid-1980s. Nearly 4,000 members of households, age 45 and older, were interviewed. The households were selected such that they represented a cross-section of all U.S. households. The researchers found relatively few age differences in the percentages of expenditures on various items. This was true, for example, for food, recreation, and giving (e.g., to charities). However, people age 65 and older did allot more of their spending to housing and health care than did younger people. By contrast, people in the 45- to 54-year age range devoted a larger percentage of their expenditures to clothing than did older adults. It seems likely that comparable results would be found for current households.

Humor

The topic of this section is not elderly people being the target of many jokes (which they are, frequently as victims of ageism; see AGEISM), but rather possible age differences in the appreciation of humor. Humor researchers have identified two basic kinds of structure in jokes and cartoons. The first involves a situation in which there is an incongruity but a resolution is offered; the second involves a nonsense situation in which there is an incongruity and either no resolution is offered or a resolution is offered only to be followed by another incongruity. Researchers have discovered that an important determinant of one's appreciation of humor corresponds with one's conservative-liberal dimension. More conservative people tend to find incongruent-resolution humor to be funnier and less aversive than do more liberal people. The opposite is true for nonsense humor. That is, it is the more liberal individual who is likely to find it funnier and less aversive. The linkage of conservatism to humor suggests that we are likely to find age differences in people's reactions to jokes and cartoons, simply because the proportion of elderly people who are conservative is greater than the proportion of younger people (see ATTITUDES [POLITICAL AND SOCIAL]).

This suggestion was tested in a massive cross-sectional study (different groups of people at each age level) by researchers in Germany. The participants in the study included more than 4,000 individuals ranging in age from 14 to 66 years. Each participant rated a number of jokes and cartoons in terms of their funniness and their aversiveness. As expected, the average funniness rating increased progressively with increasing age for incongruity-resolution jokes/cartoons, while it decreased for nonsense jokes/cartoons. The participants also took several tests to measure their degree of conservatism. As expected, conservatism was found to increase progressively after the teens. Most important, a high correlation was found between degree of conservatism and the type of reaction to humor at all age levels. Age per se does not account for age differences in appreciation of humor. It is the higher incidence of conservatism in the elderly population that is responsible for the age difference.

Huntington's Disease

Individuals with Huntington's disease (now often called Woody Guthrie's disease) have a genetically transmitted (by a dominant gene) brain disorder that causes involuntary jerky movements of the body. Children of persons with the disease have a 50–50 chance of inheriting the disease. These children are usually born before the disease is discovered in one of their parents. The disease is usually accompanied by memory problems, mental decline, and personality changes. Onset of the disease usually occurs early in middle age (35 to 45 years of age). Mental decline may reach the point of dementia as the disease progresses, and death is almost certain from 10 to 20 years after the onset of the disease.

The gene causing the disease was recently identified by a scientist at Massachusetts General Hospital. Its identification offers hope for genetic counseling in the future and perhaps even the discovery of an effective treatment or prevention of the disease.

I

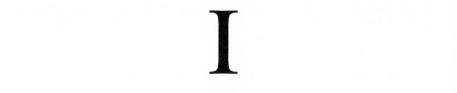

Illusions

Illusions occur when the senses are fooled in some way. They are usually associated with vision. In effect, you "see" something that isn't consistent with physical reality (as when you are tricked by a magician). Age differences are studied in the laboratory through the use of simple materials such as those used to produce the Muller-Lyer illusion. The nature of this illusion may be seen by looking at the following: ⟩——⟨ ⟨——⟩ . Which of the two horizontal lines appears longer? They are of equal length, but the one on the left probably appears to be longer. Researchers have found that the illusory experience with these lines increases in magnitude steadily from early to late adulthood. This is true of a number of other visual illusions as well (they are known as type I illusions). That is, for each, the magnitude of the illusory experience is greater for older adults than for younger adults. The increase in the magnitude of the illusion in later adulthood is the consequence of age changes in the eye, especially in the lens. The reduced amount of light reaching the retina by the "yellowing" of the lens seems to be the major reason. In fact, when young adults view the Muller-Lyer materials through goggles that reduce the amount of light reaching the retina, they experience the increased magnitude of the illusion characteristic of older adults.

There are some visual illusions, known as type II illusions, in which the magnitude of the illusory experience decreases instead of increases from early adulthood through late adulthood. An example of a type II illusion is the Uanadze illusion in which after viewing two circles of unequal diameters, you have the tendency to view two subsequently exposed circles of equal diameters as being unequal in size. It is suspected that age changes occurring at levels of the visual system beyond the eye (i.e., in the brain) are responsible for these decreases in illusory experiences.

Illusions are of interest if only because they represent a quirk in normal sensory functioning. However, they are also of interest because of their potential diagnostic value. This is especially true for type II illusions. Conceivably, older people who show virtually no illusory effect for these illusions may be experiencing some form of brain degeneration.

Imagery

Imagine a map of the United States. Now name a state that has an outline similar to that of Oregon. You surely wouldn't name Missouri or West Virginia. How would you select a state that does resemble Oregon? Many people will tell you that they are comparing "images" or mental pictures they have of various states with the image they have of Oregon. Which is bigger—a robin or a canary? To answer this question, some people will tell you they are comparing the image they form for each bird. Consider a task that psychologists call mental rotation. You see a version of the letter **R** that is either the true letter or a mirror image of the letter. Your job is to determine which it is. The problem is that the letter you see is rotated, sometimes looking like this ꓤ and on other occasions like this ꓤ. Participants performing this task, whether young or older adults, usually make few errors in judging whether the letter is true or a mirror image, although elderly adults are slower in reaching their judgments. How do you know which form of the letter it is? We know that the more the letter is rotated, the longer it takes to make the judgment, again regardless of a participant's age. It is as if you have rotated in your mind an image of the object you see until it is "straight," and the time to rotate depends on how much you have to rotate it. We also know that lists of words that are easily imagined, such as *apple* and *cigar* are easier to memorize than are lists of words that are less imageable, such as *mercy* and *justice*, regardless of the age of participants. Presumably images enhance our memory ability (see MEMORY TRAINING) of episodic events.

We do seem to possess the mental ability of forming images of objects and events in our world. However, some people report that their ability to form mental images is much greater than that of other people. To what extent is this ability affected by aging? When asked about the vividness of their mental images, younger and older people show little difference. The existence of an imagery ability in late adulthood would seemingly be apparent from the evidence that elderly adults perform well on various tasks in which imagery seems to facilitate performance. They can do mental rotations, they benefit from the presence of easily imaged words in a word list, and so on. However, there is also evidence of diminished proficiency of imagery in late adulthood. Elderly participants, for example, engage less in the spontaneous use of images than do younger participants when such use makes memorability easier. This occurs when participants are asked to learn word pairs such as *apple* and *pencil*. Young adults are likely to learn this pair by forming an image of a pencil stuck in an apple, even when they are not instructed to so. By contrast, elderly participants are unlikely to make use of such images unless they are instructed and encouraged to do so. The weaker imagery ability of elderly adults, in general, contrasts sharply with the high verbal ability of elderly adults (see VERBAL ABILITY). Some researchers believe there is a reason for this difference. Verbal ability is largely a function of the brain's left hemisphere where language centers are located for most people, whereas imaginal ability is largely a function of the right hemisphere. The argument is that the right hemisphere of the brain "ages" at a faster rate than the left hemisphere. The evidence to support this argument is conflicting; some studies suggest a differential rate of aging, but other studies do not.

Implicit Memory

Several minutes after studying a lengthy list of common words, you are asked to recall as many of the words as you can. Not surprisingly, you discover that you can recall fewer than half of the words on the list. Perhaps somewhat more surprisingly, you also discover that you are even unable to recognize some of the words you could not recall. Does this mean that memories of the nonrecalled and nonrecognized words do not exist? Did memory traces of these words fail to be registered in your memory store? Or, alternatively, were they registered but somehow were "erased" before you had the chance to test your memory? Not necessarily. Both recall and recognition are part of what memory researchers call *explicit memory*. Explicit memory is memory that requires conscious recollection of the events to be remembered in the sense of deliberately searching your memory store to find specific memory traces. Memory researchers have discovered that memories that are beyond conscious recollection may nevertheless be present and may become evident when the constraints of conscious recollection are removed. Memory without conscious recollection is known as *implicit memory*.

Suppose that *shade* was one of the words in the list you could neither recall nor recognize. To demonstrate the memory for that word's presence in the list, you are given another task to perform after your explicit memory for the list words has been tested. The task is really an indirect test of memory, but this information is not revealed to you. You are simply told that the investigator is interested in word productions to word stems (e.g., the first two letters of a word). You are given a number of word stems, such as *cl*, *tr*, and *sh*, and you are asked to produce a word beginning with each stem. The question is, what word are you most likely to produce with the *sh*? There are many words beginning with *sh* that you could give—for example, *sh*ape, *sh*ark, *sh*ame, *sh*oot, *sh*are, and even an expletive. However, the probability is quite high that you will come up with *sh*ade, the previously studied word that is not consciously recollective.

Other procedures could be used to demonstrate your implicit memory in the absence of explicit memory. For example, instead of giving you word stems to complete, words could be flashed on a screen and you could be asked to identify them. At first, the flash for a given word is too brief for you to identify it. The duration of the word's exposure is gradually increased until you are finally able to identify it. The duration of exposure is likely to be much briefer for previously studied words that are beyond recollection (such as *shade*) than for other similar words that had not been included in the study list. Again, implicit memory exists even when explicit memory does not. In this instance, it is your word recognition rather than your word production that is facilitated by the implicit memory.

Normally aging older participants frequently perform, on the average, moderately below the level of young adult participants on tests of explicit memory (see EPISODIC MEMORY). By contrast, age differences on implicit memory tests have been found to be slight and often nonexistent. That is, in the absence of the need for conscious recollection, older adults seem to manifest as much memory as do young adults. Patients with organic amnesia, such as those with Korsakoff's disease (see KORSAKOFF'S DISEASE), also show as much implicit memory as do age-matched individuals without amnesia, even though the patients with amnesia show pronounced deficits in their explicit memory. The fate of implicit memory with Alzheimer's disease in its early stages is presently unresolved. In some studies patients with Alzheimer's disease have been found to be quite deficient in implicit memory and explicit memory. However, other studies of patients with Alzheimer's disease have shown little implicit memory deficit in the presence of considerable explicit memory deficit, relative to normally aging elderly adults.

The existence of implicit memory helps to explain some puzzling memory phenomena. Have you ever had the experience of feeling you have met this person before, but you cannot recollect when it was or what the name of the person is (including not recognizing the name when you are told it). Assuming you really did meet the person before, you are probably showing implicit memory. In fact, implicit memory may account for some of our experiences we refer to as déjà vu (the feeling you have been somewhere before or have experienced a particular event before, but you cannot recall the place or the prior experience). As another possible phenomenon, consider the following scenario. You are doing your laundry, and you notice that your supply of detergent is low. So you make a mental note to buy detergent the next time you go to the supermarket. Several days later when you go shopping you make your list of items you need to purchase. Missing from the list is detergent. You failed to recollect consciously the event in the laundry room. However, at the market, as you pass through the soap department, the detergents seem to attract you to them, and you find yourself putting a box of your favorite brand in your shopping cart. Your implicit memory came through for you. It seems that implicit memory is as likely to benefit many elderly people as it is many younger people.

Influenza

Influenza (or flu) is a viral infection of the respiratory tract. There are two main kinds of viruses causing influenza, type A and type B; each type has many different strains. Type A viruses generally cause more severe illness than type B. Symptoms of influenza include muscle aches, fever, sore throat, and, in some cases, nausea, vomiting, and diarrhea. The disease is highly contagious, and it is spread by direct contact with an infected person or by airborne droplets when an infected person coughs or sneezes. It may also be caught by handling material containing infected body secretions. Symptoms usually appear from 1 to 5 days after exposure to the disease. Treatment consists of bed rest, drinking lots of fluids, and medicines to reduce the fever and discomfort from muscle aches. An antiviral prescription drug, amantadine, may reduce fever and other symptoms of type A influenza if taken when the symptoms first appear.

Influenza can lead to pneumonia, especially in older people, and become life-threatening. A vaccine is available every fall before the flu season (a new vaccine is needed every year). Elderly people should be encouraged to have the vaccination if its use causes no serious complications. People who are allergic to eggs should not get the vaccine, nor should persons with a fever or an active infection of any kind. Amantadine may be substituted for those people unable to have the flu vaccine. Vaccination is not always effective in avoiding influenza for older people, but it should make the symptoms less severe in those vaccinated people who do contract the disease. Despite the major health risk of not being vaccinated, it is estimated that fewer than 40% of people age 65 and older are immunized each year by the vaccine. Some elderly people are unduly afraid that the vaccine will make them sick, whereas many others are either unaware of the vaccine or unaware of the risks of not being vaccinated.

Intelligence

Intelligence is a frequently used term, but it is difficult to define. We refer to some people as being bright, others as being average, and still others as being dull. In what ways do these people differ from one another? More intelligent people seem to learn more easily, to have better memories, more proficient reasoning ability and problem-solving skill, and a greater store of knowledge about the world than do less intelligent people. Intelligence is made up of a number of different abilities that collectively define intelligence. However, it is the learning ability that attracted the attention of psychologists who have studied intelligence. They constructed tests of intelligence with one objective in mind, namely, to devise a test whose scores could predict scholastic success. Therefore abilities believed to be related to academic achievement were tested. The test constructors were very successful in their endeavors.

The testing of intelligence began with the work of Alfred Binet in the early 1900s. He and Theodore Simon constructed a test that could identify low-achieving children in Parisian schools and predict the success of children in general in school. Eventually Binet and Simon's test was modified and enlarged by Lewis Terman of Stanford University in 1916. The resulting Stanford-Binet test was subsequently revised several times, but its objective has always been to predict academic performances of children. The first widely used adult intelligence test was the Army Alpha test that was developed during World War I (see ARMY ALPHA AND ARMY BETA INTELLIGENCE TEST). The test was intended for use with adults rather than children, but its objective remained much like that of the Binet-Simon and Stanford-Binet tests—the prediction of academic success. However, in this case academic success referred to successful completion of army training programs. Other tests for adults, such as the Primary Mental Abilities test and the Wechsler Adult Intelligence Scale, have been similarly graded in terms of their success in predicting academic performances, whether it be in college or in an industrial or military training program. Participants in such academic or industrial training programs are likely to be young adults. But what about older adults who have been away from academic or training situations for some years? The traditional intelligence tests were not developed for them. Intelligence in the daily lives of older adults is applied to the solving of everyday problems and comprehending information relevant to their lives, and not to earning academic grades. Over the years there have been attempts to construct intelligence tests that appear to be more relevant to the everyday lives of elderly people. For example, questions are asked that probe their understanding of legal terms and documents or their ability to comprehend and follow the directions on a medicine bottle or an appliance. The objective is a worthy one. Unknown, however, is whether scores on such tests of practical intelligence relate any better to intelligence manifested in the everyday world than do scores on the more traditional intelligence tests.

Psychologists view intelligence in terms of a top-to-bottom hierarchy in which abilities are ordered in terms of their specificity. At the top of the hierarchy is a very broad or general ability that is called g (for general). The amount of g one possesses is believed to be determined largely by familial inheritance. This general ability factor is believed to influence, to some degree, more specific intellectual abilities. General ability, in turn, is "split" into two general, but distinctive, abilities that each encompass a number of specific abilities found at the bottom of the hierarchy. The two general abilities subsumed under g are called *crystallized intelligence* and *fluid intelligence.* Crystallized intelligence is influenced greatly by one's experiences, education, and social and cultural environment. The specific abilities derived from crystallized intelligence include vocabulary and general knowledge. Fluid intelligence is basically "raw" intelligence that is determined relatively independent of educational opportunity. The specific abilities derived from fluid intelligence include numerical ability and analogical reasoning ability. Traditional intelligence tests include subtests that sample abilities related to both crystallized and fluid intelligence. From scores on these subtests, separate estimates may be given of the test taker's crystallized ability and fluid ability. In addition, all of the subtests may be combined to give an estimate of that person's g ability (often expressed as an intelligence quotient [IQ] score).

In general, age-related declines in crystallized intelligence as measured by intelligence tests tend to be slight, if they exist at all, at least until very late in adulthood. However, declines in fluid intelligence test scores begin after early adulthood and progress in amount through late adulthood. When specific abilities are examined, considerable variability in age-related changes is found. Abilities identified with crystallized intelligence generally remain fairly stable throughout adulthood or may show either modest increases or modest decreases from early to late adulthood. Abilities identified with fluid intelligence generally show age-related declines; the extent of the decline is much greater for some abilities than for others.

It is important to realize that most elderly people function very well in their everyday lives despite their apparent decline in fluid intelligence abilities. Added experience, and therefore increases in crystallized intelligence, seemingly compensate for whatever declines occur in fluid intelligence. Moreover, declines in fluid intelligence often may be more apparent than real. Many psychologists in the area of intelligence believe that there is considerable plasticity or resilience among older adults in their ability to regain to some degree their earlier level of fluid intelligence performances with appropriate instructions and training on specific abilities, such as reasoning.

K

· ·

Korsakoff's Disease

Korsakoff's disease is a neurological (brain) disorder most commonly found in long-term alcoholics after 20 to 30 years of excessive drinking. The primary cause of the disease is a thiamine deficiency caused by the alcoholic's failure to eat a nutritionally balanced diet. The disease is likely to have its onset when alcoholics are in middle age or early old age, thus making it of concern to gerontologists. The primary symptom of the disease is profound amnesia, especially anterograde amnesia (difficulty in acquiring new information and storing it in memory; see AMNESIA). However, unlike patients with Alzheimer's disease, who also have severe amnesia, patients with Korsakoff's disease are unlikely to have a major loss of other mental functions, such as intelligence. However, personality is likely to be affected by the disease, as patients become apathetic and excessively passive in their behaviors.

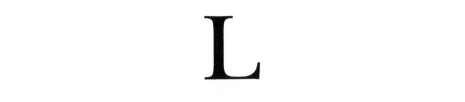

L

Learned Helplessness

The concept of learned helplessness was introduced to psychology by animal research in the mid-1970s. Dogs were subjected to intense electric shock under conditions in which there was no way to escape the shock. Eventually they encountered new situations in which electric shock could be avoided by performing a specified behavior. They were found to be very deficient in learning to avoid the shock even though they had the opportunity to do so. The researchers concluded that the dogs had actually learned to be "helpless." It was as if they had acquired a "what's the use" attitude—no matter what they did, they had earlier found there was no escape from being punished. Moreover, the dogs were observed to become distressed and passive in their behavior. The concept of learned helplessness was eventually extended to human behavior. Some people living under various negative and stressful conditions, such as poverty, may discover that there seems to be no relationship between their behavior and escape from the stressful conditions. That is, no matter how they try to cope with the negative events in their lives, they are unsuccessful in improving their lot in life, resulting eventually in a state of learned helplessness characterized by persistent passive behavior and even severe depression.

On the surface, older people might seem to be highly vulnerable targets for acquiring learned helplessness. More than younger people, they may be subjected to negative life events that are seemingly inescapable. However, various evidence suggests that older people are no more susceptible to learned helplessness than are younger people. For example, elderly people, in general, express satisfaction with their current lives that is no less than that expressed by younger people (see LIFE SATISFACTION). Nor is their incidence of severe depression greatly different from that of younger adults (see DEPRESSION [INCIDENCE, SYMPTOMS, CAUSES]). In addition, many elderly people are very effective in coping with stressful events in their lives (see STRESS AND COPING WITH STRESS).

Learning (Overview)

See also CLASSICAL CONDITIONING; CONCEPT LEARNING; MAZE LEARN-ING; MOTOR SKILL LEARNING; OPERANT CONDITIONING; SPATIAL LEARNING; VERBAL LEARNING

If all new learning suddenly stopped for you, you would have no new acquisitions of knowledge. The name of a new president or new senator would be unfamiliar to you in terms of their office every time you encountered the names. It would be impossible to acquire new words either in a foreign language or in your own native language. Strangers who were introduced to you would continue to be strangers on future encounters. There would be no hope of acquiring new recreational skills. If you did not already know how to play golf, operate a word processor, or play bridge, you wouldn't in the future either. How to operate a new kitchen gadget would have to be relearned every time you used it. Finding your way around a new neighborhood would be a brand-new adventure every time you left your home. It would also be impossible to learn the meaning of new concepts, such as that of a black hole or AIDS.

Learning is essential for adaptation to our environments, and it is just as essential for older people as it is for younger people. Fortunately, elderly people remain active learners. They do learn new information, new recreational skills, new names with new faces, and so on. Of course, this does not mean that there are no declines in learning proficiency with normal aging. Given the importance of new learning to our everyday lives, it is essential that we discover the extent of these declines, the reasons they occur, and possible ways of reducing the declines in proficiency.

Our examples of new learning should make it apparent that there are many kinds of learning. Among the kinds of learning studied by psychologists are classical conditioning, operant conditioning, maze learning, spatial learning, motor skills learning, verbal learning, and concept learning. A description of aging research on each kind of learning is found in separate entries.

The concepts of learning and memory are obviously related, and they are difficult to distinguish. Learning a task of any kind usually involves the intent to learn the task, practice on the task, and progressive improvements in performance on the task with practice. This fits nicely with what happens when you *learned* to ride a bicycle. You had the intent to do so, you practiced it, and you gradually mastered the skill. This description of learning works less well for classical conditioning (see CLASSICAL CONDITIONING). Here there is no intent to learn, but there is practice and gradual learning occurs. The fit is even poorer for the *memory* you have of the first bad spill you had with your bicycle. The memory of that spill required no intent, and practice was not needed (one occurrence only was involved). This is an example of episodic memory, that is, memory for personally experienced events in one's life (see EPISODIC MEMORY). There are many other forms of memory as well (see MEMORY [OVERVIEW]).

Legal Advice

Elderly people are often faced with problems that may or may not require the services of a lawyer. The American Association of Retired Persons has available a booklet providing information as to when legal services may be needed, as well as information on how to locate a good lawyer and how to negotiate a fee. The booklet, *Finding Legal Help: An Older Person's Guide,* costs $2 for members and $3 for nonmembers. To obtain a copy write to Legal Counsel for the Elderly, P.O. Box 96474, Washington, DC 20090-6474, and enclose a check or money order to cover the cost.

Leisure Activities

A leisure activity is usually defined as one in which individuals engage during their free time. Older people generally have more time available for pursuing leisure activities than do younger people. Of interest in gerontology is the nature of elderly adults' leisure activities and how they differ from those of younger adults. Not surprisingly, most elderly people decrease their strenuous leisure activities and increase their more sedentary activities (e.g., reading and watching television), relative to the activities engaged in earlier in their lives. A survey of people living in a small Midwestern city indicated that for people in the 65- to 74-year age range, the predominant activities were those involving social interactions and travel. Social activities were also reported by many of those surveyed who were age 75 and older, as were home-based and family-based activities. However, the percentage of those reporting travel as a leisure activity declined from 60% in the 65- to 74-age range to 40% in the 75 and older age range. In general, the variety of leisure activities in which people engage declines progressively from young adulthood through middle age and into late adulthood. The choice of activities for many elderly people is surely restricted by their changing physical health status.

Lexicon

As you read the words in this sentence, what enables you to do so? Each word in the sentence must have its own representation in your semantic, or permanent knowledge, memory (see SEMANTIC MEMORY). The printed version of the word *what* is quickly read as the word "what" because the mental operations of reading ensure automatic contact with information in your memory that corresponds to that word. These representations are stored in a part of our semantic memory known as the *lexicon* (or mental dictionary).

Adults of all ages have difficulty *not* reading a word when it is in their visual fields. That is, contact with the word's representation in the lexicon occurs automatically and effortlessly regardless of an adult's age, and it is a process that is difficult to stop. The automaticity of reading a word when it is physically present is clearly demonstrated by what psychologists call the Stroop effect (named after the psychologist who discovered it). Suppose you are given a series of color patches (red, green, yellow, red, etc.) and you are asked to name each color as you see it. Regardless of your age, you will respond rapidly to each color (and, of course, correctly). Now change the nature of the task. This time you are asked to name the color of the ink in which a word in a series of words is printed. The first ink color is red, and your response should be "red." However, the word in which it is embedded is "blue." Similarly, the second ink color is green, but it is the color ink for the printed word "yellow." Your responses of "red" and "green" will occur much more slowly than they do when you are simply naming red and green color patches (it is this slower responding in the second situation that defines the Stroop effect). The slower response occurs because you cannot avoid reading the color words, and by so doing you have to inhibit the name of the word in order to name the color of the ink. Older adults tend to show an ever greater Stroop effect than do younger adults, because the added years of reading have increased the difficulty of "turning off" the reading of a word.

Our point is that color words have representations in our lexicons that are activated whenever they are encountered in printed form. Similar representations are present for every other word in our active vocabularies. Contact with representations in our lexicons also occurs automatically when we hear spoken words. Without such automatic contact we would be unable to engage in normal everyday conversations, listen to a lecture, or understand the content of a television program. Access to words in our lexicons is as automatic for normally aging people as it is for younger adults, although access takes place a bit more slowly (at the level of milliseconds slower) in late adulthood.

Access to words is facilitated by the organized structure of our lexicons. Words are not stored randomly or haphazardly. Related words appear to be stored in close proximity to one another. The activation of a given words' representation in the lexicon spreads automatically to these nearby related words (a phenomenon known as spreading activation). When you read the word *doctor,* the activation of its representation spreads quickly to the representations of such related words as *nurse.* Spreading activation makes reading time faster for those words that have been already activated prior to their physical appearance. Consider the sentences, "The doctor gave the instrument to the nurse" and "The carpenter gave the instrument to the nurse." Identifying the word *nurse* as "nurse" occurs more quickly in reading the first sentence than in the second sentence. This is because the activation of *nurse*'s representation in the lexicon began while reading *doctor* but not while reading carpenter. Numerous laboratory studies have revealed that spreading activation takes place to the same degree for elderly adults as for younger adults, although the time required for spreading to be completed is a bit longer for older adults (and much slower for patients with Alzheimer's disease).

The existence of spreading activation is not the only kind of evidence to indicate that the lexicon has an organized structure. The other major form of evidence is derived from the nature of word associations. Our associations of words to other words tend to show regularity and commonality among people of all ages. Most important, research on word associations indicates that the structure of the lexicon changes little, if any, with normal aging (see WORD ASSOCIATIONS). In fact, the most likely change in the structure of the lexicon with normal aging is in the number of representations of words it contains. Elderly adults typically have a larger vocabulary than younger adults (see VERBAL ABILITY).

Life Expectancy

Life expectancy in any given year is usually defined as the average length of time an infant born in that year is expected to live, given that conditions present in that year stay unchanged. As conditions have changed over the years, so has life expectancy. In 1900, life expectancy in the United States was only 47 years. This does not mean that few people at that time lived beyond age 47. In fact, many individuals lived well into late adulthood. The reason that life expectancy was so low was the high mortality rate for infants at that time. Their ages at death entered prominently in the calculation of the purely statistical concept of a life expectancy. As health conditions improved over the years, the incidence of infant deaths, as well as the incidence of deaths of adults below age 40, declined dramatically. The net effect has been a progressive increase in life expectancy. During the 1980s life expectancy had reached 74.5 years. However, the likelihood of living to an advanced old age did not increase nearly as dramatically. People age 75 had a life expectancy of about 8 years (i.e., on the average they were expected to live that much longer) in 1900 and about 11 years in the 1980s. This age may increase, however, by a year or two in the 1990s as progress continues to be made in the treatments of heart disease and cancer. Consequently, life expectancy at birth may also increase by a year or two by the end of the 1990s.

The figures noted above are for the entire United States and include both men and women. Life expectancy may also be determined separately for the sexes, for different races, for different geographical regions, and for different occupations. Life expectancy is presently about 8 years longer for women (combined for races) than for men (about 78.5 years for women and 70.5 years for men). Blacks (combined for the sexes) have a life expectancy that is about 5 years less than that of whites. For white men the current life expectancy is about 72.5 years; for white women it is about 79 years. For black men it is about 66 years; for black women it is about 74.5 years. Life expectancy is also higher in some states (e.g., in Hawaii and in the northern plains states) than in other states (e.g., South Carolina). Similarly, life expectancy is higher for some occupations (e.g., judges) than for other occupations (e.g., coal miners). Life expectancy currently varies greatly among the countries of the world. In countries such as India and Ethiopia life expectancy is no greater than it was in the United States in 1900. The high incidence of infant and child mortality in these countries accounts largely for the low average life expectancy. By contrast, there are countries, such as Sweden and Japan, where life expectancy is greater than that of people in the United States.

Life Satisfaction

How satisfied are you with your present life? Do you feel that your achievements come close to matching what you hoped they would be at your present age? Do you feel as satisfied with your life now as you did, say, 10 years ago? On a 9-point scale in which 1 is very dissatisfied and 9 is very satisfied, where would you rank yourself? Your satisfaction with your life is a rather good index of your morale and your feeling of well-being. Surprisingly, life satisfaction does not seem to be related to age. That is, older adults, in general, express no less or no greater satisfaction than do middle-aged or young adults. The average rating on the 9-point scale is about the same at each age level, and, in some studies, has even been found to be greater for older adults than for younger adults. For example, in a study conducted in 1975 of more than 6,000 Americans ranging in age from 4 to 99, little variation in life satisfaction was found that could be attributed to age. Later surveys, including one of Israeli citizens ranging in age from their late teens to 65 and older, have confirmed the absence of any major effect of age on life satisfaction.

Our reference has been to present life satisfaction. Of further interest is what people believe their life satisfaction will be in the future. In the survey of Israeli citizens, the participants were asked to estimate their life satisfaction 5 years from now. From the late teens through the early 30s, future life satisfaction was estimated to be considerably higher than present satisfaction. However, beginning in the late 30s, there was a progressive decline in rated future life satisfaction, such that by late adulthood future life satisfaction was rated, on the average, no higher than present life satisfaction. This trend suggests that people become increasingly less optimistic about the future as they progress through middle age into late adulthood.

The fact that elderly people differ little from younger people in their average degree of life satisfaction does not imply that all elderly people are satisfied with their present lives. There is considerable variability in life satisfaction scores—many older people are far less satisfied than other older people. One of the most widely researched topics in gerontology is determining the reasons for this variability among elderly people in life satisfaction. What factors account for some elderly people feeling less satisfied than others? The most important factor, and one that should not be surprising, is health status. Older adults who perceive their health to be poor tend to be less satisfied with their lives than other elderly adults who perceive their health to be good or excellent. Socioeconomic status is another important factor, as is the amount of social interactions of elderly people. However, it is likely that the frequency and quality of social interactions is dependent on health status.

Numerous other factors have been related to the degree of life satisfaction expressed by elderly people. For example, older people who are married tend to express greater life satisfaction than elderly people who are divorced or widowed. Similarly, elderly people who appear to be more religious tend to express moderately higher life satisfaction than less religious elderly people. Here too, however, it may be health status that is the more important causative factor. Church attendance is likely to be greater for elderly people who are in good health than for those who are in poor health. There is evidence to indicate that elderly blacks are less satisfied than elderly whites, undoubtedly because of the larger percentage of elderly blacks living on poverty level incomes. Extroverted elderly men tend to express greater life satisfaction than elderly men who are less extroverted, and evidence indicates that elderly men high in the personality trait of neuroticism score less high in life satisfaction than men who score lower in neuroticism (see PERSONALITY TRAITS). There appears to be little difference between elderly men and elderly women in life satisfaction scores.

The critical roles played by health status and socioeconomic status on life satisfaction in late adulthood suggest that future generations of older people will have fewer members who are dissatisfied with their lives. That is, medical progress in the years ahead will ensure good or excellent health for a larger percentage of elderly people than presently. Similarly, improved pension plans and improved pre-retirement economic planning should greatly reduce the percentage of elderly people with impoverished lives.

The life events one has experienced early in adulthood are also likely to affect one's life satisfaction in late adulthood. For example, a recent study on elderly women's life satisfaction found a relationship between the hardships they experienced during the Great Depression and their present life satisfaction. These hardships seemed to be related to greater life satisfaction late in life for middle-class elderly women, but diminished life satisfaction for working-class women.

Life Span

The life span of a given species is the length of time a member of that species could live if free of disease and accidents that prevent fulfillment of that duration. It may be estimated for a species by the oldest age a member of that species has been known to reach. For human beings, that age is at least 120 years (a woman in France celebrated her 120th birthday in 1995). There have been reports of individuals who have lived longer than 120 years, but these claims have been difficult to verify. In general, other species have much shorter life spans than the human being. For some insects, the life span is only a few days. For the mouse it is about 3 years, and for the horse it is probably 30+ years (although there have been claims, difficult to verify, of horses living over 60 years). On the other hand, the life span for the Galápagos tortoise may be as high as 150 years.

The human life span has apparently been the same for centuries. However, is it possible that the human life span can be increased in the future? Some scientists believe that this is a definite possibility. They have based their belief on research with rats. Rats that live on a restricted diet from birth have been found to have a longer life span than rats living on a normal diet. Restricting food intake seems to retard aging in rats. Whether similar food restrictions could increase the life span of human beings remains highly speculative. Many scientists believe that health interventions, such as regular exercise and nutritious diets, will serve to increase the number of people who are able to attain the full life span, but they are unlikely to increase the life span itself.

Locomotion

Elderly adults, in general, walk more slowly than young adults. The age difference in velocity is already apparent by age 65. Further decreases in velocity occur after age 65 such that people in their 80s walk considerably more slowly than people in their 60s. Researchers in France have determined that the reduction in walking rate is almost entirely the consequence of the shorter strides taken by elderly people. This may be seen in the fact that the stride length averaged 1.09 meters for participants in their 60s and 0.71 meters for participants in their 80s, and speed of walking averaged 1.00 meters per second and 0.60 meters per second at the two age levels. These researchers also discovered that adults of all ages are capable of increasing their walking speed when required to do so. Regardless of age, the increase in speed is accomplished by both increasing stride length and decreasing cycle time (i.e., time from left foot placement to the next left foot placement).

Whether exercise improves the gait of elderly people is inconclusive. Researchers at Indiana University found that participants age 65 and older who received 12 weeks of dynamic resistance strength training did not differ from other participants in a nonexercise control group at the end of 12 weeks. Nor did the researchers find exercise to improve balance for participants in the exercise group, again relative to those in the control group.

Some older people do seem to walk faster than they did when they were younger. A faster gait is apparently their way of compensating for their relatively poor balance and the shift forward in their body's center of gravity.

Loneliness

Feelings of distress, separation, and isolation—these are the feelings that define loneliness. A Harris survey revealed that the proportion of elderly people experiencing loneliness is substantial. In fact, loneliness is ranked high among the most serious problems older people believe to confront them. The probable causes of loneliness for elderly people were investigated by researchers at the University of South Carolina. Information was obtained from nearly 3,000 individuals aged 65 and older. A number of conditions were found to contribute to the loneliness experienced by many elderly people. However, the most important contributor was that of a low level of social fulfillment. Reduced social fulfillment means that they do not have enough friends, they do not have enough to do to keep busy, and they do not feel needed. Among the other conditions contributing to loneliness of elderly people are changed marital status, reduced income, and poor health. However, the effects of these other contributors are largely indirect; that is, they affect loneliness largely by way of their negative influences on social fulfillment.

Longevity

Elderly people obviously differ greatly in the number of years they actually live. Viewers of the *Today* television program are reminded constantly that some lives continue well past the century mark. However, we all know older people who died long before attaining that mark. The average expected length of life for people of a given age is called their life expectancy, and the maximum number of years people are believed capable of living under the most favorable circumstances is called the life span (see LIFE EXPECTANCY; LIFE SPAN). But what about individual persons? What determines their greatly different longevities? Scientists have long believed that heredity is a major determinant of individual differences in longevity. Those people who have a long life are more likely to have ancestors who also had a long life than are people who have a shorter life.

Alexander Graham Bell conducted a genealogical study years ago of a single family that had thousands of descendants. He found that children of parents who lived to be 80 years or more lived about 20 years longer than children whose two parents died before they were

60 years old. A study in the 1950s reported that identical twins (who have identical heredities) die several years closer together than do fraternal twins (who are like ordinary siblings and do not have identical heredities). A similar difference in longevities between identical and fraternal twins was found recently for Danish citizens who were born between 1870 and 1880. Nevertheless, it should be noted that the relationship between parents and children in years lived is only slightly positive. That is, the correlation is positive, but not much greater than zero.

There are, of course, other factors that are major determinants of individual differences in longevity. Regular exercise and other good health practices are likely to add years to one's life. Obesity and smoking are likely to subtract years from one's life, as is prolonged exposure to various pollutants in the environment. There are also more subtle factors that influence longevity. For example, married people tend to live several years longer than unmarried people. There is even evidence to suggest that certain personality characteristics are related to longevity. For example, people who live to age 90 and beyond tend to have a flexible attitude toward life in general. They are also unlikely to be extreme in their habits (e.g., excessive eating of junk foods, excessive drinking of alcoholic beverages), and they tend to adapt readily to sources of stress in their daily lives.

Other possible factors have been discovered by researchers in California who have been following the lives of over 1,500 intellectually bright children who were first studied in 1921. Perhaps the most obvious factor determining longevity among these individuals is their sex. By 1991 50% of the men but only 35% of the women were known to be dead. In addition, those participants in the study who were more conscientious and socially dependable as children tended to live longer than those who were less conscientious and socially dependable, and those participants whose parents had divorced when they were children tended to die at an earlier age than those whose parents had remained married.

Longitudinal Method

John's parents have been measuring his height on every birthday through age 18. Not surprisingly, they have discovered that John has grown taller with age. John's parents may not realize it, but they were using one of the major methods employed in aging research to determine the presence and nature of age differences on whatever characteristic or behavior is being measured. That method is called the *longitudinal method.* Assuming that John is a fairly representative child, we may conclude that children grow taller as they become older. This is a true age change for every normally developing child. We could have reached the same conclusion if we examined the heights of representative 1-year-old children, 2-year-old children, and so on through age 18. In this case, however, we have conducted a cross-sectional study in which the same individual is tested only once, and all individuals are tested at about the same time (see CROSS-SECTIONAL METHOD). Our cross-sectional study, however, runs the risk of falsely concluding that the age difference in height is related to a true age change (growth) in height. There is the possibility (*very* slim, of course) that the 2-year-old was born with his or her current height, the three-year-old with his or her current height, and so on. If this were true, then the observed age difference represents a cohort or generational difference and not a true age change (see COHORT EFFECT [GENERATIONAL]). The longitudinal reassessment of the same individual ensures that the change found with increasing age is a true age change (see AGE CHANGE VS. AGE DIFFERENCE). When the interest lies in determining if an age difference represents a true age change, then the longitudinal method has a decided advantage over the cross-sectional method.

In aging research the longitudinal method uses a group of individuals rather than a single individual. The basic procedure calls simply for testing and retesting the participants in the group. Ideally, we would like to recruit participants who are young adults and test them on the characteristic or behavior in question (e.g., intelligence). We would then retest them every few years until they reach late adulthood. The change in average scores with increasing age would identify a true age change. Because all of the participants came from the same generation, the observed age difference could not be related to a cohort or generational effect. Unfortunately, there have been very few longitudinal studies in which participants have been tested and retested for a period of many years. The studies with the best retesting records have been concerned either with intelligence (see, for example, SEATTLE LONGITUDINAL STUDY) or health (see, for example, NORMATIVE AGING STUDY). Most longitudinal studies have been directed at a relatively short span of years, but often that span is a critical period when true age changes may be expected to occur (e.g., participants tested initially at age 65 and then retested at age 75).

Unfortunately, the longitudinal method is not without its problems. One problem is that many participants are likely to withdraw from the study because of death, illness, disinterest, relocation, and so on. There is often a disportionality among the dropouts in terms of ability as measured on the initial test. If the test was boring and uninteresting, the dropouts are more likely to be participants of high initial ability than participants of lower initial ability. By contrast, if the test was very challenging and demanding, the dropouts are more likely to be participants of low initial ability than participants of higher initial ability. An additional problem arises from what is called progressive error. Retesting obviously leads to increasingly greater familiarity with the test in question. Consequently, scores on that test may increase simply from familiarity and disguise what the participants would have scored at a later age in the absence of such familiarity. Finally, there is the possibility in some cases of the presence of a historical time effect. Social and cultural conditions change over the years. Consider, for example, young adults tested for the presence of depressive symptoms in the mid-1920s during a period of economic prosperity, and then retested in the mid-1930s during the time of the Great Depression. The presence of transitory depressive symptoms brought about by the sad economy of that time would not be surprising. An age difference in depression for 25- and 35-year-old people would be the likely outcome. However, it is unlikely to be a true age change. The greater number of depressive symptoms for the 35-year-old participants was undoubtedly a temporary phenomenon, and the symptoms surely decreased when economic prosperity was restored. The possibility of a historical time effect is avoided in a cross-sectional study in that all of the participants at each age level are tested at the same historical time.

M

Magazine Reading

In the most recent study to determine the magazine preferences of elderly adults, *Reader's Digest* was read most frequently by both elderly men (72% of the men surveyed) and elderly women (69%). The magazine surely received by more elderly adults than any other magazine is *Modern Maturity*. Unknown, however, is the percentage of elderly adults who read it regularly. Other popular magazines for both elderly men and elderly women are *TV Guide* and *National Geographic,* with about 40% of each sex reporting reading each regularly. There are some obvious sex differences in preferred magazines. For example, *Sports Illustrated* was reported to be read regularly by 47% of the elderly men surveyed and by less than 3% of the elderly women. By contrast, 50% of the women and only 25% of the men reported reading *Better Homes & Gardens* regularly.

Of further interest is how these preferences compare with those of young adults. A large number of young adults (college students) were surveyed in the same study. Young adults of both sexes read *Reader's Digest* and *National Geographic* far less frequently than elderly adults. Young men share with elderly men a strong interest in *Sports Illustrated* (more than 90% report reading it regularly). A major difference between young and elderly men is in the regular reading of *Playboy* and *Penthouse* (more than 70% of the young men, less than 13% of the elderly men). A comparable distinction is found in the reading of certain magazines by young and elderly women. Less than 25% of the young women read *Better Homes & Gardens* regularly. By contrast, nearly 80% of the young women, and less than 15% of the elderly women, read *Cosmopolitan* regularly.

Managerial Ability

It is not unusual to find older people in managerial positions in business and other settings. However, relatively little is known about the effects of aging on managerial ability. Studies conducted in the 1970s suggested that older managers are slower in making decisions than younger managers, but they may be more thorough than younger ones in the amount of information they use in making those decisions. A more recent study compared teams of midlevel managers of different age levels in making decisions in situations that simulated in the laboratory various situations encountered by managers in business and industry. They found the performances of young participants (28 to 35 years of age) and middle-aged participants (45 to 55 years of age) to be similar. Older participants (age 65 to 75 years) were less proficient than the younger participants in some aspects of utilizing information effectively, and they tended to make fewer decisions than the younger participants. However, the older participants handled simulated emergencies as effectively as the younger participants. The researchers who conducted this study believe that the skills that appeared to be somewhat deficient in their oldest managers could be taught by use of laboratory simulation employed in their study.

Marriage and Marital Satisfaction

There are more married elderly men than there are married elderly women. There are several reasons for this imbalance. In general, men marry women younger than themselves, and therefore married men are likely to reach late adulthood earlier than their wives. In addition, women live longer than men and therefore are more likely to experience loss of a spouse than are men (see WIDOWHOOD AND WIDOWERHOOD). Moreover, older men are more likely than older women to marry for a second (or more) time, and often to a younger woman. The most likely members of the elderly population to be married are elderly white men and the least likely are elderly black women. Elderly black men and women are more likely to be single than elderly white men and women.

Various surveys indicate that married older people have better physical and mental health than unmarried older people. Married elderly people also tend to express greater life satisfaction and to have greater social support, greater economic resources, a lower incidence of entering nursing homes, and live several years longer than unmarried elderly people. There are several reasons why marriage often has such positive effects in late adulthood. One reason is that older married people are more likely to avoid behaviors that risk their health than do unmarried elderly people. Another reason is that a spouse is available as a caregiver in times of need. Continuing marriage into late adulthood also provides continuing opportunity to work together toward shared goals (e.g., trips that had long been postponed) and to share such positive events as the births of grandchildren.

Most married elderly people consider their marriages to be happy and often very happy. In general, marital satisfaction appears to be greatest for young adults and elderly adults and least for middle-aged adults. Of course, divorces do occur among elderly married people (see DIVORCE).

Maze Learning

A maze consists of a pathway from a starting point to an end point or goal. Along the way are left-right choice-points. At each choice-point one path (e.g., left) continues in the direction of the goal; the other (e.g., right) is a blind alley or cul-de-sac. A learner moves through the maze a number of times. Gradually the number of errors (entries into blind alleys) is reduced until the learner eventually moves through the maze without making an error. Most psychologists believe that learners are, in effect, acquiring a "map" or mental representation of the maze rather than simply a series of left and right turns. When all of the choice-points have been learned, the map is complete. Thus maze learning simulates somewhat the kind of learning needed to find one's way around a novel environment (e.g., a new neighborhood) and is therefore of interest in aging research.

Most aging research on maze learning has used rats as participants and a three-dimensional maze in which the rats move their entire bodies. This research has revealed that age differences in the number of errors made while learning the maze are slight when there are only a few choice-points to master (two to four), but they are quite pronounced when there are as many as 14 choice-points. With human participants, a paper-and-pencil maze is used in which participants see only one choice-point at a time and they respond verbally with "left" or "right" at each one. Several studies have indicated that both middle-aged and elderly adults make many more errors than young adults in learning a complex (many choice-points) paper-and-pencil maze.

Maze learning has gradually lost favor with gerontological researchers as other tasks have been found to represent more closely "map" learning in the everyday world. These other tasks usually require participants to travel in some way through a novel environment (e.g., a strange neighborhood; see SPATIAL LEARNING).

Medicaid

The Medicaid program was designed to be a joint federal and state program for assisting low-income people in the payment of their medical costs. It began in 1965 as a companion program to Medicare. The intent of the program is to serve as a third-party insurance. Among its many services are the payment of nursing home care, skilled nursing care, and physician's services. More than one-third of Medicaid's funds are spent on services for elderly people.

Medical Costs (Misunderstanding)

A familiar theme heard in recent years is that elderly people are responsible for our high health costs, and they are robbing current young adults of their future Social Security benefits. Much of this new form of elder abuse (see ELDER ABUSE) stems from the view held by many younger adults that most older adults are physically disabled. In fact, most severely disabled adults living in the community are under age 65. One study conducted in the late 1980s revealed that hospital costs for people over age 80 were less than half those of other age groups. Hospital costs for people in the age range of 65 to 79 years were found to be similar to those of people under age 65 (see also HEALTH CARE COSTS).

Medicare

Title VIII of the Social Security Act established the Medicare program in 1965. From its beginning, the program was intended to prevent elderly people from suffering financial disaster produced by the costs of major illnesses. There are two parts to the Medicare program, a compulsory program, Part A, and an optional program, Part B. For Part A no premiums are charged for workers and their spouses who have had at least 10 years of employment covered by Social Security. For Part B there is a monthly premium (currently around $30) that is deducted from Social Security monthly payments or is billed quarterly for those people who do not receive Social Security payments. About every dollar in premiums is matched by three dollars of government subsidies. Most people who participate in Part A also participate in Part B. Most people on Medicare are age 65 and older. Also eligible are people with kidney disease who need dialysis or a transplant and disabled people who have received Social Security benefits for 2 years.

Part A provides coverage of hospital costs and related services. Coverage is based on the principle of a benefit period. A period begins when a patient enters a hospital and ends when the patient has been out of the hospital for 60 consecutive days. Every new hospital admission begins a new benefit period unless it occurs within 60 days of the patient's last discharge from a hospital (in which case admission is within the prior period). The patient must pay a deductible for each benefit period. If the patient stays in the hospital for more than 60 days, there are additional daily costs called copayments or coinsurance that are paid either by the patient or by the patient's supplementary medical insurance. Part A may also help to pay for up to 100 days of the care received in a skilled nursing facility for rehabilitative services (but not for custodial care received in a nursing home). The first 20 days in a skilled nursing facility are fully paid by Medicare. There is a daily copayment from the 21st day through the 100th day. Part A also pays for most of the cost of the care received in a Medicare-certified hospice center for the terminally ill, and the full costs of home visits for patients who need physical therapy, speech therapy, or part-time skilled nursing care. Part A does not cover full-time nursing care at home, Meals on Wheels, or home services that are needed for personal care or housekeeping.

Part B is designed to pay for doctor's bills, outpatient care, and medical equipment such as wheelchairs and oxygen apparatus. Patients usually are reimbursed for 80% of charges approved by Medicare after they have met a deductible of $100 yearly. Approved charges are usually (about 60% of the time) less than the amount billed by a doctor or other health care provider.

Some medical expenses are not paid by Medicare. They include long-term nursing home care, hearing aids, eyeglasses (except for the first corrective glasses needed after cataract surgery), and routine dental care (extractions, fillings, dentures). Outpatient prescriptions are covered only after an organ transplant or during hospice care. In general, Medicare provides greater support for the physical health needs of elderly people than for their mental health needs (see MENTAL HEALTH AND MENTAL HEALTH SERVICES).

Medication Compliance

Illness usually requires taking medications, the frequency and length of time for which the medications are to be taken vary for different kinds of illnesses. Compliance with the doses of medication and the schedule of administration of those doses is essential for the medication to be effective. Are older people likely to be less compliant than younger adults? The results of several surveys have not been helpful in answering this question because they have yielded conflicting results. Some surveys indicate less compliance within the elderly population and other surveys indicate comparable compliance relative to younger adults. Noncompliance usually means underadherence in the sense of taking less medicine than is needed. It is estimated that about 90% of the noncompliance by older people consists of underadherence.

There are a number of factors suggesting that elderly people are at a greater risk of harm from noncompliance than are younger people. One factor is that the incidence of diseases and illnesses requiring treatment by medication is higher among the elderly population than among the younger population. In addition, more older people than younger people need to take several different medications daily. It is estimated that as many as 25% of elderly people take three or more medications per day. The more medications needed per day, the easier it is to mismanage the schedule. The visual and hearing impairments experienced by many older people add to the possibility of their noncompliance, as does the fact that as many as 25% of elderly people live alone and therefore have no one to check regularly with their compliance. Compliance, regardless of one's age, tends to decrease the longer medications are needed. Elderly people are likely to have illnesses of longer durations than are younger people. Perhaps the most important reason, however, is that elderly people are more hesitant, in general, than younger people in asking their physicians and pharmacists for information about their medications.

The consequences of noncompliance are likely to be more serious for elderly people than for younger people, given the likely age difference in the severity of the illness being treated. These consequences include further medical complications for the noncompliant elderly person and the possibility of an untimely and needless death. It is estimated that about 15% of admissions of elderly people to hospitals result from noncompliance with a medication regimen.

Forgetfulness is a major reason for noncompliance by older people. Fortunately, steps have been taken in recent years to increase the rate of compliance from elderly people. These steps include special packaging and labeling of medications to make it easier to follow a regular schedule in their use and the application of various memory strategies to help elderly people remember when to take their medications. One memory strategy is the use of color-coded pill trays over an extended period of time. Another strategy is the use of a portable bar code reader in which the exact time the medication is taken is measured. One such recording system is the Medication Event Monitoring

System manufactured by the Apex Corporation. A microcomputer in the pill container's lid records the date and hour each time the container is opened. Data are fed to the computer, which generates a compliance report that is available to the patient's physician.

Another system is the Electronic Pill Box Timer-Clock that sells for less than $20. It has two separably programmable timers that sound an alarm at medication time. The patient then resets the timer for the time of the next dose. Researchers in California have also recently discovered that compliance may be increased by the use of a voice mail system.

Medications

Americans spend billions of dollars annually on both prescription and nonprescription medications. Older individuals account for more than a third of the dollars spent on prescription medications. A recent large-scale survey revealed that prescription drugs are used by nearly 70% of men age 65 and older and by about 75% of women age 65 and over. Moreover, the percentage of elderly people taking prescription drugs increases with age after age 65. By contrast, the percentage of elderly people taking nonprescription drugs seems to show little increase with age beyond age 65. The use of medications among the older population is greater for those who smoke and drink alcoholic beverages than for those who do not. More frequent use of medications is also associated with symptoms of depression and with impairment of physical functioning.

The use of medications may present a number of problems for elderly people. According to a study conducted in 1987 by Harvard University researchers, one of the major problems for as many as a fourth of Americans age 65 and older is the prescription of drugs that should *not* be taken. For example, nearly 2 million elderly people had prescriptions for dipyridamole, a blood thinner useful only for people with artificial heart valves, and more than a million had prescriptions for propoxyphene, an addictive narcotic, in place of aspirin. Some of the other major problems related to medication are described in other entries (see MEDICATION COMPLIANCE; MEDICATION SHARING; OVERMEDICATION).

Medication Sharing

Elderly patients are advised to take only medications prescribed by their physicians and to destroy the remaining medicine after the schedule is completed. However, too frequently this destruction is not carried out, and leftover medicines are free to be shared with other older people. A survey conducted by researchers at the University of Iowa revealed that 40% of the elderly people interviewed had shared medicines with someone else. Especially likely to have engaged in this dangerous practice were younger elderly adults, elderly adults who had frequent contact with friends, and elderly adults who had difficulty making an appointment with a physician.

Memory Complaints

Human memory is imperfect at all ages. Nevertheless, older people tend to complain more about their memory problems than do younger people (see DIARY STUDIES OF MEMORY FAILURES). It is true that episodic memory proficiency tends to decline moderately with normal aging. However, some elderly people are unusually upset about their memory ability and complain frequently about it. Others, however, take memory in stride and complain infrequently, if at all. What happens when "complainers" are compared in memory performances with "noncomplainers"? Researchers at Washington University (St. Louis) recruited a number of elderly complainers through newspaper advertisements. They found that the complainers differed little in their laboratory memory performances from those of age-matched noncomplainers. The researchers also found that memory training improved the memory proficiency of the complainers, but it had little effect on their complaints about their memories. It is apparent that some elderly people believe their memory must be functioning very poorly simply because they are old, and that memory must suffer greatly in old age. They therefore tend to exaggerate their minor to moderate memory problems.

Memory for Television Programs

Elderly adults watch several television programs daily. Do they remember less of their contents than do younger adults who watch the same programs? Memory that occurs for the content of television programs (including commercials) is almost certain to be incidental memory. People do not ordinarily watch television with the intent to remember what they are watching, nor are they likely to rehearse that content to themselves in an attempt to ensure its memorability. Nevertheless, the very act of attending to and comprehending the content ensures the automatic memory of much of what is seen. This is apparently as true for older adults as for young adults. Surely, regardless of your age, you still remember much of the content of the *Murder, She Wrote* episode you watched last night. (However, much of that content is likely to be forgotten over time, to the point that when you watch the rerun you may not remember the murderer; see FORGETTING). In several studies, young adult and elderly participants have watched television programs (with commercials inserted) in the laboratory and were then tested for memory of their contents shortly after viewing the programs. In general, age differences in accuracy of memory for the contents have been found to be slight. This should provide some comfort to those advertisers of products relevant to elderly consumers. Unknown is the extent to which elderly adults may forget the content more rapidly than younger adults. Because elderly adults, on the average, watch more television than younger adults, they might be expected to experience more interference from other programs they have viewed and therefore forget more of the content of specific programs.

Memory (Overview)

Imperfections of memory are found at all ages. Memory psychologists studying the effects of aging investigate the extent to which these imperfections increase during late adulthood, the reasons for their occurrence, and the discovery of means by which elderly adults may compensate, at least partially, for whatever declines do occur in memory proficiency. The study of memory and aging is complicated by the fact that diseases that are more often found in late adulthood than in earlier adulthood may be related to the presence of memory problems. This is especially true of cardiovascular diseases (see CARDIOVASCULAR DISEASE AND MENTAL PERFORMANCE). Most aging research on memory is concerned with normal aging's effects on memory, independent of disease complications. For this reason, most research on adult age differences in memory is conducted with older participants who report their health to be good or excellent. It is most important to realize that memory proficiency in late adulthood shows great variability, more so than in earlier adulthood. On most memory tasks, the extent of individual differences is greater for elderly participants than for younger participants. As a result, it is not unusual to discover elderly participants who perform at a level above the average level of performance of even young adults.

The most difficult problem in determining the effects of normal aging is that created by the extreme complexity of the human memory system. The memory system consists of two main components: semantic memory (see SEMANTIC MEMORY; LEXICON) and episodic memory (see EPISODIC MEMORY). (There is a third component known as sensory memory; see SENSORY MEMORY.) The distinction between the two main components is an important one in that aging has little effect on semantic memory and moderate effects, in general, on episodic memory. However, even with episodic memory there are different forms of memory that vary greatly in the extent of their age sensitivity.

Semantic memory is the permanent knowledge of information that is stored without regard to the context (where and when) in which it was acquired. Your knowledge of the capital of Illinois, the square root of 16, and the first president of the United States are stored in semantic memory. Such information is stored without personal reference in terms of when you acquired the knowledge and where it occurred. An especially important part of your semantic memory is your lexicon or mental dictionary (see LEXICON). Stored here are the representations of the words in your vocabulary that you gain access to automatically and rapidly as you read them in a text or hear them in a conversation. In general, we expect to find little change in semantic memory with normal aging. In fact, we are likely to find increases in the amount of information held in our semantic store as we progress from early to late adulthood (see VERBAL ABILITY). Gaining access to the information in the semantic store does slow slightly with aging. Consequently, older adults are likely to be a little slower in reading than younger adults, and they are more likely to have difficulty understanding sentences spoken at a rapid rate.

Episodic memory is memory for personally experienced events or "episodes" in your life. These episodes are stored in memory as memory traces that are in reference to "when" and "where." That is, the time and the location of episodes are contextual components of the information stored. What did you eat for dinner last night? What did you receive as gifts on your tenth birthday? Your correct answers to such questions are possible only because of the record (memory traces) of these events in your long-term episodic store.

When elderly adults complain of their "memory problems," they are usually referring to their episodic memory system. The extent to which episodic memory is affected by normal aging cannot be determined simply. Episodic memory has its own variations and forms. Essential to episodic memory is a piece of "mental equipment" memory researchers call *working memory* (see WORKING MEMORY). Working memory is where limited amounts of information that may either be recalled immediately or within a few seconds without forgetting are held briefly or where you may rehearse that information for transmission to the long-term store for more permanent storage. Information recalled directly from working memory is called *short-term memory* (see SHORT-TERM MEMORY). A familiar example of short-term memory is your retention of a telephone number from a directory that you remember just long enough to dial. Unless actively rehearsed, this kind of information will be lost within 15 to 20 seconds. In general, the capacity of short-term memory declines only slightly with normal aging, and the rate of short-term forgetting is about the same for younger and older people. For example, the digit span of elderly adults, on the average, is only about 5% less than that of young adults.

Information that is rehearsed, encoded as a memory trace, and stored in a long-term store makes up *long-term episodic memory*. It is the current functioning of this form of memory that is of greatest concern to elderly people ("I remember well the events of 50 years ago, but I have trouble remembering those events that happened yesterday"). How age-sensitive is long-term episodic memory, and what is responsible for declines that occur with normal aging? Again, simple answers are not possible. Some forms of long-term episodic memory are more age-sensitive than other forms. For example, recall of information is likely to show greater degrees of age differences favoring younger adults than is the recognition of the same information. This suggests that the retrieval of information from the long-term memory store is an effortful process that is especially difficult for older people. The effort required, and therefore the difficulty, is greatly reduced when only recognition is needed. It is effortful memory that is most often studied in gerontology—for example, memory for lists of words and memory for face-name pairings. In addition, some information is recorded and stored in long-term stores without much effort. It seems to be registered automatically without intent to remember and is brought about either by the simple act of the comprehension of incoming episodic events (e.g., your memory for conversations with other people, your memory for television programs watched and stories read; see, for example, CONVERSATION MEMORY) or by the execution of actions (e.g., turning off the gas on the stove; see ACTION MEMORY).

Such memory functioning is especially important in our everyday lives. The imperfections of memory are apparent at all ages. Most important, the extent of age sensitivity or decline with normal aging appears to be less, on the average, than that found when effort is needed to register information in the long-term store. Episodic memory is also distinguishable in terms of whether it concerns the content of events (e.g., the content of a specific beer commercial you watched on television) or some noncontent characteristic of the event, such as "When was it you last saw that commercial?" The age sensitivity of noncontent memory varies greatly with the nature of the characteristic involved, and is especially large for temporal memory (knowledge of the time of an event; see TEMPORAL MEMORY) and very modest for memory of the frequency with which events occurred (e.g., "How many times in the past week did you see the beer commercial in question?"; see FREQUENCY-OF-OCCURRENCE MEMORY).

There are many other important questions that have been asked (and answered to some degree) by memory researchers. For example, does physical exercise of the right kind slow any age-related declines in memory proficiency? Yes, but only if it has been exercise practiced regularly for a number of years (see EXERCISE AND PHYSICAL/MENTAL PERFORMANCE). Does intensive mental activity during late adulthood relate to the magnitude of age-related declines in memory proficiency? Here, the evidence is somewhat conflicting, and much future research on this topic is needed (see ACTIVITY AND MENTAL PERFORMANCE). Can memory training programs improve the memory proficiency of elderly adults? Probably not, at least the kinds of programs currently in use (see MEMORY TRAINING).

Memory Span

Your memory span for a given type of item is the longest series of items that you can read or listen to and then recall without an error. It is a form of short-term memory or memory over a brief interval that is sometimes used to determine the amount of information that can be held in short-term memory (see SHORT-TERM MEMORY). The most familiar tests of memory span are those for digits and for words. To test digit span, a participant starts by receiving a short series of randomly selected digits (e.g., 5, 2). Assuming this series is recalled correctly, another series is given that is one greater in length than the first series (e.g., 8, 4, 7). This procedure (adding one digit to the series) continues until the participant no longer has an errorless recall of the series. The average digit span has been found to be about 7 digits for young adults and about 6.5 digits for elderly adults (65 to 75 years of age). The age-related decline in span length is thus only about 7% (i.e., the difference between the two average scores divided by the average score made by young adults—0.5 divided by 7). A similar procedure is used to test for word span, only now common words are used instead of digits. The average word span is about six words for young adults and about five for elderly adults, again a modest age difference.

Memory Training

Can memory proficiency be improved? Memory training programs attempt to teach people ways of improving their episodic memory proficiency. Typically, such programs train the participants in the use of what are called *mnemonics* as a means of increasing the proficiency of encoding information for registration in the long-term memory store. A mnemonic is a device or procedure for changing in some way the information you wish to remember in order to make it more memorable. Most mnemonic procedures make use of translating verbal information into images. They are most likely to be applied when the material to be memorized consists of a series of words, such as *car* and *dog*. A participant in a memory training program may be taught to use the method of loci. Here the trick is to make use of a well-traveled pathway with visually distinctive locations along the way. A participant's own house usually offers such a pathway. As you open the front door, you enter a hallway. Now the participant is urged to form an image of a car stuffed inside the hallway. Next comes the living room. Now form an image of a large dog sleeping on the sofa in the living room. This continues throughout the trip through the house, with an image of a word to be remembered in each location. To recall the words, you make the trip again, this time capturing the image of each word as you encounter it. An alternative procedure is called the pegword method. Here the participant is first taught a rhyme that begins with "One is a bun," "two is a shoe," and so on. Now the trick is to form an image of each word to be remembered with the object named in the rhyme. Thus you might form an image of a Detroit (or Tokyo) sandwich in which a car (the first word in the list) is stuffed in a bun and dripping with mustard and other goodies, then an image of a dog wearing highly polished shoes, and so on. To recall the words, you simply say each number in the rhyme to yourself (e.g., "one"), recover the object named with it (e.g., a bun) and the image of the word to be remembered (e.g., a car). Elderly adults can learn to use either the method of loci or the pegword method. However, they are likely to discover that these methods have little usefulness in the everyday world. It is not often necessary to memorize a list of words, even a shopping list—why not write down the items and take the shopping list with you? Moreover, the methods rely on imagery, and elderly people are less proficient in the use of imagery than younger people (see

IMAGERY). Even memory researchers report they rarely, if ever, use these mnemonic procedures in their daily lives.

A somewhat more useful mnemonic is the keyword method. It may be used to learn either face-name pairings or foreign language equivalents of English words. In either case, imagery again is a basic ingredient of the mnemonic. Consider meeting Mr. Whalen at a party. The first step in associating his name with his face is to identify a prominent feature of Mr. Whalen's face (e.g., a large mouth). The next step is to translate the person's name into a word that is easily imagined (e.g., "a whale" in the case of Mr. Whalen). The final step is to imagine the imagined object in interaction with the prominent facial feature (e.g., a whale stuffed inside a large mouth). The idea is that on your next encounter with Mr. Whalen, you will notice the prominent mouth, recover the image of a whale, and hopefully come up with "Hi there, Mr. Whalen." As with other mnemonics, elderly adults can be taught to use the keyword method to learn new face and name pairings. However, they are likely to abandon its use rather quickly. Again, the use of imagery decreases in proficiency with normal aging. Moreover, how often can you use a large mouth as the prominent feature? Surely you will encounter other people with the same prominent feature, and confusion as to which image to retrieve for recalling the correct name will surely result.

The keyword method is probably most useful when you plan to visit a foreign country and you would like to know a few words in that country's language. Suppose you plan to visit Russia, and for some reason you would like to remember that the Russian word for mountain is *gora*. To use the keyword method, you would translate the Russian word to an English word that both sounds like a part (not necessarily all) of the foreign word and is very imaginable. In this case, the keyword word might be *garage*. Then form an image of a mountain stuffed inside a garage. When you next encounter *gora*, the image you retrieve should help you to remember that it means "a mountain."

Researchers at Washington University (St. Louis) have prepared a self-instructional manual that describes these mnemonics (and others as well, such as the use of organizational strategies to find relatedness among events to be remembered; see EPISODIC MEMORY), and practice exercises in their use. However, they have discovered that the greatest benefit from the use of the manual comes when participants also meet in group sessions with a trainer and other participants to discuss their memory problems and how mnemonics may help to reduce them.

Most problems with remembering name-face pairings are not likely to be memory problems at all. They are more likely to be attentional problems. You probably were not paying sufficient attention to fully hear the person's name when he or she was introduced to you. When you do hear the name, repeat it several times to yourself while looking at the person's face. If you are introduced to several people at about the same time, an effective way of improving your later memory of their names is to wait 15 or 20 seconds after the introductions and then recall the names while looking again at their faces. Elderly people, in general, do have long-term memory retrieval problems. The short-term retrieval of people's names should enhance later retrievability. Unfortunately, memory training programs usually offer little assistance in improving the retrieval of information from memory. The probable emphasis is on getting information into memory.

There is an important (and perhaps the most important) further potential use of memory training. Depressed elderly people frequently express great concern about their memory problems. Researchers have discovered that a number of these depressed individuals have a significant reduction in their memory concerns after completion of a memory training program. Most important, many of them also appear to have a reduction in the intensity of their depressive symptoms.

Menopause

Menopause is the end of menstruation. While in their 40s, women's menstrual cycles tend to become irregular, and they usually stop by the age of 50 to 55 years. The transition period during which ovulation stops is called the climacteric. Until recently, the end of ovulation was viewed as the end of a woman's childbearing years. This has changed drastically with the in vitro fertilization of women in their 60s. With menopause there is a decrease in the levels of the sex hormones (estrogen and progesterone) produced by the ovaries. The walls of the vagina become thinner and less elastic, and the production of vaginal lubricants decreases. The changes in the vagina may cause it to become irritated and lead to dyspareunia (painful intercourse). However, not every woman experiences these changes. For some they may last for years after menopause; for others they may occur only early in menopause. The decrease in hormonal levels often results in hot flashes, headaches, and various other symptoms. Hot flashes vary in their frequency and severity. They usually last for about a minute, and, in some women, they may occur four or five times a day. Some women experience nervousness and/or a degree of depression. Irritability may occur because of sleep disturbances from hot flashes. The decrease in estrogen level may also lead to osteoporosis (see DISEASES [CHRONIC]).

Many postmenstrual women benefit greatly from estrogen replacement therapy. One such benefit is the frequent reduction in the severity of the symptoms that accompany menopause, such as hot flashes. Moreover, there is evidence to indicate that estrogen replacement therapy may reduce the risk of osteoporosis, colon cancer, and perhaps even Alzheimer's disease (see ALZHEIMER'S DISEASE; DISEASES [CHRONIC]).

There are a number of excellent books on menopause in women and the changes accompanying it. They include *Menopause Naturally: Preparing for the Second Half of Life*, by Sadja Greenwood, M.D., *Menopause: A Midlife Passeage*, edited by Joan C. Callahan, and *Menopause: A Positive Approach*, by Rosetta Reitz.

Some men experience a form of "male menopause." There is a decrease in the male sex hormone testosterone in the late 60s. During this period, some men may display symptoms similar to those found in female menopause, such as hot flashes. However, the decline in testosterone production for most older men is much less than the decline in the sex hormone production for most older women.

Mental Health and Mental Health Services

Satisfactory mental health usually means that an individual is satisfied with his or her life, is adapting adequately to everyday pressures and stressors, is free of intense negative emotions such as anxiety, depression, and hostility, is free of psychosis and neurosis, and is free of negative personality traits like neuroticism. There is no reason to believe that the mental health status of older adults, in general, differs greatly from that of younger adults, in general. When asked to rate their life satisfaction, elderly adults express a degree of satisfaction that is about the same as that of younger adults (see LIFE SATISFACTION). Most elderly adults are fairly successful in coping with problems and stresses in their lives (see STRESS AND COPING WITH STRESS). Severe depression seems to be no more prevalent in late adulthood than in earlier adulthood (see DEPRESSION [INCIDENCE, SYMPTOMS, CAUSES]). The onset of psychosis and neurosis is rare in late adulthood (see PSYCHOSIS; NEUROSIS). Negative personality traits such as neuroticism show little increase from early to late adulthood (see NEUROTICISM; PERSONALITY TRAITS).

Nevertheless, a number of elderly adults do experience mental distress, just as many younger adults do, and they, like younger adults, may benefit from treatment by mental health professionals. Unfortunately, such treatment is less likely to be received by older adults than by younger adults. Surveys have indicated that only around 6% of the services offered by community mental health centers are provided to older adults, and an even smaller percentage of private practice mental health services is provided for older clients. Part of the problem is the fact that training programs for mental health professionals, including both clinical psychologists and psychiatrists, have often ignored training experiences with the unique mental problems of elderly people (e.g., stress from the death of a spouse). Also part of the problem is the fact that Medicare has placed financial obstacles in the way of treating elderly clients with low incomes. In the past, there has been a bias in the Medicare program against the long-term treatment of chronic mental and emotional problems. Inpatient services under Part A of Medicare were limited to a total of 190 days, and outpatient services under Part B to a 50% to 60% copayment rate in contrast to the 80% to 20% rate for physical health services. The bias also is evident in limitation of the services offered by a clinical psychologist to elderly clients. Diagnostic testing was reimbursed only if it had been requested by a physician, and psychotherapy only if it was supervised by a physician. Fortunately, these restrictions are gradually changing through the efforts of mental health professionals to influence Congress to modify the provisions of Medicare. For example, a bill passed in 1988 enabled psychologists to be paid by Medicare for services provided independently of physicians at rural health clinics and community mental health centers.

A further problem remains—namely, the reluctance of many older people to seek help for their mental and emotional problems, a reluctance much greater than that found for younger adults. This problem should diminish in the future as currently younger adults reach late adulthood. They will bring with them a greater knowledge of mental health services and a greater knowledge of what may be accomplished by such services.

Mental Status Questionnaire

The Mental Status Questionnaire is widely used as part of the diagnostic procedure used to identify individuals likely to have true dementia, as distinguished from memory problems related to normal aging or depression-induced mental problems. The questionnaire is a 10-item inventory designed to determine the effectiveness of an individual's orientation with regard to time and place. Included are questions such as: "What is today's date?" "What is the month now?" "How old are you now?" and "Who is president of the United States?"

Metamemory

"My memory is terrible—I can't even remember what I had for dinner last night." "I have trouble remembering the names of new people I meet." "My memory at age 70 is as good as it was 30 years ago."

The people making these statements are, in effect, evaluating the proficiency of their own memory capabilities. Knowledge of our own memory system is termed *metamemory*. Metamemory includes more than knowledge (correct or incorrect) about your memory proficiency. It also includes your knowledge of how to improve your memory through the use of effective strategies.

One method used to determine age differences in the knowledge people have (or believe they have) of their own memory proficiencies is completion of a questionnaire in which respondents rate their proficiency on various forms and tasks of everyday memory functioning (see METAMEMORY IN ADULTHOOD [MIA] QUESTIONNAIRE AND META-MEMORY FUNCTIONING QUESTIONNAIRE [MFQ]). In general, these ratings reveal that older adults have a lower regard for and less confidence in their memory abilities than do younger adults. However, the scores of elderly participants on laboratory memory tasks have been found to be only slightly related to their proficiency ratings, and older adults with memory complaints usually perform as well on these tasks as do noncomplainers (see MEMORY COMPLAINTS). In addition, there is evidence to indicate that individuals may not be the best evaluators of their own memory abilities. The ratings given by spouses of older people tend to relate more closely to scores earned on laboratory memory tasks than do the ratings given by the task performers themselves.

Another way to evaluate age differences in the knowledge (or lack of knowledge) of people about their memory abilities is to have them predict how well they do on a memory task they are about to receive. Suppose, for example, that you know you will have 3 minutes to study a list of 20 common words (e.g., apple, table), and that you will then be asked to recall as many of the words as possible in whatever order you wish. How many words would you predict that you would recall? Five? You don't have much confidence in your memory ability. Fifteen? Overconfident, perhaps? When faced with making this prediction, elderly participants tend to make the same prediction, on the average, as do young adult participants (usually a prediction of about

10 words). The actual number of words recalled is likely to be closer to the predicted number for the young participants than for the older participants. In other words, elderly participants tend to be somewhat overconfident in their memory ability despite the lower ratings they usually assign to their memory functioning.

Overconfidence by older participants is revealed further when the situation with a word list is changed. This time the participants are told to study the word list until they are ready to recall all of the words. Elderly participants, on the average, spend less time studying the list than do young adult participants, and therefore recall fewer words than do the young participants. Interestingly, when older participants are required to spend as much time studying as the average time spent studying by young participants, their recall scores more closely approximate those of the young participants.

Knowledge of how to use memory strategies effectively is especially important for proficient memory performances. Suppose you have been given a list of seven common words to learn in a specific order (i.e., serial learning; see VERBAL LEARNING) and without error. You have as much time as you need to master the list. An effective strategy for making certain of an observable errorless recall would be to study the list for a while and then monitor yourself to recall the words. If you found you made an error, you should study more and then test yourself again. This cycle of study–self-testing should continue until you no longer make an error. Researchers at the University of Akron discovered that this self-monitoring or self-testing strategy was used by most of their young adult participants, but by few of the older participants. When other elderly participants were instructed regarding the value of self-testing and encouraged to use this strategy, they approximated the level of performance of young adults who spontaneously engaged in self-testing.

The effective use of memory strategies is likely to be part of the content in a memory training course for elderly adults. For this reason alone, it is probably worthwhile for elderly people who seem to have a memory problem to participate in such a course.

Metamemory in Adulthood (MIA) Questionnaire and Metamemory Functioning Questionnaire (MFQ)

These questionnaires are the two most widely used tests for assessing a subject's view about how well his or her memory system is functioning in the everyday world (see METAMEMORY). The MIA has 120 items that measure eight dimensions of memory functioning. For example, one of the dimensions is labeled "Capacity," and it is measured by such questions "I am good at remembering names (yes or no)." Another dimension is labeled "Strategy," and it is measured by such questions as "Do you write appointments on a calendar to help you remember them (yes or no)?"

The MFQ has 64 items that evaluate memory functioning in terms of seven different scales. One of these scales is labeled "Frequency of Forgetting," and it is measured by questions such as "How often do these present a memory problem to you? . . . names" (then other sources of potential problems are given). Another scale is labeled "Retrospective Functioning." It is measured by questions such as "How is your memory compared to the way it was . . . one year ago?" Other time references are also given.

Metaphors

Metaphors are frequently used in both literature and everyday communication. A metaphor is a figure of speech in which a word or phrase indicating one kind of idea or object is used in place of another through the use of a comparison (analogy) between the substitute and the idea or object it replaces. A familiar example is "The ship plows the sea." Here the ship replaces farm equipment that plows the land. Thus the ship moves through the sea much the same as the farm equipment moves through the land. When given novel metaphors to interpret (e.g., "Man is a wolf"), older adults have been found to be just as insightful, if not more so, than young adults in their interpretations. This is to be expected, given the fact that verbal abilities in general are largely unaffected by normal aging (see VERBAL ABILITY).

Mini-Mental State Test

The Mini-Mental State Test is one of the several tests used in the diagnosis of dementia. It contains 11 items dealing with the orientation, concentration, and language functioning of the client. For example, temporal orientation is tested by asking the year, season, month, date, and day when the testing occurs. Language functioning is tested by such requests as asking the client to write a sentence and to repeat the phrase "No ifs, ands, or buts." Individuals with true dementia are likely to score very low on these questions. For example, they are unlikely to know what year or day it is.

Motion Perception

Sensitivity to the motion of objects takes several forms. One involves the ability to detect whether two slightly moving objects are moving in the same direction or in opposite directions. Elderly adults generally show moderately poorer discrimination of direction than do younger adults. Another form involves the ability to detect slight motion for a previously stationary object. Researchers at Case Western Reserve University have discovered that older women tend to have higher motion thresholds (i.e., it takes more movement before being detected) than elderly men and that elderly men are about as proficient as young adults in detecting motion. They have also discovered that patients with Alzheimer's disease have significantly less sensitivity than normally aging individuals in detecting motion and that their sensitivity becomes progressively worse as dementia progresses.

Motor Behavior

Motor behavior refers to muscular actions performed to fulfill some objective of the performer. Examples of everyday motor behaviors are braking a car, pushing a lawn mower, shifting gears of a car, and hitting a golf ball. Although normally aging people are perfectly capable of performing most motor behavior, nevertheless some attributes of motor behaviors are expected to be affected by aging. Most apparent is the slower reaction time in initiating motor behaviors and the longer time required to complete many motor behaviors (e.g., locomotion). For example, it is expected that elderly people generally will be slower in braking their cars than younger people when some external event signals the need for braking.

Laboratory research has revealed that there are also more subtle age differences in motor behaviors. For example, age differences have been found by researchers at the University of Wisconsin in the use of advance information to aid selection of a specific required behavior. Their participants performed simple movements of their arms that varied over trials in terms of which arm to move, the direction of the movement, and the extent of the movement. Different amounts of advance information were given over many trials. On some trials, no advance information was given as to which arm would be signaled to move, which direction would be signaled, and the extent of the movement. On other trials, only one bit of advance information was given (e.g., which arm would be signaled to move). On still other trials, two bits of information were given (e.g., which arm to move and in which direction). On the remaining trials, all three bits of advance information were given (which arm, what direction, and how far). The researchers found that the speed of movement in response to the investigator's signal was, as expected, slower for elderly participants than for younger participants regardless of the amount of advance information given. However, younger participants benefited less from advance information than did older participants. That is, their speed in responding was nearly as fast when no advance information was given as when all three bits of advance information were given. By contrast, the response speed for elderly participants was much slower without advance information than with all three bits of information. It does take older people longer to prepare for a movement than it does younger people. Therefore any early start in preparing for that movement (as in the use of advance information) provides a greater advantage for older people than for younger people. Younger people are so fast in their behaviors that there is little room for advance information to facilitate their behaviors. The Wisconsin researchers also found that elderly participants have greater difficulty than younger participants in coordinating movements of the two hands.

Motor Skill Learning

We learn many motor skills during the course of our lives and at different times in our lives. We learn to ride a bicycle, to play the piano, to drive a car, to type, to play golf, and so on. In each case, learning requires coordination between perception and muscular actions. For this reason, motor skill learning is often called *perceptual-motor learning*. Of interest is the effect of aging on both the retention of motor skills learned years ago and the acquisition of new motor skills.

Many motor skills learned years ago are retained remarkably well with considerable practice of those skills. For example, professional golfers, musicians, and typists practice their respective skills virtually daily throughout their adult lives. Jack Nicklaus continues to be a great golfer even though he is now in his 50s. Great musicians like Pablo Casals and Arthur Rubinstein gave many excellent performances at very advanced ages. Skilled typists continue to do well into late adulthood. But what about skills that have not been practiced during the intervening years? A familiar observation is that after years of not riding a bicycle, most people are able to regain their earlier skill with little practice. There is a large savings in terms of the amount of practice needed to regain the skill relative to the amount of practice needed to acquire the skill originally. There is evidence to indicate that the savings is also large for typing after some years of not doing any typing.

Of course, motor skill learning does not cease for older people. They may decide to take up golf when they are in their 60s or 70s, or they may have the need to acquire computer skills. Unfortunately, some may have to learn how to maneuver a wheelchair.

Age differences in motor skill learning have been investigated in the laboratory largely through the use of two different tasks. The first is called the pursuit-rotor task. A disk revolves fairly rapidly while a participant tries to maintain contact with a stylus on a designated part of the disk. Participants are given many trials of a set duration (e.g., 30 seconds). A number of studies have indicated that both young adults and older adults steadily improve the amount of time spent maintaining appropriate contact with the stylus as practice progresses. Learning occurs as participants acquire the visual-hand coordination needed to perform the task. However, the rate of learning is considerably slower for elderly subjects than for younger subjects.

The second task involves mirror-image tracking in which participants move a stylus through a six-pointed star cut through a metal plate while viewing the star in the mirror (i.e., what the participant sees is the reverse of the actual movements). Both young adults and elderly adults improve with practice on this task. The time needed to move through the star decreases regardless of age, as does the accuracy of movement. However, as with the pursuit-rotor task, the rate of learning the visual-hand coordination needed to perform the task is much slower for older adults. The same age difference is present even when an everyday kind of task is brought into the laboratory. In particular, elderly participants have been found to learn word processing skills, but at a much slower rate than young adult participants. However, the rate of learning differs little between young adults and middle-aged adults. Learning of new motor skills clearly is well within the capabilities of most elderly people, but, as with other forms of learning, it is likely to be at a slower rate of progress. This is true for learning word processing and other computer skills. A number of researchers have found that older adults can learn computer skills, but at a slower rate and with more errors than for younger adults. There are now computer networks that exist largely for people older than 65 years of age. The most popular is Senior Net, which has over 13,000 members. It provides useful information about health, Social Security, and other topics of great interest to older people.

Multi-infarct Dementia

Multi-infarct dementia (formerly called cerebral arteriosclerosis) accounts for 10% to 20% of adult dementia. It consists of mental impairment caused by a stroke in which the flow of blood in the brain is disrupted (called an infarct) and areas of the brain are damaged. A series of strokes may produce pronounced dementia in the form of memory loss and disorientation and, in some cases, losses in the ability to understand language or to produce appropriate language (an aphasia; see APHASIA) and/or to recognize objects (agnosia).

Multi-infarct dementia differs from that found in Alzheimer's disease in several ways. The onset is sudden, rather than gradual (as in Alzheimer's disease), and the progression in severity occurs in stages or steps rather than continuously (as in Alzheimer's disease). The extent of dementia tends to stabilize (and improvement may occur with speech therapy and other forms of therapy, and even without the intervention of therapy) until another stroke occurs. If another stroke occurs, the severity of impairment is likely to increase.

Multi-infarct dementia is more common in men than in women; the reverse is true for Alzheimer's disease. Multi-infarct disease often occurs earlier in life than Alzheimer's disease. Neurologically, patients with multi-infarct dementia tend to have fewer senile plaques and neurofibrillary tangles in neurons than patients with Alzheimer's disease (see ALZHEIMER'S DISEASE). Perhaps the most important difference between the two diseases is that multi-infarct disease may be prevented in many cases by medications for hypertension (high blood pressure), changes in diet and exercise habits, treatment of diabetes, and the cessation of smoking and alcohol consumption. Currently there is no known method of preventing Alzheimer's disease.

Myths about Aging

A myth is a widely held false belief, usually resulting from hearsay evidence and causal and inaccurate evidence. There are many myths about human aging. For example, many people believe that there have been individuals who have lived 130 and even more years. There is no carefully documented evidence to indicate that this is true (see LIFE SPAN). Another biological myth about aging is that most people age 65 and older are so physically incapacitated that they cannot function on their own. In truth, nearly 90% of people in that age range manage to function adequately in their daily living.

Perhaps the most prevalent myth about aging is that most older people become asexual, both in the sense of losing interest in sexual behavior and in the sense of losing the ability to perform sexually (see SEXUAL BEHAVIOR).

Myths are also widespread regarding the mental functioning of elderly people, including the belief that they are incapable of new learning (the "you can't teach old dogs new tricks" falsehood) and the belief that memory overall deteriorates greatly in late adulthood. Older people are indeed capable of new learning, even though it may progress a bit more slowly than it does in younger people. Memory is a complex system made up of a number of components, some of which show modest declines in proficiency for many people as they age, but other components are remarkably resistant to declines in proficiency in late adulthood (see MEMORY [OVERVIEW]). Unfortunately, myths about aging are held not only by many young adults but also by many older people. Such beliefs could have serious negative consequences. For example, those elderly people who believe that new learning is beyond their present capabilities are unlikely to make an effort to participate in new learning experiences. One of the major objectives of gerontological research is to replace myths with facts based on scientific evidence.

N

. . . .

Nails

Fingernails and toenails do not grow as rapidly for elderly people as they do for younger people, and they therefore require less-frequent trimming in later adulthood than in earlier adulthood. On the other hand, elderly adults' nails become dry and brittle, and they are more difficult to trim than they are for younger adults. Consequently, the need for assistance in trimming nails, especially toenails, tends to be greater for elderly adults than for younger adults.

National Institute on Aging

In 1974, the United States Congress passed the Research on Aging Act. The act noted the absence of any American institution devoted to intensive studies of the biomedical and behavioral aspects of aging. To remedy this problem, the act created the National Institute on Aging as the eleventh component of the National Institutes of Health. Operation of the Institute began in 1976 with Dr. Robert Butler as the first permanent director. One of the first steps taken by the Institute was the incorporation into its programs of the Baltimore Longitudinal Study that had begun in 1958 (see BALTIMORE LONGITUDINAL STUDY). Other programs soon became part of the Institute's operations. They included the Biomedical Research and Clinical Medicine Program, the Behavioral Sciences Research Program, and the Epidemiology, Demography, and Biometry Program. Some of these programs fund research by highly qualified scientists at universities and medical centers. Other programs are conducted by scientists who work directly in laboratories operated by the Institute. Throughout its history, Alzheimer's disease and geriatric medicine have been major priorities of the Institute. The Institute is generally considered to be the premier institute on aging in the world. For further information write to the National Institute on Aging at 9000 Rockville Pike, Bldg. 31 #5 C35, Bethesda, MD 20892-3100 (telephone, 301-496-9265).

Neuropsychology

Neuropsychology is the branch of psychology that deals with the relationship among the brain, mental functions, and behavior. Neuropsychologists are heavily involved in research on the effects of various brain disorders on memory performances and the reasons why these effects occur (e.g., what area of the brain is dysfunctioning to produce memory impairment). They are the most likely researchers on the impairment in memory found in Alzheimer's disease, other adult dementias, and in other amnesic conditions such as that found in Korsakoff's disease. Neuropsychologists are also likely to be part of the diagnostic team in the diagnosis of Alzheimer's disease. Such diagnosis requires the distinction between normal aging's effects on memory and dementia's effects, as well as the separation of dementia's effects on memory from those of depression's effects.

Neurosis

A neurosis is a less severe psychological disorder than is a psychosis (see PSYCHOSIS), although neurotic symptoms may certainly make everyday functioning difficult. It is unusual for a neurotic person to become psychotic as the symptoms worsen. Individuals who are neurotic simply become more intensely neurotic. There are various forms of neuroses that differ in their symptoms. These include anxiety neurosis and obsessive-complusive neurosis. Anxiety neurosis is characterized by an enduring, persistent feeling of uneasiness. Obsessive-compulsive disorder is characterized either by obsession with some trend of thought or by some ritualistic compulsive act (such as repeated hand washing to avoid contact with germs). Other neuroses are hypochondria in which a person believes he or she suffers from or may contract a particular disease and anorexia nervosa (in which individuals starve themselves). The onset of neurosis in late adulthood is rare. Well-adjusted younger people tend to become well-adjusted elderly people. However, young neurotics who remain uncured are likely to become elderly neurotics with the continuation of their symptoms.

A myth of aging is that the proportion of hypochondriacs among elderly people is greater than it is among younger adults. The incidence of hypochondriosis is no greater in late adulthood than in earlier stages of adulthood. A true hypochondriac is likely to regard physical symptoms such as irregular bowel movements as an indication of a serious disease when medical evidence shows that none exists. When many elderly adults report various physical symptoms, they are likely to be manifestations of normal aging and not of hypochondria.

Neuroticism

Neuroticism is one of the basic personality traits identified by psychologists (see PERSONALITY TRAITS). At the low extreme of this trait are individuals who are well adjusted and emotionally stable, while at the high extreme are individuals who show maladaptive behavior (i.e., self-defeating behavior that interferes with daily living) and negative emotions (e.g., anxiety and depression). Those individuals with neurosis score very high on this trait. However, neuroticism in varying degrees is one of the dimensions of normal personality. Most individuals fall in the middle between the two extremes of the trait. Of those individuals who score high in neuroticism, most are not considered to be true neurotics who possess clinically significant symptoms. As is true for most personality traits, there is considerable evidence to indicate that neuroticism is remarkably stable with normal aging. That is, current elderly people who score low, average, or high in neuroticism were likely to have scored similarly as low, average, or high when they were young adults. One's level of neuroticism at any age level is an important determinant of life satisfaction and psychological well-being. A high level of neuroticism at any age level is a likely reason for medical complaints that have no apparent physical cause.

Nightmares

A nightmare is a frightening dream, usually so intense that it awakens the sleeper. Adults of all ages are susceptible to occasional nightmares. Of interest is whether they are especially likely to occur among older adults. The results from a recent study by researchers at the University of Arizona suggest that the frequency of nightmares is actually lower among healthy older adults than among college students. The participants in their study kept a log for several weeks in which they recorded each morning the number of nightmares they had during the previous night. Only about 25% of the elderly reported having at least one nightmare during the 2-week period, in contrast to the nearly 50% of the college students. The overall number of nightmares reported during the interval was nearly twice as high for the college students as for the elderly adults.

Normative Aging Study

The Normative Aging Study is a program of longitudinal research that is supervised by the Veterans Administration. It began in 1963 with the selection of more than 2,000 healthy male participants from the Boston area who were recruited largely by newspaper and radio advertisements. At the time of the study's initiation the participants ranged in age from the 20s to more than 75 years, with an average age of about 45 years. The participants have received medical examinations and other tests every 5 years until they reached age 52. After that age they are retested every 3 years. By 1985, 84% of the original group of participants remained in the study. At that time the average age of the participants had reached 61 years.

The study has been concerned with both physical and mental health and with the factors that may lead to decline in each with aging. For example, components of the study have involved investigations of the predictors from earlier adult life of the development of hypertension in later life, the effects of smoking on health in later life, and effects of retirement on health. The results obtained in the Normative Aging Study have contributed substantially to our knowledge of the causes of health problems in late adulthood.

Norms

One of the uses of the term *norms* is in the description of the standing of individuals with respect to others their own age. Familiar to parents is the news that their child is at the 50th percentile rank in weight. This means that their child is average in weight, in the sense that the child has a "score" corresponding to the average score (i.e., weight) for children his or her own age. If the parents heard that their child is at the 25th percentile, then they would know that he or she is somewhat below average in weight. Elderly adults may similarly discover their standing in weight with respect to other elderly people. Students taking college admission tests are similarly identified in terms of where they rank relative to other students on the same test. A score of 500 usually means that they have a score at the 50th percentile.

To be useful in knowing where an individual ranks with respect to others his or her own age, norms must be derived from a representative sample of individuals that age. Thus to gather norms for weight, a large sample of children of a given age must be selected so that they are representative of all children of that age in terms of race, rural/urban residence, socioeconomic status of their parents, and so on.

Based on the average weight and the variability of weights around that average for this representative sample, norms in the form of percentiles may be established.

Norms for mental performances and characteristics are, unfortunately, uncommon, especially after childhood. The major exception is for intelligence tests, particularly the Wechsler Adult Intelligence Scale (see WECHSLER INTELLIGENCE TESTS). Large and fairly representative samples of adults at a number of different age ranges were tested in the standardization of this test. For a given age range, say 60 to 64, the average test score for the representative sample of people was assigned the intelligence quotient (IQ) value of 100. The score that was one standard deviation above average (a standard deviation is the score that when added to and subtracted from the average score gives the range of scores within which the middle third of the distribution of scores may be found; see VARIABILITY OF BEHAVIOR) was assigned the value of 115. Intelligence test scores tend to follow a normal probability (bell-shaped) curve or distribution; this means that roughly 34% of the sample had scores that corresponded to IQs between 100 and 115 and 16% had scores corresponding to IQs greater that 115. Similarly, a score that was two standard deviations above average was assigned the IQ value of 130, with roughly 2.5% of the sample having scores greater than an IQ of 130. The norms based on this sample may then be used to identify the rank of any individual aged 60 to 64 years who takes the test relative to the original representative sample. If that individual scores an IQ of 100, then he or she is at the 50th percentile (average). If the person scores 115 or 130, then he or she would be at the 84th or 97.5th percentile, respectively. Thus the norms for this test are age-appropriate norms that take into account the decline in test scores that may occur with normal aging. That is, your normative score is based on others your own age, and not on the performance of only young adults.

Unfortunately, there are few other mental tests or tasks that are normatively age-based in the same way as the Wechsler Adult Intelligence Scale. The selection of large and representative samples is a very difficult, expensive, and tedious process. The Wechsler Memory Scale that is widely used in memory dysfunction diagnosis does have norms of this kind, but they are generally considered by experts to be inadequate. Patient (and compulsive—and well-funded) researchers of gerontology are needed to provide the kinds of norms needed to interpret the performances of elderly adults on various mental tasks.

The term norms is used in another way as well, namely, in terms of incidence rates for such events as diseases, deaths, divorces, life crises, and dementia. Surveys or examinations of large samples of people are needed to determine what percentage in each age group is characterized by the event. Thus for a particular disease we may discover that the national incidence rate for people age 55 to 64 years is 10% and for people age 65 or older it is 35%. We would know immediately that the event in question is especially related to late adulthood. If we knew the incidence rate in a particular part of the country is well above the norm (e.g., 55% when the national norm for people age 65 or older is 35%), we would have reason to examine what is causing this striking disparity. Or when we know the normative incidence rates for thyroid disorders, and discover both husband and wife have the disorder, we are bewildered by the seeming defiance of the laws of probability, and we begin to wonder if the correspondence is only a coincidence. Similarly, when we know that divorce is more the norm for younger people than for older people, we have a better understanding of why it is often more stressful for the elderly people—it is less expected.

Nursing Home Staff (Resident Dependency)

Many nursing home residents become almost completely dependent on staff members to perform everyday behaviors they are capable of doing themselves (e.g., washing their faces, feeding themselves). Staff members often expect residents to be dependent on them, and they therefore fail to encourage the residents to be as behaviorally independent as possible. Residents, in turn, are often rewarded for their dependency on staff members by the attention given to them by the staff. The danger is that residents may lose skills they possess if they are not practiced regularly, thus making them increasingly more dependent on others to help them.

Researchers in Germany have developed a training program for staff members of nursing homes that enables at least some staff members to change their caregiving style in a way that encourages more independence on the part of the residents under their care—and without risk to the well-being of the residents. Nursing homes should be encouraged to train their personnel to behave in ways that are suited to the skill levels of their elderly residents. Residents who are able to perform basic behaviors without assistance should be encouraged to do so.

Nutrition and Diet

Guidelines for good nutrition and a healthy diet in late adulthood closely resemble those in earlier adulthood—plenty of green vegetables and fresh fruits, protein sources that offer balanced amino acids, whole grains, and so on. However, more proteins may be needed in very late adulthood because protein metabolism may decline in efficiency. An increase in protein intake is often recommended for people with various diseases, and the proportion of elderly people with these diseases is greater than it is for younger people. One problem facing elderly people with a low income is the high cost of meat, the common source of much of our protein intake. Poor chewing ability may also limit the amount of meat consumed by many elderly people. Dairy products and eggs may serve as a substitute, but they may, in some cases, present their own dietary problems, especially by increasing "bad" cholesterol levels. Fish and poultry are also substitutes, but they too are expensive, and difficult to chew for some elderly people. A protein balance of the essential amino acids may be approximated by casseroles of beans and rice. Such casseroles have the advantage of being both inexpensive and easy to chew.

Carbohydrates make up the major portion of diets at all ages. Aging is associated with a delay in the return of blood glucose levels to basal values after the consumption of glucose substances. It is estimated that 20% of older people have difficulty regulating glucose in their blood and have impaired glucose tolerance that is associated with an increased mortality rate from cardiovascular diseases. Such substances as nondietary candies and soft drinks should probably be avoided as much as possible by many elderly people. The vitamin and mineral needs of elderly people are about the same as they are for younger people. Vitamin supplements should not be needed for most elderly people who consume a balanced diet. When supplements are needed, they should be at the recommendation of one's physician and a professional dietitian. According to a researcher at Boston University Medical Center, elderly people with a vitamin D deficiency should compensate for the deficiency by soaking up sunshine in small daily amounts on their hands, arms, and face (without sun block) rather than by increasing the amount of their milk consumption.

Elderly people who have an inadequate diet and are malnourished, and those who are underweight, are especially vulnerable to diseases and to risk of death during surgery and stress. The mortality rate for very thin and frail elderly people has been found to equal that for obese elderly people. The mortality rate for obese elderly people is especially high when they have hypertension and some other diseases. Overweight elderly people should consider behavior modification (see PSYCHOTHERAPY) as a means of controlling their food intake and weight. Dietary restrictions and the form of exercise should be recommended by the obese person's physician.

Unfortunately, there are apparently a number of older adults who do indeed have an inadequate diet. A recent survey by researchers at the Ross Laboratories in Ohio of the food intake of nearly 500 normally aging adults age 65 to 98 years revealed that 40% of these people have energy intakes from food that were well below the recommended amount. A number of these people also had deficiencies in their mineral intake. Alarmingly, more than 20% of the participants reported that they ordinarily did not eat lunch.

Body changes that occur with simply growing older do require some adjustments in the diets of older people. In general, people over age 30 lose 2% to 3% of their lean body mass during each successive decade of their lives. This loss is accompanied by an increase in body fat. For men, increased body fat usually results in a "spare tire" (or middle-aged spread) around the middle of the body. For women, increased body fat may settle in the hips and thighs, in the buttocks, or in the middle of the body. A spokeswoman for the American Dietetic Association recently alerted men and women to the fact that if they continue eating after age 30 as they did when they were younger, men will gain, on the average 1½ pounds per year and women 1 pound. To maintain weight at the level it was at age 30, a person needs up to 5% fewer calories during each successive decade of living. However, the nutrient needs remain the same. Thus to reduce calorie intake, while maintaining basic nutrients in the diet, potato chips and other junk foods should be eliminated largely from their daily intake of food. Women, in general, have a greater problem than men in controlling their weight because they consume fewer calories and therefore have fewer calories that can be varied while retaining basic nutrients. There is limited evidence to indicate that aerobic exercise and weight lifting helps to retard the loss of lean body mass.

Proper nutrition and diet for elderly people may be impaired by conditions that interfere with normal eating behavior. Eating commonly occurs in the presence of others eating at the same time, and it therefore serves as a source of (usually) pleasant social interactions. Perhaps the most serious negative condition is widowhood. A study by researchers at Georgia State University of 50 recently widowed elderly women revealed that the loss of their spouses had negative effects on their motivation to cook and to eat. Only 24% of the widows reported their appetites to be good or excellent, compared with 92% of the elderly women in a control group whose husbands were still living. Moreover, only 18% of the widows selected foods for their good nutritional content compared with 62% of the women in the control group.

The higher risk of heart and circulatory problems in late adulthood than in earlier adulthood makes it especially important for older people to control the amount of cholesterol in their diets. Cholesterol is a waxy, fatlike substance that is found in all animal tissues and is needed in small amounts for many of the body's chemical processes. The two most important forms of cholesterol are low-density lipoprotein cholesterol (LDL) and high-density lipoprotein cholesterol (HDL). LDL increases the risk of heart disease when present in a large amount, whereas a high level of HDL may help to prevent heart disease. LDL collects on the walls of arteries, leaving less space for blood to flow through them. The consequence may be atherosclerosis and an eventual heart attack (see DISEASES [CHRONIC]). The body produces most of the cholesterol it needs for its chemical processes. To avoid harmful levels of LDL, elderly adults (and younger adults as well) should limit their intake of high-LDL foods, such as butter, whole milk, cheese, egg yolks, and fatty meats, and replace them with such foods as cholesterol-free margarine, skim milk, egg whites, and lean meats.

Certain fats in one's diet may change the blood's cholesterol level even more than the cholesterol consumed in foods. Limiting the intake of foods high in saturated fats (e.g., bacon grease, poultry skin) is essential for maintaining a healthy level of LDL. By contrast, polyunsaturated fats, found in such oils as safflower and soybean, are recommended because they tend to lower the level of LDL in the blood. In addition, recent European studies found evidence to indicate that the drugs simvastatin and pravasatin may be effective in lowering cholesterol levels, thereby delaying the onset of heart disease.

To make certain they consume a healthy diet, elderly people should consult their physician and a dietitian at a local hospital. Alternatively, a good source for planning healthy meals is *The American Heart Association Cookbook* (published by Ballantine Books).

O

. . . .

Old (Defining Late Adulthood)

All researchers in gerontology share the problem of defining what is meant by "older." Phrased somewhat differently, the question becomes "What defines the onset of old age?" A firm definition is virtually impossible to attain. The difficulty rests in the fact that old age is a relative term. The aging process actually begins at birth and continues throughout the remainder of the life span. The onset of "oldness" has no set physical marker, and the definition of *old* becomes arbitrary. In an important way, "old" depends on what physical ability or psychological ability is of concern. An Olympic-class gymnast is "old" at age 25, whereas a professional baseball player is not "old" until past age 35. By contrast, an Olympic-class yachting participant is "young" at age 45 (e.g., Sir Eyre Massey Shaw won a gold medal in the 1900 games at the age of 70) as is a candidate for the presidency of the United States.

Clearly, aging affects various abilities at different rates. Moreover, there is a wide range of ages along the adult life span at which the onset of aging for specific abilities and functions becomes apparent. That range occurs later for the ability to hit successfully against a major league pitcher than for the ability to perform complex gymnastic exercise, and still later for the ability to maneuver a yacht. Similarly, physiological functions age at different rates. Relative to young adults, the basic metabolic rate shows little change even at age 70, whereas the maximum breathing capacity shows considerable decline by age 60 and younger. Such variability among different abilities and functions and among individuals at a given age for those abilities and functions has led to the concept of *functional age* as a way of defining old. The concept, however, has many problems, and it has not been widely used (see FUNCTIONAL AGE).

In the absence of a firm biological or psychological criterion for defining the onset of old age, most laypeople and gerontologists have turned to an arbitrary criterion. That criterion is the setting of a specific chronological age (i.e., years since birth) as being the onset of old age. In recent years that age has been 65 years. Why age 65? Until 1979, attainment of this age signaled forced vocational retirement for most people. Retirement at age 65 is a relatively recent event. It originated in Germany in 1889. Otto von Bismarck's statisticians determined, on an actuarial basis, that 65 was the ideal age for establishing a not-too-costly retirement pension plan. Retirement at age 65 eventually reached the United States and became the standard practice in 1935.

Now that the retirement age has been advanced to 70 years for many people by an amendment to the Age Discrimination in Employment Act, an interesting possibility is that old age will eventually be redefined as having its onset at age 70. In practice, however, gerontological researchers usually set their own age criteria for selecting samples of elderly participants in their studies. It is not unusual to discover studies in which membership in the "old" group is set at age 60 or even in the 50s.

Older Americans Research and Services Questionnaire

The Older Americans Research and Services Questionnaire (OARS) is used to gather information about the functional status and service needs and uses of adults age 18 and older. Its major use, however, has been with older adults. OARS has two main parts. The first assesses functional status in five areas, including physical health and the activities of daily living (see ACTIVITIES OF DAILY LIVING). The second part assesses the need for and use of 24 services (e.g., transportation, financial assistance, and meal preparation). OARS is widely used in national health surveys and in assessing the functional status and service needs of people with diseases such as arthritis.

Operant Conditioning

The basic principle of operant conditioning (or operant learning) is that the event following a response determines either the frequency or the speed of that response's future occurrences. If the event is something positive (e.g., food to a hungry rat, candy to a child, money to an adult), then positive reinforcement occurs, and the consequence is an increase in the frequency or the speed of the behavior. If the event is negative (e.g., electric shock to a rat, a spanking to a child, loss of money to an adult), then punishment occurs, and the consequence is a decrease in the frequency or the speed of the behavior.

B. F. Skinner, the famous American psychologist who discovered the principle in the 1930s, found that both human beings and animals are susceptible to behavior modification by either positive reinforcement or punishment. Older adults are no exception. For example, positive reinforcement has been found to increase their speed of performing various tasks (e.g., memory scanning and digit symbol substitution; see SHORT-TERM MEMORY; WECHSLER INTELLIGENCE TESTS). Ethical issues limit research on the use of punishment to effect the behavior of older adults. However, when money is used for positive reinforcement of a fast response, then taking away that money may be used as a mild punishment for a slow response. This form of punishment after a slow response on a task has been found to decrease future occurrences of slow responses for both older and younger adults.

Positive reinforcement has been found to be effective with some patients with Alzheimer's disease in increasing the frequency of behaviors relevant to their own grooming and caretaking. Positive reinforcement has also been demonstrated to decrease the frequency of excessively aggressive behaviors of institutionalized elderly people. Here the treatment consists of positively reinforcing nonaggressive behaviors. Operant conditioning is also frequently used as a form of therapy (called behavior modification) to promote greater occurrences of behaviors that are advantageous to the individuals receiving the therapy, such as quitting smoking and managing pain (see also PAIN MANAGEMENT; PSYCHOTHERAPY; PSYCHOTHERAPY WITH NURSING HOME RESIDENTS; SMOKING).

Originality

If you were asked to list six uses for a newspaper other than its main use (for reading, of course), what would you say? "To start a fire" is highly likely—and it would be an answer given not only by you but by many others as well. Would you have included "To provide the words for constructing a kidnap ransom note"? This is the type of question included on an "Unusual Uses" test. The purpose of this test is to measure individual differences in originality. Originality calls on what psychologists term *divergent or productive thinking*, in which the objective is to give a unique solution to a problem (e.g., what to do with a newspaper). By contrast, most of our everyday problem solving calls on *convergent thinking*, in which the objective is simply to find the most appropriate solution to a problem, regardless of the originality of that solution. Starting a fire with a newspaper would not be very original, whereas constructing a ransom note from it would be quite original (i.e., given by very few people) and dependent on divergent thinking. The more such unique (but rational) answers you give on the Unusual Uses test, the higher your originality score.

Research with the Unusual Uses Test, along with a number of other tests of originality, has revealed that older adults display moderately less originality than do younger adults. The most comprehensive study was conducted with participants in the Baltimore Longitudinal Study. More than 800 men ranging in age from 17 to 101 years received a battery of six tests, each designed to measure originality in some form. For example, one of the tests required imagining the consequences of unusual situations. The correlation between age and scores on this test was negative (that is, there was a trend for scores on the test be lower for older than for younger participants) and statistically significant (i.e., unlikely to be related to chance). However, the magnitude of the correlation was modest. The implication is that originality is by no means the exclusive province of young adults. Many elderly adults show as great, if not greater, degrees of originality than do many much younger adults.

Overmedication

One of the problems confronting many elderly people is their underadherence to their medication regimen (see MEDICATION COMPLIANCE). A different, but equally serious, problem is the risk of overmedication. It is estimated that one-fourth of the more than 1 billion prescriptions issued annually are for elderly people. Moreover, about 25% of older adults are required to take at least three prescription medicines. This should not be surprising, given the incidence of various diseases in late adulthood. The health risk exists because medicines often interact with each other, and their interaction may produce memory problems, dizziness, and bladder problems, along with a number of other potential problems, as side effects. Some medicines, such as certain ones for treating arthritis, may interact with coffee or alcohol to damage the lining of the stomach. The effects of these various interactions are estimated to result in nearly 17% of hospital admissions for people over age 70. Many hospitals now have geriatric services that are available for older people to evaluate their medicine regimen and to advise them in ways of reducing these potential risks. They are services that should be consulted regularly by elderly people, especially those over age 70.

P

. . . .

Pain

Pain is a major source of discomfort regardless of one's age. Of course, it may also play an important role in alerting a person to the presence of life-threatening circumstances. What happens to the sense of pain as we age is poorly understood. A number of researchers have examined age differences in pain sensitivity by determining age differences in the pain threshold (i.e., the minimal intensity of a pain-provoking condition that is felt as being painful). A variety of conditions have been used, with a variety of body parts receiving the conditions. For example, in some studies radiant heat has been applied to an arm, and in other studies electrical stimulation has been applied to an unfilled tooth. Several of these studies have reported sensitivity to decrease with increasing age, whereas others have reported either increasing sensitivity with increasing age or no age difference in sensitivity. It seems likely that the extent of change in sensitivity with aging is likely to be modest. On the other hand, clinical evidence from patients with real-life pain-provoking injuries and diseases suggests that older people feel pain less intensely than do younger people and that elderly people have a greater tolerance of pain than do younger people. Conditions, such as appendicitis, that produce intense pain in younger adults often produce little pain in elderly adults. This, of course, is a mixed blessing in that some elderly adults may be unaware of an impending illness. Tolerance of pain is only partly a physiological function. It also depends on a person's attitude toward pain and whether an event is expected to increase or decrease the pain.

Chronic pain is usually defined as pain from an illness or injury that persists for 6 months or longer and has not responded to treatment. Elderly adults are more likely than younger adults to experience chronic pain associated with such diseases as rheumatoid arthritis and gout. Conversely, older adults may experience less pain than younger adults from such conditions as headaches and backaches.

Pain Management

Health practitioners are finally realizing that chronic pain (see PAIN) need not necessarily be tolerated—it can be managed or controlled. Pain treatment centers that offer a number of ways for managing pain are now located in many hospitals (usually affiliated with universities) around the country. Unfortunately, people over age 70 tend to be underrepresented as clients at these centers. Many elderly people seem to accept pain as simply being part of being old.

A number of approaches to minimize pain are now available. For example, much of pain comes from muscles. It may be largely relieved by training the patient to relax through the use of biofeedback (see PSYCHOTHERAPY) or to perform certain exercises. Exercise has been found to be a critical means of managing pain for many people with arthritic pain. Appropriate exercise keeps their joints flexible and protects them from undue stress. Patients with cancer or postsurgery patients with intense pain can have narcotics delivered to their bodies by a computerized pump that administers patient-controlled analgesics (PCA). Patients may administer pain-relieving drugs to themselves whenever they experience pain. Postsurgery patients have been found to administer less of these drugs than doctors would have prescribed for them. Another approach involves the injection of a nerve-deadening solution (called a nerve block) into the spinal cord. It blocks pain from traveling by spinal nerves to the brain. Behavior modification (see OPERANT CONDITIONING; PSYCHOTHERAPY) has also been used effectively to manage some types of pain. Patients are reinforced during periods of pain for visualizing pleasant images and repeating positive words.

For more information on pain management, write to the National Chronic Pain Outreach, 7979 Old Georgetown Road, Suite 100, Bethesda, MD 20814, or to the International Pain Foundation, 909 Northeast 43rd St., Suite 306, Seattle, WA 98105. Informative books about pain management include the *Handbook of Chronic Pain Management*, by Dr. C. David Tollison, and *Management of Pain*, by P. P. Raj.

Pain Medications (Analgesics)

An analgesic is a pain-relieving medication. A wide variety of such medications are available without prescription to relieve mild to moderate pain. Many of these are of a general class known as NSAIDS (nonsteroidal anti-inflammatory drugs). They can be effective by decreasing the level of inflammation at the site of tissue injury. Among these drugs are aspirin (the original NSAID drug). For some older people, aspirin may cause uncomfortable gastric side effects. A noninflammatory alternative drug is acetaminophin, but anyone suffering liver disease must be careful to avoid excessive use of this drug.

Opiate analgesics, used for moderate to severe pain, require a prescription. Included among these drugs are codeine, morphine, methadone, and demerol. One of these drugs is likely to be the one used in a patient-controlled pain management program (see PAIN MANAGEMENT).

Parapsychology

"Hey, I know what you are thinking!" If this is really true, you are demonstrating extrasensory perception (ESP). That is, you are receiving information from someone without the use of any of your senses. Extrasensory perception is one of the phenomena studied in parapsychology (the prefix *para* means outside the boundaries of traditional psychology). Another phenomenon belonging to parapsychology is that of clairvoyance. It refers to an awareness of an event occurring that is far away and transmitting no information to the senses of the person experiencing the event. For example, someone may claim that he or she sensed an accident happening to a relative at the time it occurred.

There is no scientific evidence to support the reality of ESP and clairvoyance, as well as the other phenomena studied by parapsychologists. You may make a good guess as to what someone is thinking—but what about the many times your guesses are wrong? Similarly, you may, by coincidence, have had a feeling of something happening to someone—but what about the many times that feeling is wrong? Of course, scientific evidence to the contrary does not prevent many people from believing that on occasion they have had some mystical experience that is beyond scientific explanation. To determine how many people have had various mystical experiences, psychologists ask people to rate on a scale of 1 to 4 (1 = never; 4 = often) the frequency with which each has occurred to them. Surveys of adults of all ages have indicated that the percentage of adults of all ages who report at least one occasion of experiencing ESP has increased during the past 20 years from 58% to 65%. Similarly, the percentage experiencing at least one occasion of clairvoyance has increased from 24% to 28%. Especially striking is the increase in the percentage of people who report at least one experience of spiritualism, that is, contact with someone who was dead (from 27% to 40%). An increase also occurred for the experience of déjà vu (feeling you were somewhere you have been be-fore even though you know it is impossible). There must have been something strange in the air during the past 20 years.

The one mystical experience that showed a decline in percentage (from 35% to 31.5%) is the feeling of being close to a powerful force that lifted you out of yourself (an out-of-body experience). Re-searchers at Eastern Virginia Medical School who analyzed the more recent survey found that the percentage of older people having mys-tical experiences was less than that of younger people. Wisdom does come with aging.

Parent Care Advisor

This is a monthly newsletter for caregivers. It gives advice on com-pleting Medicare and Medicaid forms, financial and legal matters, low-cost services, and many other concerns of caregivers. For a sub-scription, write to American Health Consultants, 3525 Piedmont Road, Building Six, Suite 400, Atlanta, GA 30305.

Parenthood

This entry deals only with parenthood at middle age and beyond. By then women have passed the childbearing years. By contrast, some middle-aged men do become fathers, perhaps for the first time. There is evidence to indicate that men who become fathers in middle age are likely to experience more companionship with their children than men who become fathers at an earlier age.

Middle age, however, is most commonly associated with parents whose children have grown up and are independent, thus creating an "empty nest." The consequences of an "empty nest" are varied. Long of interest to family researchers has been the development of "empty nest" symptoms in some mothers who have lost their role as a care-giver to a child or adolescent. They perceive their lives as now having little purpose. The most common symptom is depression. However, many mothers react to the independence of their children quite dif-ferently; they experience relief and satisfaction. They now see them-selves as having more time for travel and the pursuit of other leisure activities than was previously possible. This is especially likely for mothers who have worked. Unfortunately, the impact of an "empty nest" on fathers has not been widely investigated.

Of course, in recent years a number of middle-aged parents (and some elderly parents) have seen the "empty nest" refilled as unmar-ried adult children and even married children have returned to live in their parental home, thus creating an "extended family." This is especially likely to happen when the "child" has lost his or her job or has to accept a very low-paying job. A survey in 1990 revealed that 16% of young adults age 25 to 29 years were living with their parents—and the percentage is probably even higher today. A recent study conducted by researchers at Brown University revealed that unmarried children were much more likely than married children to live with parents. They also found that it is the children in the extended family who are most likely to benefit from the shared living, especially in terms of the parents being the main contributors to living expenses.

Middle age also presents the danger of divorce for parents whose main roles in life centered on their children. Now that they no longer share the responsibility of child rearing, they may discover that they have little else in common.

Older women are likely to have a closer relationship with their daughters than with their sons. After a divorce or the death of their husbands, they are more likely to share a residence with a daughter than with a son.

During late adulthood, parents usually assume a new role as grandparents (see GRANDPARENTING), as well as continuing in their roles as parents to their adult children. In most cases, contact and mutual help between older parents and their adult children are at a high level, even when they live far apart. The positive relationships may be strained, however, by a number of factors. Included are the high time and resource demands placed on the adult children as they raise their own families and the reliance of some older parents on their adult children for financial aid and health care.

Parkinson's Disease

Patients with this disease have a deficit in one of the chemical transmitters (dopamine; see BRAIN AND AGING) found in the area of the brain controlling motor or muscular behaviors. Among the symptoms of the disease are the presence of tremors, difficulty initiating movement, and loss of postural reflexes. It is an age-associated neurological (brain) disease in that its incidence below age 40 is very low, and the incidence increases steadily after that age. The average age of onset is believed to be in the late 60s. However, the onset may go unnoticed for a number of years. Both depression and amnesia occur in a fairly large proportion of patients with Parkinson's disease as the disease progresses in severity. A surgical procedure known as pallidotomy has been found to relieve tremors for some victims of the disease. However, it is unknown how long the relief will last. In addition, transplanting fetal brain tissue into the brain of a Parkinson's patient has been found by a doctor at Mount Sinai Medical Center (New York) to produce clinical improvement. The transplanted cells survived and supplied the patient's brain with new nerve connections. The possibility of such transplants serving as an effective treatment depends on the results of clinical trials on many patients.

Participation in Research

Advancement in gerontological research necessarily requires the participation of older people in biological, psychological, and sociological studies. A major problem confronting gerontological researchers is the reluctance of many elderly people to serve as participants. The National Center for Health Statistics reports a participation rate of 75% for adults age 21 to 60 years but less than 60% for adults over age 60. Obviously, many older people view such participation negatively. The participation rate is usually higher when potential participants perceive their participation in a study as personally beneficial (e.g., taking part in a study on urinary incontinence) than when they see no personal benefit (e.g., taking an intelligence test). Paid participation is a common method used to recruit older participants for their part in a study.

Participation in a research study involves informed consent in which potential participants are fully informed in advance of what will happen to them during their participation and what potential risks may be involved in their participation. They are also offered the opportunity to withdraw from the study at any time without receiving punitive action (e.g., nonpayment for their services).

Participation in Voluntary Organizations and Volunteer Work

Millions of Americans belong to seemingly countless numbers of voluntary organizations and clubs. Memberships and active involvement in these organizations are low for adults in their 20s but quite high for adults in the age range of 35 to 44 years of age. Of great interest to gerontologists is the degree to which older adults withdraw from participation in voluntary organizations. A significant reduction, relative to middle-aged adults, could be taken as a sign of the preference for many elders to withdraw from active lives.

Evidence from a survey of 200 people age 65 and older in an Ohio community indicates that participation in organizations remains high in late adulthood. Of those surveyed, 87% reported belonging to one or more organizations, and 74% reported attending meetings at least once a month. Moreover, 69% stated that they were very involved in the activities of their organizations. Men were as likely as women to be members of organizations. However, women were more likely to be involved actively than men. There was only a slight tendency for those age 73 and older to be less involved than those in the 65- to 72-year age range. Unless this Ohio community is a unique place, there is good reason to believe that most older people prefer activity rather than inactivity. However, there is also evidence to indicate that formal activity (as in organizations) is less of a contributor to the life satisfaction of elderly people than is informal activity (e.g., with friends and relatives; see ACTIVITY THEORY).

Volunteerism may also involve working in some capacity (usually unpaid, such as staffing an information desk at a hospital). It is estimated that more than 40% of elderly people participate in volunteer work. This percentage is considerably higher today than it was 25 years ago (about 11%). Moreover, the percentage of volunteer workers is likely to increase in the future as the educational level and the health status of new generations of elderly people increases.

Partners in Caregiving: The Dementia Services Program

This program provides technical assistance and some funding to adult day-care centers. It has supported 50 centers in 28 states and the District of Columbia, and it has provided models and advice for other centers. The program is sponsored by the Robert Wood Johnson Foundation. Its national office is located at the Bowman Gray School of Medicine at Wake Forest University. For further information write to the Dementia Services Program at Department of Psychiatry and Behavioral Medicine, Bowman Gray School of Medicine, Wake Forest University, Winston-Salem, NC 27157-1087 (telephone, 910-716-4941).

Personality (Overview)

See also CONTROL OF LIFE'S EVENTS; PERSONALITY STAGES; PERSONALITY STYLE; PERSONALITY TRAITS

"Sally has a sparkling personality." "Joe's personality really turns me off!" These statements show how people usually refer to personality in their everyday lives. They are referring to how one person perceives another person. Sally is perceived by the person who made the statement as someone who is lively and perhaps even bubbly, whereas Joe is perceived as someone who is irritating and perhaps boorish. To psychologists, however, personality has a different meaning. It refers to the collection of traits, beliefs, motives, values, style of behavior, and so on, that characterize any given individual. It is the unique organization of these attributes that defines that individual's personality. Every individual seemingly has a different organization than everyone else. Nevertheless, the different components of personality may be separated and studied independently of other components.

Traits may be measured as one component of personality. This is accomplished by the use of questionnaires in which respondents answer questions about themselves (often true-false questions). From the answers given, the subjects are scored on a continuum on such traits as introversion-extroversion. Interest in gerontology centers largely on the question of age comparisons on the different components of personality. For example, how do adults of different ages compare on the trait of introversion-extroversion? These age comparisons are usually directed at answering the question of whether personality remains stable (i.e., basically unchanged) or altered in some significant way from early to late adulthood. In terms of the trait of introversion-extroversion, do young adults become increasingly introverted as they grow older? This would be a major change in personality with aging. Alternatively, do those individuals who are extroverted when they are young remain basically extroverted when they become old?

Personality Stages

A stage theory is one that views life span development in terms of a series of major transitions that everyone undergoes and in the same order of stages. A successful transition from one stage to the next means that the individual has moved from one level of functioning to another, qualitatively different level of functioning. The ease of making a transition from one stage to the next depends on how successfully an individual has made earlier transitions. Stage theories have been applied to both cognitive (mental) life span development (see COGNITIVE [MENTAL] STAGES OF DEVELOPMENT) and personality. The most prominent stage theories of personality are those of Erik Erikson, whose theory dates back to the late 1950s, and of Daniel Levinson, whose theory was developed in the late 1970s.

Erikson's theory states that personality development over the course of the life span is determined by the interaction between biological and psychological forces within an individual and the external demands of society. There are eight stages assumed to be encountered during the entire life span, beginning in infancy and ending with old age. Each is characterized by a struggle between two opposing tendencies that create a crisis for the individual.

Erikson is perhaps best known for giving us the term "identity crisis" in reference to the stage and crisis confronting adolescence (fifth stage in his theory). Here the issue is whether the adolescent will find an identity for himself or herself. If not, the presumed consequence is that of an identity confusion. Failure to successfully resolve this crisis is likely to affect negatively the resolution of crises at later stages of development. Our interest rests in the seventh and eighth stages of Erikson's theory. The seventh stage is found in middle age and is characterized by the crisis between generativity and stagnation. Generativity refers to the caring for the young and working to improve the living conditions for future generations. Failure to achieve generativity (i.e., stagnation) should result in the individual becoming directed only at self-interests with little concern about society's future. Successful resolution of the generativity versus stagnation crisis is deemed necessary if an individual is to adjust satisfactorily to old age and to avoid dwelling on a meaningless life. The eighth and final stage is characterized by the crisis between integrity and despair. The crisis begins with awareness of an old person that death is near. Integrity refers to the evaluation of one's own life and finding that it had meaning. Without such meaning, one faces impending death with despair.

Levinson's theory is based on the concept of a life structure that is created by an individual. This structure defines the individual's goal at a particular period of life and the various roles that individual must assume in regard to family, work, and society at large in order to attain that goal. This life structure must experience transitions as the individual progresses through life and the roles expected of him or her are altered. For example, during mid-life the individual evaluates past accomplishments within earlier life structures. If these accomplishments are not viewed satisfactorily, then a mid-life crisis is likely to occur, and the individual feels the need for creating a very different life structure.

Personality Style

Personality style refers to the manner in which individuals perceive the events occurring in their environments. For example, how sensitive are individuals to the context (i.e., things going on in the background and where they are taking place) that surrounds the events important enough to attract their attention? To what extent do individuals perceive irrelevant events (events not related to their immediate objective) while attending to relevant events (events directly related to their immediate objective)? Psychologists view individual differences in sensitivity to contextual events and irrelevant events in terms of a broad personality style dimension called *field dependence–field independence*. In general, people classified as field-dependent are believed to rely primarily on external stimuli and events in making perceptual judgments and to experience their environments in a global, relatively undifferentiated way. By contrast, people classified as field-independent are believed to rely largely on internal stimuli (e.g., their own thoughts about events) in making perceptual judgments and to experience their environments in a relatively differentiated way. Field-dependent people are therefore more likely than field-independent people to be distracted by irrelevant events and to have attentional problems when confronted by multiple stimuli or events.

A standard test for measuring a person's dependent-independent dimension is the rod and frame test. The person is tested in a darkened room with an apparatus composed of a luminescent rod surrounded by a luminescent square. The person's task is to move the rod until, on some trials, it is vertical with respect to the floor or, on other trials, it is horizontal with the floor. The task is made difficult by tilting the square background, thus making accuracy (as measured by deviation from verticality or horizontality) contingent on the person's ability to ignore the distorting background offered by the square.

Several cross-sectional studies have compared the performances of young adults and older adults on the rod and frame test. Accuracy scores are greater for young adults than for elderly adults. The implication is that elderly adults are, on the average, more field-dependent than are younger adults. Comparable outcomes have been found in other cross-sectional studies employing different tests for field dependency and field independency. This evidence is consistent with laboratory evidence indicating that older participants have greater difficulty than younger participants in ignoring irrelevant information when they have to search a display to find some specified relevant information (see SELECTIVE ATTENTION). Unknown, however, is the extent to which this age difference is the consequence of a true age change; that is, do people really become more field-dependent as they progress from early to late adulthood? Conceivably, these cross-sectional age differences reflect a difference among generations.

That is, members of earlier generations may be more field-dependent throughout their lives than are members of later generations.

Researchers at Duke University found that elderly men and women who are open and trusting had better health and a greater sense of well-being than those who were more cynical and suspicious of others. They also found that those with an optimistic style of thinking had greater life satisfaction than those with a pessimistic style of thinking.

Personality Traits

Personality psychologists view a trait as a component of personality that accounts for relatively permanent dispositions and consistencies in an individual's behavior over time. Each trait is regarded as being defined by bipolar opposites, such as introversion and extroversion. A trait is therefore a dimension that ranges between two extremes, with different individuals scoring at different points on that dimension. Thus individuals may be characterized as being highly introverted, moderately introverted, mildly introverted, and so on, through being highly extroverted. Individuals who are highly introverted are likely to behave in a withdrawn manner across a wide range of situations and circumstances. Similarly, individuals who are highly extroverted are likely to behave in an excited, somewhat boisterous manner across the same situations and circumstance in which the introverted person behaves in a withdrawn manner.

Traits are identified by psychologists through the use of personality tests and questionnaires in which people answer questions about themselves and their behaviors. On the basis of answers to different questions, the respondents are scored on the traits believed to be measured by the specific test. The number of personality traits measured may vary from several to more than a hundred, depending on the specific personality test. The personality test currently of interest in gerontology is called the NEO Inventory, a test containing 144 items. The inventory measures three broad traits. The first is neuroticism, which is defined by the extremes of emotional stability and instability. The second is extroversion, defined along the introversion and extroversion dimension. The third is openness, which is defined by the extremes of openness and closedness in feelings and ideas. Considerable research, both cross-sectional and longitudinal, has indicated that these traits show little change from early to late adulthood. That is, older adults differ little from younger adults in their trait scores, and scores on each trait remain about the same when respondents are retested after a period of years. A number of other studies with other personality tests measuring a greater number of traits have provided similar evidence. Thus personality traits do seem to remain relatively stable from early to late adulthood. Your traits as a young adult are likely to be the same as you grow older. It should be noted that some early studies on age differences in personality indicated that elderly people did differ from younger adults on such traits as introversion-extroversion, with older people scoring as being more introverted than younger people. We know now that the cross-sectional age differences found in these studies were the result of cohort or generational effects, and were not the result of people changing from extroversion to introversion as they grow old. People from earlier generations appear to have been more introverted than people from later generations. It is members of these earlier generations who served as the elderly participants in the early studies on adult age differences in personality traits.

Pet Therapy

The relationships between human beings and their pets have long been recognized as providing many benefits for the human beings, such as unconditional love and companionship. It has been only in the last 20 years, however, that the potential therapeutic value of pets on nursing home residents has received attention. Residents of geriatric nursing homes are frequently adversely affected by institutionalization. They tend to become increasingly emotionally flat, socially withdrawn, and solitary in their behavior as their stay in the nursing home becomes prolonged. The hope is that the presence of a pet, either a dog or a cat, in the nursing home will delay the occurrence of these negative symptoms of institutionalization. In effect, resident interactions with a pet are hoped to provide a kind of therapy.

Two kinds of pet therapy programs have been introduced for elderly nursing home residents. For the first, residents are permitted to have brief occasional visitations with a dog or cat. The available evidence indicates that this type of program has little benefit for the residents. The other kind of program requires the dog or cat to become a permanent resident of the nursing home, with freedom to visit individual rooms, dining halls, meeting rooms, and so on. In this situation, the therapeutic value of the pet is likely to be greater. The most comprehensive study of the impact of a resident pet on the behavior of the human residents was conducted in an Australian nursing home. It was found that a dog did increase social interactions and decrease solitary behaviors among the residents, but only for a month or two after the dog entered the home. After 5 months or longer the residents had largely reverted to the behaviors characteristic of them before the dog's arrival. Part of the problem in retaining the improved functioning of the residents over a longer period was related to the dog herself. She spent more time with staff members, and less time with the residents, during the 5-month period. To ensure maximum benefit from pet therapy, some way of avoiding the "staff drift" must be implemented in the nursing home.

Interactions with pets are not limited to residents of nursing homes. Many older community-dwelling adults have a pet in their homes with whom they have many pleasant interactions. A reasonable belief is that such interactions should enhance the psychological well-being of the older adults and thereby enhance their physical health as well. This seems to be the case for older adults who have been experiencing severe stress in their lives. For most older adults, however, the evidence indicates that pleasant interactions with a pet at home have little effect on physical health and little effect on longevity.

Physicians (Communication with)

One problem confronting health care for older people is the barrier many elderly patients face in communication with a physician. Physicians realize the importance of effective communication with their elderly patients, but they often complain that their busy schedules do not permit such time to discuss the problems of their patients in any great detail. The total time spent in communication during an office visit is not the only important element in aiding elderly patients. Perhaps more important is how the available time is spent. Researchers at the City University of New York–Brooklyn College examined the flow of communication for a group of elderly patients making their first visit to a specific physician. The physicians tended to dominate the conversations. Responses to patients' questions were more likely to be responded to effectively if the questions were related to topics raised by the physicians than if the questions were related to topics raised by the patients themselves. In addition, the physicians were likely to communicate better with elderly patients who expressed less concern about control of their own health than with elderly patients who expressed more concern about the control of their own health.

Physiological Functions

One way of expressing age-related changes in physiological function of some organ or system of the body is in terms of the percent of proficiency of average functioning in a given age range, relative to the functional level at age 20. These percentages reveal both the magnitude of declines in functioning with age and the considerable variability in magnitude for different functions. For example, the velocity of nerve signal transmission is about 95% (of what it is at age 20) at age 60 and about 90% at age 80. The kidney filtration rate is about 85% at age 60 and about 75% at age 80, and the maximum breathing capacity is about 62% at age 60 and 42% at age 80. These are average figures, and there is considerable variability or dispersion about these averages at each age level (see FUNCTIONAL AGE).

Maximum breathing capacity is the maximum amount of air taken into the lungs with a single breath. The decline in capacity results in the more frequent shortness of breath (a condition called dyspnea) experienced by older people than younger people and in the greater fatigue likely to be experienced during exercise by older than by younger people.

Digestion is usually not greatly impaired by aging, but many elderly people do experience irritable bowel syndrome, diverticulosis (pouches in the walls of the intestines), and constipation. Laxatives are often used by elderly people, but they often reduce the efficiency of digestion and lead to nutritional deficiencies. Constipation and diverticulosis are most effectively treated by a controlled diet, certain drugs, and exercise. Older people with these digestive dysfunctions should consult their physicians regularly for the treatment most likely to benefit them.

Kidney function declines in efficiency in late adulthood as the number of nephrons (the kidney's functional units) declines to about half the number present at birth. As a consequence, stress is more likely to produce kidney failure in elderly people than in younger people. Normally aging elderly people are likely to have an increase in the frequency of urination, relative to younger people, and a larger residual amount of urine after urinating, as a result of age-related changes in the elasticity and responsivity of the bladder.

Pick's Disease

Pick's disease is a form of dementia that is often indistinguishable from Alzheimer's disease in terms of impaired mental functioning. The disease may be associated with a single dominant gene, a gene also suspected by some researchers to be associated with Alzheimer's disease. Some of the changes occurring in the brains of patients with Pick's disease resemble those found in patients with Alzheimer's disease. These changes include the destruction of brain centers deep inside the brain that are essential for the production of an important neural transmitter (acetylcholine; see ALZHEIMER'S DISEASE). However, the high frequency of senile plaques in the brains of patients with Alzheimer's disease and the many neurofibrillary tangles found in the neurons in Alzheimer's disease are not characteristic of Pick's disease. In addition, there is a behavioral difference commonly found between patients with Alzheimer's disease and patients with Pick's disease. Patients with Alzheimer's disease tend to be neat and sociable, whereas patients with Pick's disease tend to be sloppy and unsociable.

Picture Memory

When young adults have their memories tested for pictures of scenes or pictures of common objects that are presented in a lengthy series, their accuracy in identifying old pictures (i.e., they were included in the series) as old and their accuracy of identifying new pictures (i.e., they were not in the series) as new are both quite high. In fact, their accuracy is much higher than it is for similar identifications of words seen in a lengthy series. This difference in accuracy between recognizing pictures and recognizing words is known as the *picture superiority effect*. Older adults also show the picture superiority effect. However, the accuracy of picture memory has generally been found to be less for elderly participants than for younger participants. Nevertheless, the age difference in memory proficiency favoring younger adults has generally been found to be less for pictures than it is for words.

Plasticity Theory

Some degeneration of the brain occurs with normal aging. Some neurons are lost while others decline in their functioning. However, positive changes also occur in the brain; for example, the number of dendrites connecting neurons with other neurons may increase, as may the complexity of the connections. Of great interest is the discovery of means of increasing the plasticity of the brain, that is, its capability of compensating via positive changes for the negative changes. Research with rats has discovered that old animals given an enriched environment (e.g., placing colorful and manipulable objects in their environments) show greater plasticity of their brains than do other old animals who remain restricted to their colorless and sterile environments. Most important, old rats in enriched environments display greater learning proficiency than old rats without such enrichment.

Plasticity theory suggests that comparable effects should occur for the older human brain. Stimulating environments and stimulating mental experiences and activities should increase the amount of plasticity occurring in the brain. To date, the evidence indicating that high levels of mental activity relate positively to higher levels of performances on various mental tasks is somewhat ambiguous (see ACTIVITY AND MENTAL PERFORMANCE), but research in this area is in its infancy. More supportive of plasticity theory is evidence that practice and training on some mental tasks lead to improvement in performances on those tasks for elderly people. Such experiences may be regarded as stimulating the brain's plasticity.

Pneumonia

Pneumonia is an infection of the lungs that affects either a section of a lobe of the lungs (lobar pneumonia) or patches scattered throughout both lobes (bronchial pneumonia). There are more than 30 different causes of pneumonia but the three main causes are bacteria, viruses, and mycoplasmas. *Pneumococcus* pneumonia is the most common form of bacterial pneumonia (accounting for about one-fourth of all cases of pneumonia). Pneumonia-producing bacteria are present in some healthy throats. When a person's resistance to disease is low, as it may be in many elderly people, the bacteria may work their way to the lungs, causing part of a lobe or even an entire lobe or several lobes to fill with liquid. The infection may then spread through the body by way of the blood stream. Symptoms of bacterial pneumonia may include chills, severe chest pain, a cough that produces rust-colored or greenish sputum, lips and nails with a bluish cast, and fever (as high as 105 degrees).

Viral pneumonias account for nearly half of all pneumonias. Early symptoms may include headache, a dry cough, fever, and muscle aches. Primary influenza virus pneumonia is especially severe and may be fatal. Most cases of viral pneumonia occur in people with pre-existing heart or pulmonary disease, which make older adults especially vulnerable.

Mycoplasma pneumonia is caused by small organisms with characteristics of both bacteria and viruses. The disease occurs mainly in older children and young adults, and it is usually mild and rarely fatal.

Prompt treatment with antibiotics may cure bacterial and mycoplasma pneumonia. The specific antibiotic is determined by the nature of the organism causing the pneumonia. It is important to continue taking the medication as instructed by the physician after the fever has subsided, or the pneumonia may recur in a more severe form than the original form. Full recovery from the disease may take a number of weeks for older adults. They should make certain that they have adequate rest during this period, but usually they may perform their normal daily activities. A vaccine is available for pneumococcal pneumonia, and it should be given once to those with the greatest risk of pneumococcal pneumonia, including people age 65 and older. It is estimated that the vaccine is effective in preventing pneumococcal pneumonia for about 40% to 60% of older adults who receive it. The vaccine is especially useful in reducing the severity of the symptoms and decreasing the risk of death for elderly people who do contract the disease. It is unfortunate that fewer than 20% of people age 65 and older receive the vaccine.

Posttraumatic Stress Disorder

It is not unusual for individuals who have survived a traumatic event in their lives to experience a form of long-lasting anxiety known as posttraumatic stress disorder (PTSD). There are three main symptoms: reexperiencing the traumatic event, avoiding situations that are reminders of the event, or diminished responsiveness. The event may be a natural disaster or military combat. A natural disaster, such as a severe earthquake, may be experienced by individuals of any age. In terms of military combat, PTSD is most commonly associated with combat veterans of the Vietnam War, veterans who have yet to reach late adulthood. Of particular concern in gerontology is the possibility that some combat veterans of World War II and the Korean War may still have PTSD. These veterans are now members of our elderly population. According to a 1987 survey by the Department of Veterans Affairs, nearly 65% of men over age 50 at the time of the survey served either in World War II or the Korean War. More than half of those in World War II and over a third of those in the Korean War experienced combat. It is estimated that there will be 9 million veterans age 65 and older by the year 2000. Several studies have revealed that the presence of PTSD in elderly combat veterans is relatively low, but somewhat higher in veterans of the Korean War than in veterans of World War II. A probable reason for this difference is the greater unpopularity of the Korean War and the general lack of recognition given to veterans of the war, relative to veterans of World War II (and even the Vietnam war). PTSD is treatable with appropriate psychological and medical therapies.

A related issue concerns the effects of the disruption of an individual's life by entry into military service. Unique to World War II was the higher upper age limit of the draft (the upper 30s) than in other wars. Researchers at the Carolina Population Center found that older men in their study sample have had a greater risk of physical health problems than men who entered military service at a much younger age. The researchers attributed the effect of age at entry to the greater disruption of their social and occupational lives for the older men than for the younger men. Consequently, distress and its negative effects on health after service were likely to be greater for the men who were older at the time of entry.

Postural Change and Orthostasis

Orthostasis refers to the rapid decline in blood pressure that occurs when there is a rapid change in body position from a supine (lying) to an erect posture or even from a sitting to an erect position. Most people have experienced one of the possible consequences of orthostasis, at least occasionally, in the form of lightheadedness when they stand up rapidly from a sitting or reclining position. Normal changes with aging in arterial flexibility and in the nervous system make the reflexive raising of blood pressure during a position shift especially difficult for older people. The risk of fainting from orthostasis is therefore greater than it is among younger adults. Physicians commonly recommend that elderly people who are prone to more severe declines in blood pressure after standing avoid diuretics as much as possible and wear support hose. Researchers at the University of California–Los Angeles recently discovered that some elderly people may be trained to use behavioral techniques as a means of preventing severe blood pressure declines during orthostasis. The techniques involved in their study were either squeezing a handgrip device or performing a mental arithmetic task (summing numbers). The mental arithmetic task was found to be somewhat more effective than the handgrip task. As noted by the researchers, physicians should be alerted to the potential positive effects of these behavioral techniques and be prepared to train their elderly patients to use them, especially those patients who are especially vulnerable to orthostatic hypotension.

Fainting may also occur among older adults for reasons other than simple orthostasis, particularly for nervous system dysfunctions of unknown origin. Such dysfunctions are fairly common and are considered benign. Usually recovery from fainting begins quickly after the person falls to the floor, and consciousness is regained after a brief period. Elderly persons are advised by physicians to sit or recline at the first sign of dizziness. They may avoid the loss of consciousness by doing so. Frequent changes of body positions are believed to reduce the chances of fainting. Of course, elderly people who experience episodes of fainting should seek medical evaluation to determine whether a more serious medical problem is causing the fainting.

Posture

The control of body posture, as revealed by swaying while standing up, decreases with aging. The decline in postural control is sufficient to be a contributing factor to the high incidence of falls experienced by elderly people (see FALLS). Researchers in Australia recently demonstrated that the degree of swaying while standing on a firm surface is associated with the amount of sensory information received by the brain from the lower legs (proprioceptive stimulation), especially the ankles. The age-related decline in visual functioning and inner ear (vestibular) functioning appears to play only a minor role in determining the degree of swaying. It is a different matter, however, when the elderly person is standing on a less firm surface. In such cases, the amount of sensory information from the lower legs is reduced, and the degree of swaying is associated largely with the elderly person's visual proficiency and muscular strength in the lower legs. Elderly people should seek physical support of some kind when standing on less than firm surfaces (and to be on the safe side, even when standing on firm surfaces). This is especially true for those with poor vision and diminished muscular strength.

Primary Mental Abilities (PMA) Test

The Primary Mental Abilities (PMA) Test is a widely used group intelligence test in research on adult age differences in intelligence. It is the test used in the Seattle Longitudinal Study (see SEATTLE LONGITUDINAL STUDY), and it has been the major source of information about longitudinal changes in intelligence as measured by a standardized test.

The PMA was introduced in 1941 as a test of seven different factors or primary components of intelligence. The original seven factors were number, word fluency, verbal meaning, memory, reasoning, space, and perceptual speed. Eventually the test was reduced to measuring only five factors: number (numerical ability), word fluency, verbal meaning (vocabulary), reasoning, and space (spatial ability). A total score may be obtained from all five separate tests, as may separate scores for each of the five components. Cross-sectional studies generally indicate substantial decline in total tests scores from early to late adulthood. The decline is much less when the longitudinal method has been used. However, the extent of the decline varies greatly across the five separate abilities being measured. The age-related decline is slight for the number, verbal meaning, and word fluency components, and, in general, is found only after age 60. The decline is fairly large for the reasoning and space components and occurs before age 60.

Problem Solving

Your car won't start, and you are trying to figure out why. This is an example of a problem (the car won't start) and problem-solving behavior (figuring out why). The problem solver has a goal in mind—coming up with a solution to some situation for which there is no immediate correct behavior. Laboratory research with rather abstract problems, such as those involving a variation of the old "Twenty Questions" game, has typically revealed that older participants have greater difficulty in finding appropriate solutions than do younger participants. On the Twenty Questions task, the participant's goal is to discover the object the investigator has in mind among a series of pictures of objects in plain view of the participant (e.g., a picture of a hammer, a cup, a cow, a child, and so on). The participant is allowed to ask questions that may be answered only by a *yes* or *no*. On the average, elderly participants tend to ask fewer constraining questions of the kind "Is it living?" than do younger participants. A constraining question is one that by its yes or no answer immediately eliminates a number of objects from consideration as the one to discover. As a result, older participants generally average more questions to find the solution than do younger participants. However, with practice and training, elderly participants are found to approximate the level of performance by younger participants.

Of greater importance to our understanding of age differences in problem-solving proficiency are those studies in which participants are presented with everyday problems and are asked what they would do in these situations. For example, "You come home late at night and discover that your front door is unlocked and opened somewhat. You are surprised because you know you locked the door when you left home. What should you do?" The quality of solutions to problems of this kind has been found to be the highest for people in their 40s.

Older participants typically score only moderately below the level of middle-aged participants and as well as young adult participants. Moreover, when the problems given to participants are ones dealing with interpersonal relations, problem-solving proficiency has been found to increase progressively from early to late adulthood. That is, the most effective solutions are those offered by elderly adults. This is the kind of problem solving generally associated with the concept of wisdom (see WISDOM). For normally aging individuals, there is no reason to believe that their everyday problem-solving ability declines from early to late adulthood. In fact, with the experience they accumulate during a lifetime of confronting problems, they may even gain in proficiency.

It is a different matter, however, when very unique solutions or highly creative solutions to problems are required. Here, there is evidence of declining ability with normal aging (see CREATIVITY; ORIGINALITY).

Progeria

Progeria is a rare, fatal childhood disease that is characterized by a precocious senility of a severe degree. An 8-year-old child with the disease is likely to have the physical appearance and the bodily functioning of an 80-year-old person. The child is likely be susceptible to heart attacks and arthritis as the disease progresses. However, other diseases associated with aging, such as cancer, are usually absent. The cause of the disease is unknown, and there is presently no known cure.

Prospective Memory

Memory research has typically concentrated on what may be called *retrospective memory* (memory for past things and events). Consequently, we know a great deal about what happens to retrospective memory as people age (see EPISODIC MEMORY and other memory-related entries). In the everyday world, however, there is another form of memory that plays an important role in our everyday lives. Our failures in executing this form of memory are often referred to as "absentmindedness." To psychologists, however, the failures involve what they term *prospective memory*. Prospective memory requires performing some action at an appropriate time. For example, we intend to stop at the market on the way home from work, to drop a letter in the mailbox as we pass it on the street, to take prescribed medicine at designated times, and so on. However, we often discover that we forgot to stop at the market and must do without coffee the next morning, that the letter to be mailed is still at home, and that the night has gone by without taking the medicine. One of the more famous lapses of prospective memory occurred some years ago when a prominent professional golfer forgot to sign his card after completing a round at a major tournament, a lapse that cost him winning the tournament (and much money). Prospective memory, like retrospective memory, is obviously imperfect. Our interest is in the extent to which its imperfection increases during late adulthood.

Testing for age differences in the proficiency of prospective memory requires giving young and older adults a series of tasks to perform, each at some designated time. One way of accomplishing this is to send research participants home from the laboratory with a number of postcards. The first card is to be mailed to the investigator on the following Tuesday, the second on the next Friday, the third on the following Monday, and so on. How many times will they remember to mail the card at the right time? Alternatively, subjects may be asked to call the investigator at designated times on designated days over several weeks. With either procedure, the results have been rather surprising. Elderly adults return the cards or make the calls at the right times more often than do young adults. There is a problem, however, in concluding from this evidence that prospective memory proficiency, unlike proficiency for most forms of retrospective memory, actually increases from early to late adulthood. The problem stems from the strong possibility that elderly adults are more motivated to conform to the request of the investigator than are young adults (typically college students) in research of this kind. In fact, the evidence indicates that when young adults fail to perform the action it is not always because they did not remember to do it. Instead, when they remembered they were often preoccupied with some other activity and did not want to interrupt it.

Fortunately, there is some laboratory evidence to support further the possibility that one form of prospective memory, called *event-based prospective memory* by memory researchers, does not decline greatly, if at all, with normal aging. The evidence is derived from a study in which young adults and elderly adults were asked to memorize a number of words presented one at a time on a computer screen. They were also asked to watch for a certain word (a target) to appear from time to time on the screen. With each appearance they were to press a certain key on the computer keyboard. Pressing the key at the right time (the target's appearance) does qualify as an operation of prospective memory. Although the older adults did not outperform the young adults, they nevertheless performed as well as the young adults (i.e., the number of their prospective memory failures was no greater than that for the young adults). The implication is that prospective memory proficiency is not greatly affected by normal aging. This form of prospective memory occurs when there is some kind of external event present to serve as a reminder to perform the designated activity. There is another form of prospective memory, *time-based prospective memory*, in which the designated activity is not cued by some physically present event. Here the activity is to be performed at some designated time, such as keeping a 10 A.M. appointment with a physician. Laboratory evidence indicates a moderate decline with normal aging for this form of prospective memory.

Adults of all ages should be aware of the imperfection of prospective memory and take steps to avoid its failures. One obvious way is to make external cues available to help you remember what you need to do. This is the technique represented by the old gimmick of tying a string on your finger. The idea is that looking at the string triggers the action. The problem, however, is that you may no longer remember what action is to be performed. A more effective technique is to make clearly visible a cue that is more directly related to the action itself. Thus why not place the empty instant coffee jar on the front seat of your car when you need to buy more coffee? The sight of the jar on the way home from work that evening should remind you of the need to stop at the store. Such reminding cues are especially important for older adults. They are more likely to need prescribed medicines than are younger adults. Failure to conform to a prescribed regimen could have a serious outcome; thus it is very important that they should not be forced to rely on their prospective memories without environmental support. Fortunately, pharmaceutical companies are becoming increasingly aware of this problem, and they are introducing aids to ensure conformity to a prescribed schedule.

Prostate Gland
See also DISEASES (CHRONIC); SEXUAL BEHAVIOR

The prostate gland is a walnut-sized structure that is located just below the urinary bladder and through which the urethra passes. The prostate gland secretes a substance that aids the flow of sperm. The gland increases in size in older men, and it may eventually press against the urethra, hindering the passage of urine. A more serious problem is the risk of prostate cancer, especially in elderly men.

Proverbs (Interpretation)

"Don't cry over spilt milk." "A stitch in time saves nine." These are examples of familiar proverbs. A proverb offers a concrete analogy for a more general set of circumstances that the interpreter attempts to describe (e.g., "Once something is over there is nothing you can do to change things" as an interpretation of the "Don't cry over spilt milk" proverb). Interpreting the meaning of a proverb requires a form of reasoning. A test of adult age differences in the ability to reason through the analogy between a proverb and its meaning in everyday life requires the use of proverbs that are unfamiliar to participants of all ages. There is only limited evidence of age differences in this reasoning ability. The results of several studies indicated a moderate age difference in the ability to interpret such proverbs, with older adults giving more literal interpretations than younger adults. This outcome is surprising in that older adults are usually found to be at least as proficient as younger adults in the adequacy of the interpretations of metaphors. Interpreting a metaphor seemingly requires the same kind of reasoning through analogy required in interpreting proverbs (see METAPHORS). However, the evidence on age differences in proverb interpretation comes only from cross-sectional studies. The extent to which the age difference is the result of a cohort or generational effect (see COHORT [GENERATIONAL] EFFECT) is unknown. It is possible that members of earlier generations simply give more literal interpretations of proverbs than do members of later generations.

Psychosis

A psychosis is a severe mental disorder that greatly impairs the life of the individual affected by it. The two most common psychoses are schizophrenia and clinical depression.

The major symptom of schizophrenia is a thought disturbance characterized by intrusions of irrelevant, and often bizarre, thoughts when the disorder is in an active state. There are other symptoms that are present in different forms of schizophrenia. They include a flattened emotional state in one form and a heightened, "silly" state in another form, hallucinations in some forms, and delusions (intense and persistent false beliefs, such as a delusion of persecution) in still other forms. Schizophrenia, regardless of its specific form and symptoms, usually has its onset in early adulthood. The incidence of its onset in late adulthood is quite low. When it does occur in older people, it is likely to be expressed largely by delusions of persecution, with few other thought disturbances. Of great interest is what happens to long-term schizophrenics as they age. It is estimated that there are about 300,000 people age 65 and older in the United States who have schizophrenia. In general, the symptoms found earlier in the lives of schizophrenics become less pronounced during late adulthood.

Clinical depression is an intense and persistent state that greatly hinders everyday functioning (see DEPRESSION [INCIDENCE, SYMPTOMS, CAUSES]). Like schizophrenia, it is uncommon for clinical depression to have its onset in late adulthood. In general, when clinical depression does occur in late adulthood, its symptoms differ somewhat from the symptoms present earlier in adulthood. Affective symptoms (feelings of sadness, despair, hopelessness) are likely to be less intense for elderly depressed individuals than for younger individuals, whereas the reverse is true for somatic symptoms (complaints about physical functioning, e.g., sleep disturbances).

A less frequent form of psychosis is paranoia. It is characterized by a persisting and dominating false belief, often one in which the affected individual believes he or she is being persecuted and that other people are "out to get them." The delusion is likely to lead to very bizarre behaviors and suspicious attitudes about events and persons in the individual's world. As is true of schizophrenia, the onset of paranoia among elderly people who are aging normally is rare. However, it is not unusual to find individuals with Alzheimer's disease who have some symptoms of paranoia.

Psychotherapy

Emotional and behavioral problems occur for adults of all ages. One form of treatment of these problems for normally aging adults is psychotherapy. Psychotherapy consists of many different forms, and the appropriate form depends on the nature of the problem to be treated.

One form of psychotherapy is called behavior modification. It consists of the application of either classical conditioning or operant conditioning learning principles (see CLASSICAL CONDITIONING; OPERANT CONDITIONING) to modify a specific or habitual behavior of an individual. Classical conditioning enters into several specific forms of behavior modification. One form is called aversion therapy; another is systematic desensitization. *Aversion therapy* has been used to treat bad health practices such as excessive drinking of alcoholic beverages and smoking. The objective of the treatment is to condition an averse reaction to what had been previously a regular behavior of the client (i.e., drinking or smoking). For drinking, tasting an alcoholic beverage is accompanied by the intake of a drug to induce severe nausea. The idea is to form a conditioned reaction of nausea to the taste of the beverage. For smoking, the client is forced to smoke one cigarette after another until nausea results. The idea is to associate smoking with nausea.

Systematic desensitization is used in the treatment of phobias (intense fears provoked by specific objects, such as a snake, or conditions, such as being in an enclosed area [claustrophobia]). During the treatment the client is first taught to relax as much as possible. In later sessions with the therapist, the client is gradually introduced to the phobic object or condition while in a relaxed state. The objective is to condition a feeling of relaxation to the phobic object or condition to replace the feeling of intense fear. Classical conditioning has also been used in some cases of intense hypertension. The client is placed under physical conditions (e.g., listening to soft music in a darkened room) that lead to a lowering of blood pressure. At the same time a conditioned stimulus (e.g., the sounding of a bell) is present. The goal is to associate a lowering of blood pressure with the sound of the bell. There is evidence of successful treatment of at least some younger adults with these forms of behavior modification. However, evidence regarding successful treatment with older adults is sparse. Such methods may not work well with elderly clients. Elderly people are much slower in acquiring conditioned responses in the laboratory than are younger people, and in each of these forms of behavior modification the acquisition of a conditioned response is essential to the success of the therapy.

Operant conditioning is often used in behavior management to aid an individual to rid himself or herself of an unwanted and unhealthy habit, such as excessive eating or smoking. The objective of behavior modification with obese individuals is to help them control their weight through changes in basic eating habits. For example, they are trained to avoid eating while engaged in some other activity, such as watching television, when eating has become automatic for most obese people. The objective of behavior modification with smokers is to help them control their smoking through changes in their smoking habits. For example, they may be trained to reinforce or reward themselves (e.g., a trip to a mall) whenever they go through a period of nonsmoking or to find substitutes for smoking (e.g., taking a walk instead of smoking). These methods work for some individuals, but not for all. In addition, relapses (returning to the old habits) do occur. Nevertheless, the success rate should be as high for older adults as it is for younger adults. Unlike classical conditioning, operant conditioning has been found to be well within the capacity of elderly adults. A unique form of behavior modification is through the use of biofeedback. *Biofeedback* consists of information that informs a client that a change has taken place in some physiological function. For example, brain waves may be monitored with the client receiving feedback every time their frequency has increased. Elderly adults have been found to increase their brain wave frequencies through this method. Most important, those who have been successful often show an improvement in their reaction time or speed of responding.

Other forms of psychotherapy are designed to help clients handle their emotional problems and to enhance their feelings about themselves, rather than to change their observable behaviors. The oldest, and best known form, is psychoanalytic therapy. The objective is to enable clients to discover and deal with their unconscious guilts, impulses, and conflicts. The therapy often takes years to complete, and it is expensive. Both of these factors usually make it unavailable to elderly adults. Sigmund Freud, the pioneer psychoanalyst, doubted the success of the therapy with elderly adults, and he himself treated few patients as old as the 40s and 50s. Some later psychoanalysts have questioned the inapplicability of their therapy for older clients, but there is little evidence to indicate its successful application. It is through their efforts, however, that the technique of allowing elderly clients to reminisce about their past life and review their major life events has been incorporated into various other forms of psychotherapy (e.g., group therapy; see REMINISCENCE).

One currently popular and more successful form of psychotherapy is called *cognitive therapy*. Cognitive therapists believe that the way an individual thinks largely determines how that person feels. The therapist then helps the client to alter his or her maladaptive thinking habits. The technique is frequently used to treat such emotional disturbances as depression, anxiety, and hostility. Like other forms of therapy, the treatment is not always successful, and even when it is, clients may return to their old, maladaptive ways of thinking about themselves. However, the success rate does seem to be about as high for elderly clients as it is for younger clients, especially when it is used in combination with drug therapy to treat severe depression. Older adults often think of themselves in ways that are inaccurate (e.g., thinking that they are no longer useful human beings and that they have become totally incompetent), thus making them ideal clients for cognitive therapy.

Another currently popular form of psychotherapy is *family therapy*. It is useful when one or more elderly people are members of a dysfunctional family. The family is regarded by family therapists as being a system in which the members mutually influence one another. If the behavior of one member of the system could be changed, then the behavior of other members should change as well. The treatment is useful for families in which there is a conflict between elderly spouses (e.g., over one spouse's physical disability) or a conflict between older parents and their adult children (e.g., over the child-rearing practices of the adult children with their own children). The treatment stresses more effective communication among family members so that each member may express more clearly his or her feelings and concerns. The therapy seems to be effective for many older adults. It is also a form of therapy that may greatly benefit caregivers of physically or mentally disabled elderly adults (see entries involving caregivers).

Group therapy has long been used with older clients. It may take several different forms, but the most familiar form consists of life discussion groups. In life discussion groups, members discuss their own problems, enabling elderly people to discover that they are not alone in their problems. The groups are usually smaller in size, and the durations of the discussions are shorter than when the groups are composed of younger adults. Group therapy is especially valuable as an alternative to cognitive therapy in the treatment of depression. It may be given in various settings, including hospitals, community mental health centers, and even senior centers and retirement communities.

Unfortunately, elderly adults are less likely to benefit from psychotherapy than are younger adults, simply because they are less likely to seek help when they are confronted by behavioral and emotional problems than are younger adults (see MENTAL HEALTH AND MENTAL HEALTH SERVICES). Efforts have increased in recent years to familiarize elderly adults with mental health services through radio and television commercials. This effort would be even more successful if there were more television programs, both dramas and documentaries, that centered on the emotional problems of older adults and the ways they may be treated successfully.

Psychotherapy with Nursing Home Residents

Nursing home residents are commonly found to be apathetic, disoriented, and to have feelings of isolation. Their behavioral and emotional problems have required psychotherapies that differ greatly from those used among community-dwelling elderly adults. A number of such therapies have been introduced in recent years, and they have generally been found to be fairly successful in increasing the well-being of nursing home residents.

One form of treatment is called *reality orientation*. Its objective is to keep residents in touch with the world. To accomplish this, numerous clocks are placed in the nursing home, and calendars are located in prominent places. Name cards are used to identify each other at meals, birthdays of residents are individually recognized, visiting hours are made as liberal as possible, and independence is stressed as much as possible. To aid in orientation, halls and residential rooms are often painted in different colors. *Remotivation therapy* is intended for residents who seem understimulated in their current environments. Basically, it is a form of group therapy (see PSYCHOTHERAPY) in which small groups of residents meet to discuss shared topics of interest, such as food and clothing. The idea is to create a climate in which the residents may appreciate the contributions of the other residents. Group therapy may also include activities performed in groups, such as singing, playing bingo, and so on, that help to decrease the feelings of social isolation. *Sensory training* is a form of therapy for those older residents who are highly disoriented and unlikely to benefit from other forms of treatment. The residents are given body awareness exercises and sensory stimulation by observing, touching, smelling, and sometimes tasting common objects.

Some patients with mild mental impairment who also are affected by depression have benefited from some form of cognitive therapy for their depression (see PSYCHOTHERAPY). The therapy does not alter the mental impairment, but it does enable the patient to make fuller use of his or her mental abilities. The patient's diminished mental functioning is otherwise limited to an even greater degree by the debilitating effects of depression.

Behavior modification through the use of positive reinforcement (i.e., rewarding specific behaviors to increase their frequency of occurrence; see OPERANT CONDITIONING; PSYCHOTHERAPY) has been found to be successful in some cases in increasing such behaviors as participation in rehabilitative and recreational behaviors and in increasing self-care and social behaviors. Some institutionalized older people exhibit excessive aggressive behavior that may be harmful to both themselves and other residents. The positive reinforcement of nonaggressive verbal behaviors by following their occurrences with praise has been found, in combination with other forms of treatment, to lead to a decrease in verbal aggressive behaviors for some patients.

Quackery

Elderly adults are the most likely victims of medical quackery and fraud. It is estimated that they make up as much as 60% of such victims. Billions of dollars are spent every year on so-called remedies that are not only unhelpful to their users, but may actually be harmful to their health. People with arthritis are among the most frequent victims; many bogus remedies have been introduced over the years. Patients should check with their physician before purchasing some advertised remedy.

R

· ·

Race and Ethnic Differences in Aging

Even social and biological scientists disagree as to what defines a race or an ethnic group. Nevertheless, our society has widely accepted viewing our population as consisting of a white majority group and such racial-ethnic minority groups as blacks, Hispanics, and others.

Our concern is with the possibility that aging may have different effects on members of minority racial and ethnic groups than on whites. The reason for this possibility is one that has little, if anything, to do with inherent biological differences among races. Instead the possibility arises from the fact that proportionally more members of minority groups live in impoverished environments, have lower economic resources, and have fewer cultural and educational opportunities than do the white members of our society. These factors expose many more minority members than majority members to high-risk health conditions and to less utilization of health care facilities. Not surprisingly, life expectancy at birth is about 5 years less for blacks than for whites. This difference is related to the higher mortality rates for blacks than for whites at all ages except very late adulthood. At about 80 or 85 years of age there is a crossover effect in mortality rates; blacks at this age and older average living as many and perhaps more additional years than do whites. This is true even though disability and morbidity is significantly greater for elderly blacks than for elderly whites, as indicated, for example, by the greater number of average annual sick days experienced by elderly blacks. Most important, the incidence of heart disease is significantly higher among elderly blacks than among elderly whites (although there has been a striking reduction in the presence of hypertension among elderly blacks in recent years). Health statistics indicate that the crossover in mortality rates occurs at a much earlier age for Mexican-Americans than it does for blacks, but the incidence of morbidity is, nevertheless, higher for elderly Mexican-Americans than for elderly whites. By contrast, Native Americans have mortality rates comparable to those of whites, and Asian-Americans appear to have even lower mortality rates than the general population of elderly adults.

The overall poorer health of elderly blacks and members of some other minority groups is an outcome predicted by what sociologists call the *double jeopardy hypothesis*. According to this hypothesis, the negative effects of living for years in an impoverished environment and living under the burden of racism add to the negative effects that accompany normal biological aging for people of all races and therefore amplify the problems experienced by minority group members. Seemingly in conflict with the double jeopardy hypothesis is the fact that the incidence of elderly blacks living in nursing homes is from one-half to three-fourths of that of elderly whites. However, there are reasons other than health that seemingly account for this disparity. Elderly people who are forced to live alone are the most likely candidates for becoming nursing home residents. Elderly blacks are less likely to live alone than are elderly whites, and they are therefore less likely to enter nursing homes. Moreover, elderly black women are more likely to be heads of households than are elderly white women, meaning that they are also more likely to serve as caregivers of family members and less likely to be recipients of caregiving. However, an analysis of a survey conducted in 1987 and 1988 revealed that elderly blacks are no more likely than elderly whites to receive instrumental support (e.g., for housekeeping and transportation) and social support from others. In addition, Hispanic elderly people are less likely than elderly white people to receive instrumental support.

The double jeopardy hypothesis is strongly supported by evidence revealing, on the average, a lower level of life satisfaction among elderly blacks than among elderly whites (see LIFE SATISFACTION). Dr. Neal Krause of the University of Michigan, a prominent researcher in the area of life satisfaction, has concluded that the lower level for elderly blacks is the result of various factors. For example, elderly blacks often experience a greater gap than do elderly whites between their earlier educational goals and their educational attainment and between their retirement plans and what their economic conditions permit after retirement. In addition, elderly blacks usually are more dependent on financial assistance from family members than are elderly whites. These factors, combined with the overall poorer health status of elderly blacks, inevitably lead to lower life satisfaction. Fortunately, these factors can be overcome by greater allocation of our country's health services and financial resources to the needs of elderly minority group members.

There are other, less obvious, factors that are likely to contribute to the lower level of life satisfaction among elderly blacks. For example, married elderly people tend to be in better health and to have a higher level of life satisfaction than unmarried elderly people. Elderly married black women are in a minority (about 25% compared with about 41% of elderly white women), as are elderly married black men (about 54% compared with about 76% of elderly white men). The probability of having a spouse to serve as a caregiver is therefore greater for elderly whites than for elderly blacks. In addition, the quality of housing remains less satisfactory for elderly blacks than for elderly whites, even though the quality of housing has increased during the past two decades for both whites and blacks. A less livable home is likely to make daily living less satisfactory than does a safe and comfortable home.

With one exception, there has been little research on racial differences in mental abilities. The one exception is in the area of intelligence. There is no doubt that blacks score lower than whites at all age levels, including late adulthood, on intelligence tests such as the Wechsler Adult Intelligence Scale. Hispanics tend to score somewhere between blacks and whites, and Asian-Americans often score above whites, in late adulthood as well as at younger ages. Please note that the lower scores by blacks and Hispanics are exactly that—lower *scores* on tests that place them at a considerable disadvantage, and certainly not necessarily in intelligence as it concerns coping with problems in the everyday world. Intelligence tests have typically been constructed to predict academic achievement in a white-oriented society. They may therefore have little validity for individuals who are outside that society. Interestingly, the difference in average test scores between whites and blacks on most intelligence tests is lowest for people of relatively little formal education. It is here that blacks are least disadvantaged relative to whites of the same educational level. That is, with increasing education, the advantage of whites over blacks in average intelligence test scores increases progressively. The picture clearly indicates that blacks receiving the same quantity of education as whites are also receiving less quality of education.

Do the races differ in such basic mental functions as learning and memory? Probably not. There is no reason to expect such differences except for tasks in which the greater opportunities provided for whites in our society provide them with greater familiarity with the tasks to be mastered. There is, however, no scientific evidence to indicate whether there are real differences among the races in learning and memory abilities—or, for that matter, in reasoning and problem-solving abilities. Researchers rarely report information about the racial composition of participants in their studies of learning, memory, reasoning, and so on. If they did, it is doubtful that any significant racial differences would emerge.

Reaction Time

You are the first one in line at a stoplight. As the light turns from red to green, you press down on the accelerator of your car to proceed. How much time elapsed between the appearance of the green light and the movement of your foot on the accelerator? That time is an example of a *reaction time*. Reaction time is the time separating the appearance of a signal and the initiation of a response to that signal. If you are an elderly driver, your reaction time in the stoplight situation is likely to be some seconds slower than if you are a younger driver. The slowing down of reaction time to various sources of stimulation does seem to be an inevitable consequence of normal aging, and it is part of a general slowing of physical and mental activities that accompanies normal aging (see SLOWING DOWN PRINCIPLE). Although slower reaction times may be characteristic of older people in general, the amount of slowing does vary considerably. Reaction time, for example, is one of the abilities affected by long-term regular exercise. Elderly people who have been regular exercisers for many years have been found to have faster reaction times than elderly people who have had less physically active lives. In fact, many regular exercisers have been found to have reaction times that are as fast as many younger adults.

Age differences in reaction time are studied in the laboratory by having participants of various ages perform different kinds of reaction time tasks. A simple reaction time task is one in which participants execute a response, such as pressing a button, each time a signal (e.g., a tone or a light) occurs. Reaction time on this task increases progressively from young adulthood to late adulthood. The slowing with aging is more pronounced, however, on a choice reaction time task. Here two different signals are used, each requiring a different response. For example, when a high-frequency tone is sounded, the participant presses one button; when a low-frequency tone is sounded, the participant presses a different button.

Of great interest in gerontology is whether interventions of some kind (other than long-term physical exercise) can be found that will facilitate an older adult's response to signals (i.e., reduce reaction time). There is some limited, but promising, evidence to indicate that such interventions may be possible. Extensive practice on a video game has been found to have a positive effect on reaction time. Elderly participants who played the game for 2 hours per week for 7 weeks had faster choice reaction times on a laboratory task at the end of the practice period than other elderly participants who had received no prior practice on the video game.

Reading Skills

Although the evidence is somewhat conflicting, elderly adults, in general, appear to be somewhat slower readers than younger adults. Nevertheless, their reading strategy seems to be similar to that of younger adults. For example, both younger and older readers increase their reading time when they encounter major and minor clauses in sentences. There do seem to be some moderate adverse effects of aging on the comprehension of paragraphs but only when the content is fairly complex and requires making inferences of some kind about the events being described. Most reading material, however, is not of sufficient difficulty to present any real problems to older readers.

Reasoning

Through reasoning we are able to draw valid conclusions from facts that either are known to be true or are assumed to be true. A reasoning problem is one in which logical relationships between events are given and a solution based of these relationships is sought. A common laboratory task used to study age differences in reasoning ability involves problems called syllogisms. A *syllogism* is an argument composed of two (or more) premises or assertions. From those premises, a logical conclusion is to be derived. Consider, for example, two premises: (1) all psychologists are scientists; and (2) all scientists are computer experts. Now consider the conclusion that "All psychologists are therefore computer experts." Is it true or false, based only on the information given in the two premises? (Assume the premises to be true, even though they are not.) A correct conclusion in this case is "true." In general, older participants perform at a lower level on syllogism problems than do younger participants.

Comparable outcomes (i.e., lower scores by older than by younger participants) have been found for other tasks that evaluate other forms of reasoning, such as functional reasoning or reasoning through the use of analogy and inferential reasoning. *Functional reasoning* is the kind of reasoning needed to give interpretations of proverbs (see PROVERBS). It is also the kind of reasoning needed to solve this problem: **A,** *a;* **B,** *b;* **C,** *?* What should fill in the question mark? You need to discover what change occurred to the **A** and **B** in the series, and then apply that change analogously to the **C** to reach the solution of *c. Inferential reasoning* is involved when participants receive a series of rule-based items and then must infer or deduce what should be next to continue the series. For example, the series might be **2   8   32**—what number should be next? To respond with **128,** you must discover the rule that relates the first three numbers to each other (namely, each successive number is four times the preceding number).

The decline in average scores found with normal aging on reasoning tasks may well exaggerate the extent to which everyday reasoning abilities decline. The laboratory tasks used in studies of age differences in reasoning abilities are quite artificial, and likely to be quite different from the kinds of reasoning tasks encountered in the everyday world (e.g., deducing what your partner meant by that last bid in playing bridge, deducing which stock purchase is best at this time; see ECOLOGICAL VALIDITY). Moreover, the mental skills needed to solve laboratory reasoning problems are not necessarily beyond the capabilities of most normally aging elderly adults. There is convincing evidence to show that older adults improve their scores greatly on inferential reasoning tasks after they have had instructions on what kind of mental operations are needed to solve them and after they have had practice on similar problems (see TRANSFER OF LEARNING TRAINING). Thus elderly adults demonstrate considerable plasticity in their ability to overcome apparent deficits in mental skills (see PLASTICITY THEORY). In addition, many older adults continue to perform exceptionally well on jobs and hobbies that demand reasoning abilities as part of their expertise (e.g., executive management, playing bridge), despite the fact that they score well below the level of younger people on laboratory tests of reasoning ability (see EXPERTISE).

Recognition Memory vs. Recall Memory

Is the title of this entry (a) Recognition Memory, (b) Recall Memory, (c) Recognition Memory vs. Recall Memory, or (d) Recognition Memory and Recall Memory?

The correct answer, of course, is *c.* This is an example of a question on a multiple-choice test, a testing format familiar to millions of students. Multiple-choice tests evaluate the students' memories for recently studied (and hopefully acquired) information. Instead of being asked to recall all the information recently studied, students are asked simply to recognize it and discriminate that information from distractors (i.e., information somewhat similar to the studied information, but not identical) that are present.

A multiple-choice test is one of the methods often used by memory researchers to test for age differences in recognition memory. The procedure consists of presenting younger and older participants with a series of items or episodic events, with each item presented individually for several seconds. The items may be familiar words, pictures of objects, or pictures of scenes. The participants then receive a series of test items in which each of the previously studied words or pictures is presented along with several distractors, and participants are asked to select from each test item the "old" (previously studied) word or picture. An alternative testing procedure is to present in a random order a series of words or pictures in which half are "old" (previously studied) and half are "new" (distractors not previously studied). As each test item is encountered, the participants respond "old" or "new." Correct identifications of old items as old and new items as new are called "hits." Incorrect identifications of new items as old are called false alarms.

Regardless of the recognition testing procedure used, age differences in memory scores favoring younger participants are usually found to be much smaller than when participants are asked to recall the previously studied items. That is, older participants more closely match the performance of younger participants on a recognition memory test than on a recall memory test. In fact, in some instances the age differences found on a recall test all but disappear when a recognition test is used. This is the case, for example, when the episodic events are actions performed in the laboratory (see ACTION MEMORY).

Recognition and recall differ in an important way. To recall previously studied information, you have to conduct a vigorous search of your long-term memory store to find the memory traces of the previously studied items. Once a trace is found, then you need to recognize that it is indeed one for a just-studied item. Such a search is an effortful one that is more difficult to conduct, on the average, for older adults than for younger adults. Older adults tend to have a greater retrieval problem than do younger adults. The intensity of the search, and therefore the difficulty of retrieval, is reduced greatly when participants face a recognition memory test. The old items are reinstated at the time of the test, thereby directing the search to specific memory traces. The fact that the memory performance of elderly adults more closely approximates that of younger adults on a recognition test than on a recall test suggests that much of the difficulty experienced by older adults in episodic memory stems from their diminished retrieval proficiency. However, the fact that an age difference favoring younger adults often persists even on a recognition memory test suggests that at least part of the episodic memory problem of elderly adults is related to their less proficient encoding of the information studied.

There is another interesting outcome of research on age differences in recognition memory. Elderly participants typically have more false alarms (calling new test items old) than do younger participants. Cautious people would seemingly be more reluctant than less cautious people in identifying new test items as old. This is further evidence to indicate that older adults should not be viewed as possessing a general characteristic of cautiousness to a greater extent than do younger people (see CAUTIOUSNESS).

Religion and Church Attendance

The results from four large national surveys indicated that nearly all older people have a religious affiliation of some kind. Elderly people generally are highly religious. It is estimated that from 60% to 95% of older adults pray daily. A longitudinal study of older Mexican-Americans revealed that the frequency of religious activities may remain fairly constant as people age from their late 60s to their late 70s. On a number of indices of religiosity (e.g., frequency of prayer), elderly women are more religious than elderly men, and blacks are more religious than whites.

Older people frequently use prayer as a means of coping with stressful events in their lives. One common source of stress late in life is physical illness. A study conducted in North Carolina revealed that a large percentage of the older participants reported the use of prayer when they had symptoms of illness they believed to be serious. Other researchers in North Carolina indicated that nearly half of the elderly people they surveyed reported using religious activities as a means of coping with other kinds of stressful events. In general, morale and satisfaction with one's life have been found to be greater for elderly people who report frequent religious activities than for elderly people who report less frequent activities.

Despite the apparent religiosity of older people, there is evidence indicating that they participate less frequently in organized religious practices compared either with themselves when they were younger or with current younger people. A study conducted some years ago in New York state revealed that only 43% of the older adults surveyed attended church regularly. A more recent study of older adults living in central Missouri also indicated that fewer than 50% of those surveyed were regular church attenders. The percentage of younger people attending church regularly is considerably higher. However, the decline in church attendance does not mean that there is a decline in religiosity with normal aging. The study in Missouri revealed the reasons that older people do not attend church more regularly—poor health, bad weather, and lack of transportation—not a declining interest in religion. Religiosity obviously needs to be measured at a more personal level, such as the regular use of private prayer. As noted above, when measured in this way, it is apparent that most older people do indeed keep their religious convictions; they simply have to express them less formally than in the past.

Reminiscence

Thinking and talking about the "good old days" and your life events at that time is a phenomenon known as reminiscence that is commonly associated with elderly people. A particular form of reminiscence in which a participant is asked to review his or her life is sometimes used as a component of psychotherapy with older people with depression and with nursing home residents to help them reduce their feelings of isolation. Reminiscence is also used in some senior centers to help participants cope with stress.

The therapeutic value of reminiscence has been questioned by some gerontologists. However, it does appear that some forms of reminiscence are more characteristic of elderly people who are aging successfully, defined in terms of both positive physical health and mental health status, than of those older people who are aging less successfully. Canadian researchers recently asked a number of elderly people to reminisce about their lives. They found that most of the statements given by less successfully aging people were simple narrations about events in their lives without interpretation of their significance. Successfully aging participants gave fewer narrative statements and more integrative statements than less successfully aging participants. An *integrative reminiscence* is one indicating acceptance of one's life as having been worthwhile. Other forms of reminiscence include *escapist reminiscence* (glorifying past achievements and yearning for the "good old days") and *obsessive reminiscence* (statements revealing guilt and bitterness about the past). Escapist reminiscence was found by the researchers to occur rarely for either successfully or less successfully aging participants. Obsessive reminiscence occurred moderately often for less successfully aging participants and not at all for successfully aging people. It seems apparent that successfully aging people have succeeded in integrating life experiences positively and feel little despair about their current life status (see PERSONALITY STAGES). The treatment of depression in some older adults may be successful to the extent that the clients are successful in reevaluating their lives and finding that they have been worthwhile. Reminiscence itself may not be therapeutic, but it may serve as a useful index of how successful elderly clients have been in the reevaluation of their lives. As discovered by a researcher at the Medical University of South Carolina, a structured reminiscence of one's life history from birth may also increase one's self-esteem.

Respite Care

Respite care is intended to provide caregivers (usually relatives) of disabled elderly people (see CAREGIVERS [FAMILY MEMBERS AND FRIENDS]) periods of rest and relief away from the person receiving care. The objective is to reduce the strain and stress experienced by caregivers in prolonged service. By so doing, it is also hoped that admissions of persons to nursing homes may be delayed or even avoided completely, thereby reducing the heavy financial cost of nursing home residence. Respite care may be accomplished in several ways. Disabled recipients of the care may spend part of their time away from their homes and caregivers. Such possibilities include periods of time spent in a day-care center or periods of time spent in a nursing home. Alternatively, a substitute caregiver may be contracted to serve on occasions in the recipient's home during the day or evening or during weekends. Such respites enable the family caregiver to recover from an illness, to attend an important function, or simply to have time for relaxation.

A yearlong study conducted at the Philadelphia Geriatric Center compared caregivers who received respite care with caregivers who did not receive the service. Respite care was found to delay admission of disabled recipients to a nursing home by an average of several weeks. Although the caregivers receiving the respite care expressed great satisfaction with it, at the end of the year there was little difference in their mental health status compared with caregivers who did not receive respite care. Researchers at the University of Nebraska at

Omaha also have found that the greater the use of respite care by caregivers, the lesser the probability that the recipients of their caregiving will be placed in a nursing home.

Retirement Communities

Retirement communities in the United States are either subsidized by a government agency, most frequently by the Department of Housing and Urban Development (HUD), or nonsubsidized by private sources. The subsidized communities are for low-income retirees; the nonsubsidized communities are for those with larger incomes. The nonsubsidized housing varies from modest mobile homes to luxurious homes.

Retirement communities vary in their size, the level and kinds of services offered, and profit or nonprofit governance. They comprise five basic categories. The first consists of new retirement towns. These are large communities (e.g., Sun City in Arizona), usually constructed by private developers, that cater to younger and active retirees and have large recreational facilities, health services, and commercial facilities. Retirement villages make up the second category. They are of medium size and are usually privately developed by an organization (e.g., a union). They tend to have more limited recreational, health, and commercial services than does a new town. The third category consists of retirement subdivisions that are located in a section of a large city. They, too, have limited services, and they cater largely to younger retirees who wish to be near a large city. Retirement residences, the fourth category, consist of clusters of apartments that are usually found in high-rise, large-city buildings. Their residents are likely to be older and less active people. Their facilities are limited, but they may include daily meals. The final category consists of continuing care centers that are small in size and are designed to offer comprehensive health care and sedentary leisure activities for older and more frail people.

Retirement communities offer retirees social interactions with other retirees, and they are an alternative to the age isolation often experienced by older people who remain in their original residences after retirement. There is evidence to indicate that people living in planned retirement communities express greater life satisfaction and have better health status than other older people living in communities that are more heterogeneous in regard to the ages of the residents. However, residents of some retirement communities should be prepared to conform somewhat to the rules and regulations of their community.

Retirement (Life After)

A popular theory suggests that retirees are likely to progress through several stages after their retirement. The first stage is called the honeymoon stage, in which the retiree does the things that had been largely ruled out by full-time work (e.g., extensive travel). This stage may then be followed by one of disenchantment, in which the retiree must adjust to the realities of retirement, such as reduced income that may restrict many of the activities planned during retirement. During this stage the retiree needs to discover appropriate new activities. If successful, then the retiree enters the final, and satisfactory, reorientation stage, in which he or she accepts the limitations incumbent with aging and settles into a retirement routine.

Considerable research has indicated that these are not inevitable stages. Some retirees do not experience all of the stages, and others may encounter the stages in a different order than that proposed by the theory. Thus some retirees may not have sufficient funds for a true honeymoon phase, whereas others pass from the honeymoon stage to the reorientation stage without experiencing disenchantment. In some cases, retirees have a period of relaxation either immediately after retirement or after the honeymoon stage. This usually leads to boredom, and the retiree enters the reorientation stage and begins establishing a daily routine. Evidence indicates that the enthusiasm of retirees is usually high immediately after retirement and that some emotional letdown occurs during the second and third postretirement years. Some retirees do experience a prolonged disenchantment stage, but many others do not.

Studies indicate that individuals who had satisfying hobbies and recreational activities before retirement are most likely to enjoy their retirement years. A number of retirees who become bored and disenchanted attempt to solve the problem by joining a senior center or by either developing new interests or finding part-time work. Near retirement communities, such as those in Florida, it is not unusual to find elderly retirees working as gas station attendants, supermarket baggers, retail store clerks, and so on, usually for minimum- or near-minimum-wage pay. It is estimated that more than 25% of retirees accept some type of employment within 4 years after retirement. Nearly half of the retirees in the United States have Social Security as the primary source of income, and Social Security is often their only income.

In general, people who retire involuntarily have been found to adjust to retirement more poorly than do people who retire voluntarily. Involuntary retirees have also been found to have poorer physical health status and to experience more symptoms of depression than voluntary retirees. Interestingly, involuntary retirement is reported more frequently by individuals classified as having a type A behavior pattern than by individuals classified as having a type B behavior pattern. A type A individual is a person who attempts to control his or her environment and appears to be aggressive and ambitious in "getting ahead" on the job. Type A individuals have been commonly viewed as people who are especially susceptible to coronary diseases. A type B individual is a person who takes events more calmly and is not very assertive and ambitious in job-related situations. A survey conducted in California revealed that people in their 60s who retired voluntarily were likely to have lower stress levels and engaged in regular exercise more often than others in their 60s who had not retired. In addition, retired women reported fewer alcohol-related problems than nonretired women.

Most studies have indicated that there is no trend toward increased marital strife after a husband's retirement when his wife is not employed. In fact, in many cases the relationship between spouses is likely to improve as they find they now have time to pursue common recreational interests. However, in a recent study in Florida, slight negative effects on marital satisfaction were found for wives who were still working after their husband's retirement. An apparent reason for this dissatisfaction is the failure of many retired husbands to assume a fair share of household duties. In general, women tend to perform three-fourths of the household chores, even after they continue to work and their husbands have retired. Researchers at Old Dominion University found that employed wives were unable to elicit more household help from their retired husbands than they did before they retired. This is especially true for what are generally considered to be women's chores (e.g., washing dishes).

It is estimated that 20% to 30% of retirees in the United States cite ill health or disability as the reason for their retirement. However, it is likely that some retirees cite their health as the reason simply to justify their voluntary retirement. There is no apparent trend for retirement to result in diminished physical health, once preretirement health status is considered. On the other hand, there is some evidence to indicate that psychological symptoms, such as anxiety and depression, appear more frequently in retirees than in age-matched people still in the workforce. In addition, some evidence suggests that psychological symptoms may be present more frequently in both early and late retirees than in retirees who retire at the more standard age of 65.

For past generations, retirement usually meant adjusting to a very low income. However, the number of retirees with incomes well above the government-defined poverty level has increased steadily. These financially advantaged individuals are ones who are likely to have income sources in addition to Social Security benefits (e.g., private pensions, investments). Contrary to popular belief, the majority of retirees do not relocate geographically after their retirement.

Retirement Locations

Where do people go to live after they retire? According to a survey by a researcher at Wake Forest University, most people actually prefer not to move during their retirement years. At least that is what 84% of the participants (age 55 and older) in his survey indicated. For those retirees who do relocate, Florida and California continue to be the most popular choices, although their popularity has been declining in recent years. States that have been gaining rapidly in popularity for relocation are Georgia, North Carolina, and Virginia.

Retirement Planning

For a satisfying life after retirement, workers should begin to plan for retirement long before they actually retire. This includes establishing a pension program of some kind so that Social Security payments will not be the only source of income. The fact that retirement may be forced on an individual earlier than planned makes it especially important to begin this financial program as early as possible. Equally important is the preretirement development of interests, hobbies, and multiseasonal leisure activities that will sustain the retiree long after the likely honeymoon period of retirement has ended (see RE-TIREMENT [LIFE AFTER]).

An important issue concerning retirement is how people in their 50s feel about their eventual retirement. Of interest are the results of a survey conducted in the Boston area of a number of professional people (physicians, lawyers, professors, etc.). The professionals who least looked forward to retirement were those who anticipated that their work agendas would be incomplete before retirement, those who had a high current level of job satisfaction, and those who believed that retirement would create a financial strain. Of the professors in the survey, only about 30% viewed their future retirement positively. About 20% of the professionals surveyed revealed that they had not thought about retirement.

Of further interest are the results of a survey conducted on participants in the Normative Aging Study (see NORMATIVE AGING STUDY). Two-thirds of the people surveyed predicted correctly (within 1 year) when they would retire. This means that one-third of the participants did not foresee their date of retirement and either had to extend their work life by some years or had to retire prematurely.

Especially important are the results of a large survey of workers in the age range of 50 to 64 years. More than 60% of those surveyed stated that they had not planned sufficiently for retirement. In fact, about half of the people surveyed admitted that they had not thought about the income they would need after retirement, and that they did not even know what their Social Security and other pension payments would be. In general, living expenses are reduced after retirement, meaning that retirees need about 75% of their preretirement income to maintain their preretirement standard of living. However, the present average retiree has an income that is only about two-thirds of his or her preretirement income. Clearly, more early financial preretirement planning is needed for the majority of workers in the United States.

Some industrial companies, businesses, and universities offer formal programs to assist their employees in planning for retirement. However, in a survey conducted in the 1980s fewer than 5% of retirees reported participation in such a program, and only 12% believed they had the opportunity for participation. It is primarily economically advantaged employees who have the opportunity to participate in a preretirement program, meaning that those employees who may most need assistance have little or no opportunity. Employees should be made more aware of the benefits to be gained from participation in a preretirement program (e.g., financial planning), and they should urge their supervisors to introduce such programs if they do not already exist.

Rigidity
See also ATTITUDES

One of the commonly held beliefs about aging is that people tend to become more rigid and inflexible as they become older. One type of rigidity refers to the ability to make shifts and changes in one's behavior, especially when conditions seemingly call for such changes. Rigidity may be contrasted with its opposite, namely, flexibility of behavior. The belief that rigidity in behavior increases with aging received support from studies conducted in the 1950s. Both younger and older participants received problems to solve that involved pouring water into various size jars to obtain a set amount of water. The first sets of problems all involved application of the same, rather complicated, procedure in which several different pourings between jars were required. The final problem could also be solved by this same complicated procedure. However, a simpler procedure that could be applied to reach the same solution was also available. Younger participants made the switch to the new procedure more frequently than did older participants, thus suggesting greater rigidity on the part of the older participants. Later research compared participants of various ages on paper-and-pencil tests of rigidity. These studies indicated that age itself is an unlikely determinant of age difference in rigidity. The more likely determinant is the cohort or generation to which one belongs. That is, members of earlier generations were found to demonstrate greater rigidity in their behaviors on the tests than did members of later generations. In the earlier study with the water jars, the older participants were not only older than the younger participants, they were also members of an earlier generation. There does not seem to be good reason to subscribe to the belief that most people become increasingly inflexible in their behaviors as they grow older.

Rigidity has also been applied to social and political attitudes. Here, the common belief is that older adults are less flexible than younger adults in changing their attitudes as the social and political climate and mores change. However, evidence indicates that older adults tend to show flexibility rather than rigidity in regard to such attitudes.

S

. . . .

Seattle Longitudinal Study

The Seattle Longitudinal Study is one of the major sources of information about the effects of aging on intelligence. It was begun in 1956 by Dr. K. Warner Schaie and has continued until the present. In 1956, a large sample of adults in the Seattle, Washington, area was tested on five of the subtests of the Primary Mental Abilities test, a widely used text of adult intelligence (see PRIMARY MENTAL ABILITIES [PMA] TEST). Many participants who took this test were subsequently retested every 7 years. In addition, new subjects from the same population of adults in Seattle were tested in 1963, 1970, 1977, and 1984. These new groups permit comparisons among individuals from different generations or cohorts in scores on an intelligence test. A wealth of other information has also been gathered about the participants in the study, including work histories, social interactions, and so on.

The longitudinal reassessments of intelligence (i.e., the same individuals are retested at various ages) have indicated that intelligence does not change uniformly with aging. Fluid intelligence abilities (e.g., reasoning) tend to decrease in proficiency at an earlier age than do crystallized abilities (e.g., verbal ability). Women appear to experience decline earlier than men in fluid intelligence abilities, with the reverse being true for crystallized intelligence abilities. It is also unlikely that individuals will show declines in all of the intellectual abilities measured in this study. Perhaps the most striking observation in the study was that fewer than half of the individuals tested at age 81 showed any significant decline in the abilities from the previous testing (i.e., when they were 74 years of age). Large differences in scores among generations have also been found. In general, with age at the time of testing held constant, members of later generations (e.g., people born in 1959) score higher on reasoning than members of earlier generations (e.g., people born in 1917). The reverse appears to be true, however, for number ability; the members of earlier generations score higher.

Selective Attention

Suppose you are a participant in a miniature golf tournament. Throughout your play a radio in the background blares out the broadcast of a major sporting event. Would the broadcast affect your play? Research in Sweden (where miniature golf tournaments are very popular) suggests that it would, but only if you are an older player. Older players (in their 50s) were sufficiently distracted by the irrelevant event (i.e., the broadcast) that their performance on the relevant event (the golf game) deteriorated. By contrast, younger players (average age of 28 years) were unaffected by the broadcast. They played as well in the presence of the broadcast as they did in its absence. This study demonstrates that older people, under some circumstances, have greater difficulty in selectively attending to relevant information in the presence of irrelevant information than do younger people. Some information in our environment is relevant to what we are presently doing (e.g., the location of the ball relative to the cup in playing miniature golf). By contrast, other information present at the same time is irrelevant to our objective (e.g., the broadcast of the sporting event). *Selective attention* refers to focusing attention on the relevant information while inhibiting our attention of the irrelevant information. In the Swedish study, the irrelevant information was auditory, and the relevant information was visual. Moreover, the irrelevant auditory information was meaningful and interesting in its content. Despite this, the younger players were able to "tune it out."

However, there are other circumstances in which irrelevant auditory information is clearly of little interest to the persons receiving it. Under these circumstances, older individuals appear as capable as younger individuals in inhibiting attention of the irrelevant information. This is the case when research participants listen for the occurrences of tones of one pitch as the relevant information and tones of a much different pitch as the irrelevant information. Although adults of all ages are distracted slightly by the irrelevant information, the amount of distraction is no greater for older adults than for younger adults.

Most research on age differences in the proficiency of selective attention has made use of relevant and irrelevant events that are both visual. The materials usually consist of letters of the alphabet. A popular task in gerontological research is to ask participants to examine index cards to determine which of two target letters (e.g., **A** or **Y**) is present on each card. Thus the target letters make up the relevant events. The cards vary in the number of distracting letters (i.e., letters other than the target letters) that serve as irrelevant events. The time required to complete the task for a stack of such cards increases as the number of irrelevant letters present on the cards increases. However, the increase in sorting time is much greater for older adults than for younger adults. Older adults do have greater difficulty than younger adults in inhibiting their attention to the irrelevant events. They probably pay more attention to the irrelevant letters than is needed to determine that they are indeed irrelevant to the task at hand (finding if it is an **A** or a **Y** on each card). Suppose, for example, that one of the irrelevant letters is **Q**. This letter should be quickly identified as being a nontarget letter in that it differs greatly in its physical features from either of the target letters. Older adults, however, appear to attend to it to the point where they unnecessarily identify it as the letter **Q**. By contrast, younger adults end their attention to the **Q** much earlier once they determine that its basic form eliminates it as one of the target letters.

There are other tasks involving visual relevant and irrelevant events that have been used in research on age differences in visual selective attention. Some of these tasks share one important feature with the card-sorting task, namely, they require searching an array of relevant and irrelevant information. Studies with these tasks have yielded results much like those obtained with the card-sorting task. Older adults have been found to be moderately less proficient in selective attention than younger adults. However, there are other tasks in which a search is not needed to focus on the relevant event. Consider, for example, a task again involving two target letters, **A** and **Y**. On each of a series of trials only one of the target letters is presented on a computer screen—and always in the exact center of the screen. Participants simply identify which of the target letters is in view on any given trial. In the absence of any irrelevant letters, the decision time for older participants averages moderately greater than the decision time for younger participants. On some trials irrelevant letters are added to the left and right of the target letter at the center of the screen (e.g., **J   U   A   U   J**). Note that a search of the letters is not needed to find the target letter—it is always in the center. Under these conditions, both young and older participants show a slight increase in decision times. However, the increase, relative to the condition in which there are no irrelevant letters, is no greater for elderly participants than for young adult participants. The evidence seems to be clear. An age difference in the ability to ignore irrelevant events is present only when a visual search is a task requirement.

A visual search is required many times in the everyday world. For example, consider your attempt to follow the actions of your favorite player during a basketball game. When that player (the relevant event) is surrounded by other players (irrelevant events), a visual search is required to focus your attention on him or her. The laboratory evidence implies that the older spectator may have greater difficulty than the younger spectator in inhibiting attention of the other players. There are also many situations in the everyday world in which a search is not required to "tune out" irrelevant events. For example, while you are watching a television program (the relevant event), someone in the same room reaches for the potato chips in front of you (the irrelevant event). Here the laboratory evidence implies that the irrelevant event should be no more distracting if you are an older adult than if you are a younger adult.

Self-Concept

Your self-concept is the collection of perceptions you have of yourself; that is, it is a self-image. It includes your knowledge of your family and social roles, your knowledge of your personality characteristics, your knowledge of your abilities and limitations, your knowledge of your body and your physical appearance, and so on. Also included is an affective or evaluative component known as self-esteem (see SELF-ESTEEM). These components influence people's self-concepts at all adult age levels. Most people are able to give a fairly accurate assessment of what they are like. These assessments are expected to change from early to late adulthood as individuals' social roles, abilities, and physical condition and appearance change. In general, older adults are well aware of these changes, and they modify their self-concepts accordingly. By contrast, their personality characteristics are likely to change relatively little from those of early adulthood. Such stability is usually reflected in the constancy of this part of the self-concept with normal aging. Researchers at the University of Wisconsin–Madison have found that a positive self-concept in elderly people has a beneficial effect on their mental health.

Self-Esteem

How do you evaluate what you are in relation to what you would like to be? In asking this kind of evaluation, you are referring to a part of your self-concept or self-image known as *self-esteem* (see SELF-CONCEPT). Self-esteem may vary from positive to neutral to negative. Of interest in gerontology is whether self-esteem is lower during late adulthood, relative to earlier periods of adulthood. Cross-sectional studies have compared groups of younger and older adults in their self-esteem ratings. Most of these studies have revealed little difference in self-esteem between younger and older adults, with an occasional study reporting that, if anything, older adults have more positive self-esteem ratings than younger adults. However, the self-esteem of older women tends to be somewhat less positive than that of older men. The results from several other studies have also suggested that the individual differences in self-esteem among older adults are related to the same basic factors that are related to individual differences among younger adults. These factors include occupational success, educational attainment, and success in relating to family members and one's peers.

Semantic Memory

You possess a vast store of knowledge, even if it is not at the level of a *Jeopardy* champion. You know the names of the days of the week, the names of the months of the year, the names of the states of the United States, the names of most (if not all) European countries, the multiplication tables, the rules of long division, and so on. This is all part of information permanently stored in what memory researchers call *semantic memory,* a major part of your total memory system (see MEMORY [OVERVIEW]). A very important component of what is stored in semantic memory is your knowledge of words in your native language. This component is known as your *lexicon* or mental dictionary (see LEXICON). You have the ability to retrieve well-established information held in semantic memory quickly and seemingly effortlessly (i.e., "automatically"). What is the largest city in England? Notice how quickly and automatically "London" occurred to you. Notice how quickly you read and identified the word "quickly" in the previous sentence.

Unlike episodic memory, semantic memory holds information that is stored without reference to the context in which it was acquired. Information about when and where you learned that London is the largest city in England, or when and where you learned the meaning of the word *quickly* is usually lost from storage. You also have the ability to make inferences and reach decisions on the basis of the information stored in semantic memory. For example, if you were asked "What was Napoleon's telephone number?" you would surely respond with "He couldn't have had a telephone!" Your semantic memory contains information informing you that Napoleon died in the early 1800s and that the telephone was not invented until years after his death. To respond, you simply had to put the two facts in relationship to each other.

In general, semantic memory is remarkably resistant to declines in its functioning with normal aging. Gaining access to its information does tend to slow down a bit in late adulthood, and temporary failures to access information in it (known as tip-of-the-tongue states) occur somewhat more frequently in late adulthood than earlier in adulthood (see VERBAL ABILITY). More important, the amount of knowledge held in semantic memory tends to increase from early to late adulthood. This is apparent, for example, in the higher vocabulary test scores generally obtained by older adults than younger adults. Whatever declines that occur in semantic memory functioning with normal aging are much less pronounced than declines that may take place in episodic memory functioning. Interestingly, a reasonable argument may be made that semantic memory develops earlier in childhood than does episodic memory. There is an old developmental principle that states that functions that develop earlier in childhood are subject to later and less age-related declines than are those functions that develop later in childhood.

Senile Dementia

Senile dementia is characterized by severely impaired mental functioning in late adulthood. The symptoms include poor memory functioning, poor intellectual functioning, and poor orientation in regard to time and place. Senile dementia is found in patients with Alzheimer's disease and often in patients who have had strokes. It may also be found in individuals with other diseases, such as Huntington's disease. Presenile dementia is a similar mental dysfunctioning that occurs earlier in life, usually in middle age; it also may be found in some cases of Alzheimer's disease and multi-infarct dementia and in those with Creutzfeldt-Jakob disease.

Senior Centers

Senior centers, as places for education, recreation, and social interactions of senior citizens, began to appear in the early 1940s. With the expansion of the elderly population since the 1940s has come a similar expansion in the number of senior centers. It is estimated that there are are now between 10,000 and 12,000 senior centers in the United States and that the number of people aged 60 and older who participate in center activities is between 5 and 8 million. In a 1984 report by the National Center for Health Statistics it was estimated that 15% of the population 65 years old and older had attended a senior center during the preceding year.

Additional analyses of the data available in the survey conducted by the National Center for Health Statistics have revealed information about the most likely users of the services available at a senior center. For example, women are more likely than men to attend a center, and residents in suburban areas and rural nonfarm areas are more likely to attend than residents of other areas. In addition, attendance increases with age through the early 80s and then declines. People living alone are more likely to attend than people with other living arrangements. Race does not seem to be a factor in determining attendance. Perhaps the most important determinant is an individual's need for social interaction. Individuals reporting more frequent social interactions during the preceding year are more likely to attend than individuals reporting fewer social interactions.

Sensory Memory

A familiar experience is to listen to someone and before you respond to the content of that person's statement you find yourself saying, "Uh, what did you say?" You then find yourself responding without having the statement repeated. A probable reason for not needing repetition of the spoken words is that the words actually persisted in the form of an "echo" for several seconds after the speaker had finished saying them. This persistence enabled you to continue analyzing the words spoken until they were fully comprehended. In other words, your hearing has its own form of memory in which sounds persist as sounds for at least several seconds after the source of the sound has ended. This is one form of *sensory memory*. The other senses have similar memory components that enable sensory information to be extended in time beyond the time the source of that information is physically present. In the case of auditory information, the memory component is called *echoic memory*. The exact duration of echoic memory is unknown, but it seems to be at least several seconds for adults of all ages. It may even persist slightly longer for older adults than for younger adults. This seems likely from evidence indicating that sensory stimuli, in general, persist longer for older than for younger individuals (see STIMULUS PERSISTENCE). Of further interest is the capacity of echoic memory. How many different sounds (e.g., spoken words) may be held in echoic form at any one time? There is evidence to indicate that the capacity diminishes moderately with normal aging. However, in general echoic memory seems to function quite well in late adulthood, assuming there are no major hearing impairments, and it helps to explain why speech perception under normal conversational conditions is relatively unaffected by aging (see SPEECH PERCEPTION). This is true even though older adults require slightly more time to analyze and identify individual spoken words than do younger adults. Echoic memory allows them extra time to identify those words.

Of the other senses, only visual memory has been widely studied. In this case, it is called *iconic memory* in which "icons" (images) of visual information persist after their physical sources cease. The persistence of the information prolongs the time that visually presented information can be analyzed and identified. It also compensates for the fact that our eyes are in constant motion, and during periods of movement no image is being projected on the retina of the eye. The iconic memory of the image registered on the retina just before a movement persists long enough to enable us to see the events in our visual environment without interruption. Without iconic memory, our vision would consist of a series of flashes. The duration of iconic memory is much briefer than the duration of echoic memory, and it is probably no longer than half a second. As with echoic memory, iconic memory seems to be relatively unaffected by normal aging. The duration may even be slightly longer for elderly adults than for younger adults. However, as with echoic memory, the amount of information held in iconic memory is probably less for older adults than for younger adults.

Sequential Method

The sequential method is an alternative to the traditional cross-sectional and longitudinal methods of studying adult age differences in behavior. It was introduced by Dr. K. Warner Schaie in the mid-1960s and has been applied primarily in studies of intelligence and personality. The method is intended to avoid the problems associated with the traditional cross-sectional and longitudinal methods in determining the extent to which observed age differences are actually attributable to a true age change. These problems occur through the possibility of cohort and historical time effects that cause age differences in the absence of true age changes (see CROSS-SECTIONAL

METHOD; LONGITUDINAL METHOD). The sequential method combines the simultaneous examination of cross-sectional and longitudinal age differences, together with time-lag comparisons (see TIME-LAG COMPARISONS), all on the same behavior or characteristic.

Services (Formal)

Formal services for elderly people are to be distinguished from the informal services provided by family members and friends. How much use do elderly people make of these formal services? A recent survey of people age 60 and older in Albany, New York, revealed that the most frequently used service is the multipurpose senior center (used by about 19% of those surveyed). Other services were less frequently used. For example, fewer than 5% of those surveyed reported using Meals on Wheels, fewer than 3% reported using financial or personal counseling services, and fewer than 2% reported using telephone check-in calls. Moreover, the survey indicated that the use of formal services showed little relationship to their availability or accessibility. Understandably, they were used more frequently by those people with a disability than by those without a disability. Nevertheless, it appears that only a minority of older people take advantage of the services that exist for them. A greater effort needs to be made to make such services known to older people and to make them realize the advantages they offer.

Sexual Behavior

One of the most prevalent myths about aging is that elderly people are basically asexual and that the domain of sexual behavior is limited only to younger people. Perhaps even more disturbing beliefs held by some people are that sexual activity in late adulthood is either silly or sinful. On the other hand, statements like "He's a dirty old man" are not uncommon. The implication seems to be that many older men are too preoccupied with sex. Our knowledge about what really happens to interest in sex and to sexual behavior itself has greatly increased in the last few decades as Americans have become more open about talking in regard to their sexual behavior. It is important to distinguish between interest in sexual activity and actual participation in sexual activity. The two do not always coincide, especially in late adulthood.

Interest in continuing sexual activity during late adulthood is related to several factors. For example, in general, elderly people from the middle and upper socioeconomic classes are likely to be more interested in continuing sexual activity than people from the lower socioeconomic class. Evidence also indicates that the amount of education is related positively to the sexual interests of elderly people— the greater the amount of education, the greater interest is likely to be. However, interest in sexual behavior remains fairly constant throughout most of adulthood, and is unlikely to show any pronounced decline until after people reach their 70s.

Interviews of adults of varying ages have revealed age-related declines in the frequency of intercourse reported by married couples. For couples in their 20s, the reported average frequency is slightly greater than three times per week. For couples in their 40s, it is an average of twice per week, and for couples in their 50s, it has dropped to about once per week. The next major decrease in frequency occurs for couples in their mid-60s and older. It is estimated that at least 60% of spouses who are both in the 60- to 70-year range have intercourse at least occasionally, and 25% to 30% of couples past 75 have intercourse. In a large-scale survey of men in the age range of 66 to 70 years, 24% reported that they no longer had intercourse, another 48% reported once a month, 26% once a week, and 2% two or three times a week (no one reported a still greater frequency, possibly because they thought they might be regarded as being "oversexed"). For women in the same age range, 73% reported no intercourse at all (women in this age range are often widowed and have no available sexual partner), 16% reported once a month, and 11% once a week (no one reported a frequency of two or more times a week). If these percentages are accurate, it would appear that intercourse for men in the 66- to 70-year age range is often occurring with women younger than age 66. The frequency of intercourse by older people is likely to be greater for those who had experienced greater enjoyment from it earlier in life than for those who experienced less enjoyment.

Although sexual behavior does continue well into late adulthood (there are reports of men in their 90s having intercourse occasionally), there is undoubtedly a decline in the frequency of intercourse and in the incidence of total impotence (estimated to be about 15% of men age 70 compared with 5% of men age 40). However, researchers in Massachusetts found that in their large sample of men ages 40 to 70 more than half were impotent to some extent.

The biological aging of the sex organs accounts for only part of this decline in the frequency of discourse. Other reasons for elderly men include feelings of monotony in intercourse with the same partner, physical fatigue, preoccupation with work, fear of impotence, depression, diabetes, heart disease, and hypertension. The monotony problem surely is resolvable by the realization that variety is the spice of life, and a little variety in the form of intercourse may relieve the monotony. Preoccupation with work is likely to diminish as increasing numbers of older people retire at younger ages. The fear of impotence is likely to be greatly reduced if elderly men are made fully aware of the normal changes that are occurring in them, especially the increase in the refractory duration. A decline in physical health is likely to become decreasingly important as the health status of future generations of older people shows substantial gains. There is the common belief that intercourse is likely to precipitate a heart attack in elderly men. However, deaths during intercourse are rare, and they accounts for only 1% of sudden deaths from coronary failures. Even adults who have had heart attacks are usually able to resume sexual activity eventually.

When intercourse ceases for elderly couples, it is usually at the wish of the male partner. In fact, there is evidence indicating that the percentage of women age 65 years and older engaging in sexual activity, including masturbation, is greater than for women ages 18 to 26 years. For elderly women, the major reason for the absence of intercourse per se is the lack of a male partner. This may change in the future as increasing numbers of older women are in the labor force. Job preoccupation and fatigue may become reasons as prevalent for older women as for older men.

Changes do occur in sexual behavior during intercourse for both older men and women. For elderly men the time required to attain a penile erection increases (and the time needed for foreplay increases), the force of ejaculation and the volume of seminal fluid released decreases, the duration of orgasms decreases, and, perhaps most important, the refractory period (the time before the next erection can be attained) increases with advancing age. These changes are not really manifestations of sexual dysfunctioning, but rather manifestations of normal aging. Sex therapists believe that one of the reasons for a reduction in the frequency of intercourse by older couples is the failure of older women to understand these changes in their male partners. For older women the production of vaginal lubricant takes longer (with an increased need for longer foreplay), the vaginal opening decreases in size, the vaginal walls become thinner (resulting possibly in greater pain during intercourse), and the duration of orgasms become briefer with advancing age, even though the frequency of orgasms increases in each decade of life through the eighth decade. These changes, like those for older men, have a negative psychological effect on sexual interest. These changes are manifestations of normal aging, not sexual dysfunctioning. Other reasons include prostate problems in older men, declining health for both partners, and adverse effects of some medications for both partners.

Shepherd's Centers

The first Shepherd's Center was started in Kansas City, Missouri, in 1927 by Catholic, Protestant, and Jewish congregations. The name refers to the Bible's 23rd psalm. Older adults in good health were recruited by the congregations for the purpose of delivering services to others in need of those services. The benefits of these services extended to their deliverers as well as to their recipients. By helping others and by making new friends, deliverers greatly enriched their lives. The concept of older people helping other older people grew until there are now such centers in 100 different locations. An administrative office, the Shepherd's Centers of America, has been established in Kansas City to coordinate these centers. For more information about Shepherd's Centers, or to obtain information about starting one in your community, write to Shepherd's Centers of America, 6700 Troost, Suite 16, Kansas City, MO 64131-4401 (telephone, 816-523-1080).

Shingles

Shingles is a painful skin and nervous disease that affects nearly a million people in the United States annually. Most of the people affected are over age 50, with the peak incidence occurring between ages 60 and 70. In addition, the severity of the disease increases with age. The disease is caused by the virus varcella-zoster, and it appears first in early childhood as chickenpox. The virus then remains dormant until it is reactivated as shingles later in life. The reason for the reactivation is not known.

The first symptoms of shingles are numbness, a tingling pain on or under the skin somewhere on the body, and mild flulike symptoms. Later a rash appears on the skin. A doctor may prescribe antiviral medicines and steroids such as prednisone. Recently, the Food and Drug Administration approved the drug Famvir as a possible means of relieving the pain that often follows shingles. Treatment within the first few days of the rash's breaking out may reduce afteraffects of the disease, such as chronic pain or visual and hearing problems (if the rash appears near the eyes or ears).

Anyone who has had chickenpox and has a weakened immune system is at risk of having shingles. This combination, of course, includes many elderly people.

Short-Term Memory

You have just looked up a telephone number in the telephone directory, and you have begun to dial it. Will you remember all of the digits you need to dial? This is an example of *short-term memory*, memory of information that lasts only for seconds. Without rehearsing the information in short-term memory, most, if not all, of it is likely to be lost from memory within 20 to 30 seconds. If you are distracted for several seconds before you can dial the telephone number, you will probably find that you have forgotten several of the digits. If the distraction lasts much longer, you will probably forget most of the digits. To maintain information in short-term memory you need to repeat it to yourself constantly.

Short-term memory (also called *primary memory*) is memory for information that is presently in consciousness. Short-term memory is distinguishable from long-term memory (also called *secondary memory*) that is not in consciousness but has the potential for being retrieved and made part of consciousness (as in the retrieval of a frequently called telephone number that no longer requires you to look it up in a directory before you dial it—you have retrieved it from long-term memory). There is frequent confusion for many people between the concepts of short-term memory and long-term memory. Many older people may often say that their short-term memory is poor. They probably mean that their long-term memory for recent events ("short-term" to them means recent, but well beyond the realm of seconds) that are stored in memory (but not in consciousness unless they are successfully retrieved; e.g., the name of a new neighbor they met recently) is seemingly giving them problems. When most elderly people refer to their "long-term memory," they probably mean their very long-term or remote memory for events from years ago (see VERY LONG-TERM MEMORY). In fact, an older person who complains about "short-term memory" probably has a good short-term memory as the term is used in memory research.

Short-term memory is part of the functioning of what memory researchers call working memory (see WORKING MEMORY). *Working memory* has a capacity for briefly storing a limited amount of information. Regardless of a person's age, the information held in working memory's store is in the form of the sounds needed to reproduce it.

Thus the number "8" as one of the digits in the forementioned telephone number is stored briefly as the sound "ate." If necessary, however, the working memory is flexible enough to store information in forms other than sound. This is obviously the case in that congenitally deaf individuals have short-term memory in which information is stored either in visual form or in the form of the motions needed to reproduce the information in sign language.

Are there age differences in the amount of information that can be stored briefly and recalled completely without error? That is, does the capacity of working memory's store decrease from early to late adulthood? The capacity of the short-term store may be measured by several different procedures. The most common procedure is to determine a person's memory span for either digits or words (see MEMORY SPAN), that is, the longest series of digits or words that can be retained immediately after hearing or seeing them without making an error. When capacity is measured in this way, there is little difference between young adults and older adults in span length. For example, it is about 7 digits, on the average, for young adults and about 6.5, on the average, for elderly adults. In general, the capacity for short-term storage is only 5% to 10% less for older adults than for young adults.

The amount of information that can be stored briefly can be expanded considerably by a process known as chunking. Suppose a telephone number contains the successive digits "1   4   9   2." If you immediately identify this sequence as the year Columbus discovered America, then the four numbers may be stored as a single "chunk" rather than as four separate "chunks" (one chunk for each number). Similarly, the word sequence "turtle," "neck," "sweater" may be stored as a single chunk ("turtleneck sweater") rather than as three separate chunks (one for each word). Ordinarily you may not be able to hold more than five unrelated words in short-term memory. However, if there are 15 words and every three words forms a chunk (e.g., like "turtle," "neck," "sweater"), then you should be able to span all 15 words. There is evidence to indicate that elderly adults are less likely than young adults to spontaneously use chunking to expand their short-term memory capacity.

As noted earlier, information held in the short-term store is forgotten quickly unless it is repeated or rehearsed. To demonstrate the rapid rate of short-term forgetting, participants are given a series of trials in which they receive on each trial an item to be remembered, such as three letters of the alphabet that do not form a word (called a nonsense syllable). After hearing or seeing the item, they have a retention interval that varies in duration over the trials. For example, it may be 3 seconds on some trials, and 6, 9, 12, or 15 seconds on other trials. During the retention interval, they are prevented from rehearsing the nonsense syllable by being forced to perform some activity that blocks the opportunity to rehearse (e.g., counting backwards by 3 from a given number—363: 360, 357, and so on. Most of the syllables will be recalled when the retention interval is only 3 seconds, but most will be forgotten when the retention interval is 15 seconds. The rate of forgetting is rapid regardless of one's age, and it occurs at about the same rate for older adults as for young adults.

We have the ability to search or scan information in the short-term store to answer questions about it. For example, suppose you heard on the television news that today's winners in the National League were Los Angeles, San Diego, Philadelphia, Chicago, and St. Louis. Shortly after hearing this, someone in the next room asks you, "Did Atlanta win today?" After a very rapid search of the contents of your short-term store, you find yourself saying "No." The search didn't locate "Atlanta" in your store. If the question had been, "Did Chicago win today?", your rapid answer would have been "Yes." You would find "Chicago" to be part of the information held in your short-term memory store. The nature of searching short-term memory shows little change from early to late adulthood. Elderly adults are just as capable as young adults, but the speed of the search is a bit slower in late adulthood, in agreement with the slowing down principle (see SLOWING DOWN PRINCIPLE).

In summary, short-term memory is fairly robust in regard to declines in its functioning with aging. Its capacity for storage changes only slightly, its rate of forgetting is about what it is in early childhood, and its ability to search its own contents remains highly functional and reliable.

Sibling Relationships

A recent survey revealed that of the people older than age 60 surveyed, more than 80% reported being close to at least one brother or sister. The closeness usually dates back to childhood or adolescence, and it persists throughout adulthood. Siblings who were close during the preadulthood years are highly likely to remain close when they are both older adults. In general, however, the closeness is greater between sisters than between either brothers or sisters and brothers. Sibling rivalry often intensifies in midlife, but it usually disappears before late adulthood is reached. However, it may resurface under some conditions, especially those involving an inheritance.

Dr. Victor C. Cicirelli of Purdue University recently studied a group of elderly persons who each had at least one living sibling. He discovered those individuals, both men and women, who had a close relationship with a sister had less depression than individuals who did not have such a relationship. By contrast, elderly women who experienced poorer relationships with a sister had a greater degree of depression. In general, sisters are viewed by both elderly men and women as playing a greater role as potential sources of help and comfort than are brothers.

In general, older people are more likely to believe that a sibling will come to their aid if they have more than one sibling than if they have only one. Moreover, there appears to be some reason for this belief. There is evidence to indicate that elderly people are more likely to receive assistance from a sibling when they have more than one sibling.

Sleep

"To sleep, perchance to dream." If Hamlet had been an elderly man, he would have had some concern about the likelihood of dreaming. Dreaming usually occurs during a particular stage of sleep known as REM sleep. REM is an acronym for rapid eye movement. This stage of sleep is characterized by the eyes darting about, as well as other characteristics such as the complete relaxation of the muscles, the insensitivity of the senses to external stimulation, and the presence of brain waves that resemble those present when one is awake and alert (for this reason REM sleep is also often called paradoxical sleep). If awakened during one of the several periods of REM sleep during a night's sleep cycle, the probability is very high that the person awakened will report dreaming. That probability is much lower if the person is awakened at a time other than REM sleep. The amount of time in REM sleep decreases steadily from infancy through late adulthood. Researchers at the University of Florida found that their participants in the 20- to 30-year age range averaged 25 to 30 minutes per REM period, whereas their participants in the 50-year to 60-year age range averaged 10 to 20 minutes. Consequently, dreaming does occur less often in older than in younger adults (see also NIGHTMARES). The decline in amount of REM sleep in late adulthood may have negative effects on the mental functioning of elderly adults. A University of Washington researcher reported a fairly substantial correlation in her elderly research participants between average REM sleep time per night and scores on an intelligence test.

REM sleep is one of the five stages of sleep that occur in repeated or partially repeated cycles during a night's sleep. The four stages other than REM are often grouped together and referred to as NREM (non-REM) sleep. Of particular interest is the stage reached at the end of the first nightly cycle. It is called stage 4, or deep sleep. Recordings by an electroencephalogram reveal slow, high-amplitude waves (known as delta waves) during this sleep stage. In late adulthood, the amplitude of these waves diminishes, and the amount of time spent in deep sleep diminishes. A study at the University of Washington found that participants between the ages of 76 and 90 averaged only 25 minutes per night in deep sleep, compared with the average of 63 minutes by their young adult participants.

These changes in sleep occur even though older adults tend to spend more time in bed (10 to 12 hours) than younger adults. They also spend more time in bed with their sleep commonly disrupted by difficulty in getting to sleep and frequent awakenings once they are asleep. As a result, older adults average less sleep per night than do younger adults. The diminished nightly sleep often results in drowsiness and lack of mental alertness during the daytime hours. Interestingly, researchers at the University of Florida discovered that their elderly participants who napped less than an hour during the day did not experience any added difficulty in getting to sleep in the subsequent night.

Sleep has been related to longevity and life expectancy. In general, people who sleep 10 or more hours per day or less than 5 hours a day die younger than people who sleep between 6 and 9 hours per day. The optimal life expectancy has been found among people who sleep about 7 hours per day. Thus sleep joins other characteristics (e.g., years of education; see EDUCATIONAL LEVEL) as a predictor of life expectancy, and is likely to be one of the variables included in tables that predict life expectancy at any given age. The relationship of the amount of sleep and longevity is not fully understood. Conceivably, those people who sleep too much are doing so because they are in poor health which, in turn, would lead to decreased longevity. In addition, prolonged sleep results in diminished activity which, in turn, could be another contributor to a shorter longevity. Too little sleep may add to a person's tension level and lead to a decrease in physical health.

Researchers at the University of Pittsburgh School of Medicine recently compared three groups of elderly men (61 to 89 years of age). As diagnosed by various criteria of sleep quality, the groups consisted of good sleepers, relatively impaired sleepers, and poor sleepers. The poor sleepers, relative to the others, were found, in general, to have had more recent negative life events and less support from family members and friends. The poor sleepers were also largely the oldest participants in their study.

Sleep Disorders

Surveys of community dwelling, normally aging elderly people indicate that more than a third of them state they have problems with their sleep. Sleep problems occur among both older men and women, but the incidence may be somewhat greater for men. One of the most common forms of sleep disorder is insomnia. There are two forms of insomnia. The first is *sleep-onset insomnia,* in which the individual has difficulty getting to sleep. The second form, and the one more frequent in late adulthood, is *sleep-maintenance insomnia.* In this situation the individual awakens several times during the night, and has difficulty going back to sleep once awakened. Elderly adults who report insomnia have been found to report more symptoms of anxiety and depression and to have greater fear about losing control over their sleep than do elderly adults who are not complainers. Researchers at the Medical College of Virginia found that older insomniacs have much stronger beliefs about serious negative consequences of insomnia than do elderly self-defined good sleepers. Most of these beliefs are inaccurate. Unfortunately, these beliefs may prolong periods of insomnia and lead to a vicious circle. Older insomniacs should consult sleep therapists not only for help in improving their sleep habits (see SLEEP THERAPY) but also for information that could ease their minds about the dangers of insomnia. However, the incidence of medical disorders and the use of drugs other than sleeping pills appears to be about the same for complainers and noncomplainers.

A third of all sleeping pill prescriptions are written for people older than age 60. Sleeping pills, however, have only a short-term effectiveness in treating insomnia, and, if taken regularly, they can have many side effects. For example, individuals with sleep apnea (see below) may experience an increase in both the frequency and the duration of its episodes. Sleeping pills may also reduce the duration of REM sleep periods and increase the incidence of cardiac dysrhythmia. Moreover, some degree of sleep loss on some nights may actually improve the quality of sleep the next night by increasing the amount of stage 4 (deep) sleep.

It is estimated that at least one third of the elderly population have sleep apnea. *Sleep apnea* consists of periods lasting 10 seconds or longer in which there is a cessation of air flow in breathing. Apnea and other abnormal respiratory events during sleep are considered pathological conditions if they occur at a rate of five episodes per hour. Some elderly people may have hundreds of such episodes during a night's sleep. Apnea is usually accompanied by blood oxygen desaturation (hypoxemia), a condition that may cause mental dysfunctioning. However, researchers at the Medical College of Virginia found only negligible differences in mental functioning of older adults with mild to moderate apnea compared with those without apnea. On the other hand, pathological apnea may be associated with such health problems as obesity and hypertension.

Nocturnal myoclonus also increases in late adulthood. It is characterized by the "restless leg syndrome" and the urge to move the legs repeatedly with rapid and stereotyped flexions. Its presence both prolongs the time needed for sleep onset and increases the number of awakenings after falling asleep. A common treatment of myoclonus is the administration of the drug benzodiazepene. However, the drug has not proved to be very effective in controlling myoclonus.

The incidence of some sleep disorders in late adulthood is low. One of these disorders is narcolepsy. *Narcolepsy* is characterized by the inability to control wakefulness, with the narcoleptic individual experiencing periods during the normal waking hours in which he or she suddenly falls asleep. Another uncommon sleep disorder in late adulthood is *sleep walking*.

Several surveys of nursing home residents have revealed that they have greater sleep problems than community-dwelling adults. They rarely spend a single hour completely in sleep. In general, both brief periods of sleep and wakefulness are observed during every hour of the 24-hour day, although sleep is least likely near sunset. Their sleep pattern is greatly distorted by frequent daytime napping caused largely by lack of activity and by frequent awakening at night by loud roommates.

Some sleep researchers believe that sleep measures may provide an effective early diagnosis of Alzheimer's disease. The sleep of patients with Alzheimer's disease is usually greatly distorted. The time in bed actually sleeping is likely to be diminished considerably, and the fragmentation by awakening periods is especially pronounced. Some patients with Alzheimer's disease display what is called the *sundown syndrome*. It is characterized by agitation and confusion during the awakening periods, often accompanied by straying from bed and wandering about the residence. There is also evidence indicating that patients with Alzheimer's disease have less deep sleep than normal aging adults and that it takes patients longer to reach the REM stage of sleep.

Sleep Therapy

Sleep centers are now located at many universities and hospitals across the United States. They provide diagnostic tests of individuals who report sleep disorders. Most important, they also offer behavioral methods of treating sleep disorders, especially insomnia. These methods are greatly preferred over the excessive use of sleeping pills.

A popular behavioral therapy is called the *stimulus control* method. Clients are trained to use their beds only for sleep, to establish a regular sleep schedule, and to get out of bed after every 10-minute period of sleeplessness and do something else. Researchers at Washington University (St. Louis) have demonstrated that this method is as effective for insomniacs over age 60 as it is for younger insomniacs.

Another behavioral therapy is called the *countercontrol method*. Clients are trained to engage in a nonarousing activity during sleepless periods without leaving the bed. For example, they are to read a dull book or listen to the radio. The researchers at Washington University have also discovered this method to be as effective for older insomniacs as for younger ones. Researchers at Duke University have found another variation of a therapeutic program that seems to be especially effective for elderly people who awaken during the night and have difficulty going back to sleep. The program calls for both education about the effects of aging on sleep, the effects of sleep deprivation on later sleeping, and the application of a modified stimulus control procedure (e.g., go to bed only when sleepy, leave the bedroom if awake for more than 20 or 30 minutes and return when sleepy).

Slowing Down Principle

Many components of human behavior are slower in their execution for older adults than for younger adults. This slowing down principle applies to reaction times and the times needed to perform various behaviors. It also applies to the speed of conducting mental operations, such as those involved in perceiving and identifying visual forms. Consider the time it takes to determine whether two letters have the same name. When the two letters are physically the same (e.g., both uppercase *A*s), younger adults usually require less time to decide they have the same name than older adults. When the two letters no longer are physically identical, but still have the same name (e.g., an uppercase *A* and a lowercase *a*), the time needed to make the same name decision increases for both younger and older adults, but disproportionately more for older adults. If young adult participants averaged about 100 milliseconds to perform with physically identical letters, we would expect elderly adults to average about 150 milliseconds. If the average time for young adults to perform the name identity task in the absence of physical identity is 200 milliseconds, we would expect the average time for older adults to be about 350 milliseconds. The mental operations time for elderly adults averages about 1.5 times that of young adults.

Smell

The epithelium (tissue lining the inner surface) of the nose becomes thinner with increasing age over the adult life span. This thinning is accompanied by a loss of olfactory (smell) receptor cells that enable us to detect the presence of an odorous substance; therefore diminished smell sensitivity occurs during late adulthood. As with all of the other senses, sensitivity refers both to the threshold sensitivity and suprathreshold (above the threshold) sensitivity.

Threshold sensitivity refers to the ability to detect a weak odorous substance. The minimum concentration of a given odorous substance that must be present before the odor is just barely noticed defines the threshold value for that substance. Different odorous substances have different threshold values, with greater concentrations of some substances needed for detection than for other substances. Regardless of the substance, a greater concentration is needed for detection, on the average, by elderly adults than by young adults. For some odorous substances, the threshold value may be nine times greater for older adults than for young adults. Overall, the age-related decline in threshold sensitivity is much greater for smell than for taste.

Suprathreshold sensitivity refers to the ability to discriminate among varying intensities of an odorous substance, all of which are well above threshold value. As the concentration of the substance doubles or triples, do we also perceive the intensity of the odor as doubling or tripling? There is evidence that elderly adults have less suprathreshold sensitivity than do younger adults and that this is especially the case for sweet-smelling substances. A related problem for older people is their diminished ability to identify odorous substances (e.g., banana, lemon) by name. Odor identification peaks around the early to mid-30s and then declines steadily with increasing age. Some indication of the extent of this decline is evident from the results obtained by researchers at the John B. Pierce Foundation Laboratory. Both young and elderly adults were given a number of familiar odorous substances to identify. The young adults correctly identified about 50% of the substances; the elderly adults correctly identified about 30%. There are exceptions, however—some odorous substances are more readily identified by elderly than by young adults. This is especially true for odors that were more prevalent when current elderly people were younger than they are now (e.g., lye soap).

The age-related decline in smell sensitivity and discriminability is a major factor in affecting elderly adults' ability to identify food substances. Smell plays a greater role in discriminating among foods than does taste (see TASTE).

Smoking

According to a 1988 survey published by the U.S. Department of Health and Human Services, about 20% of men and 14% of women age 65 and older smoke cigarettes (hopefully, these percentages have decreased since 1988). Another recent survey indicated that the number of female smokers over age 65 increased by about 900,000 in the last 10 years, whereas the number of male smokers over age 65 decreased by about 140,000. About 33% of men and 30% of women in the 45- to 64-year age range smoke cigarettes. The incidence of smoking among older adults is greater for blacks than for whites, Hispanics, and Asian-Americans.

The lower rate of smoking for older people than for younger people is related to the fact that many former smokers have been forced to quit smoking in late adulthood because of their poor health status and the occurrence of emphysema, heart disease, and cancer that are only worsened by continuing to smoke. The mortality rate for elderly smokers is about twice that for elderly people of the same age who never smoked. The major health problems related to smoking for older people are cancer and heart attacks. Smoking cessation is advantageous to the health of people of any age, including those in late adulthood. The mortality rate for elderly people who quit smoking is between that of those older people who never smoked and those who continue to smoke.

Behavior modification programs (see PSYCHOTHERAPY) have become popular in the United States as a means of helping people to stop smoking. These programs are offered at many medical centers and psychological clinics across the United States. The use of nicotine patches, as prescribed by a physician, has also been a popular external aid for people to stop smoking. However, a survey by the U.S. Surgeon General's Office indicated that as many as 95% of the smokers who do quit do so without external help. Older adults who are still smoking after years of doing so are probably smokers who have not been able to stop smoking on their own. They represent difficult cases for behavior modification programs to produce a cure (i.e., stopping smoking). Nevertheless, it is well worth the effort for elderly smokers to try these programs to break the cigarette habit.

Social Exchange Theory

What do elderly people attempt to accomplish in their social interactions with other people? Social exchange theory states that adults of all ages attempt to increase their personal rewards while minimizing financial, physical, and psychological costs to themselves. However, many elderly people believe that their personal resources may have diminished to the point that they have little power left to accomplish these objectives. They may instead direct their social interactions in areas other than seeking personal rewards, such as participating in volunteer work and in making contributions to their communities. Evidence indicates that altruistic behaviors are more characteristic of older adults than of younger adults (see ALTRUISM).

Social Gerontology

Social gerontology is an area of study that is part of both sociology and psychology. Social gerontologists are concerned with the role of society on affecting the course of normal aging and on the effects of various social institutions on aging. Research by social gerontologists is conducted on such topics as family relationships and aging, living arrangements and aging, health facilities and aging, demographics of aging, racial and ethnic differences in aging, marital relationships in late adulthood, and gender differences in aging. Of particular interest in social gerontology are the many variables that relate to life satisfaction in late adulthood (see LIFE SATISFACTION).

Source Memory

"I heard that Senator Smith is retiring from the U.S. Senate." "Oh, where did you hear that?" "On the radio."

This exchange illustrates what memory researchers call source memory. Note that is it not the content of a memory (Smith is retiring) that is pertinent, but rather the source from which the content was acquired (the radio). *Source memory*, like that of some other forms of memory (e.g., temporal memory; see EPISODIC MEMORY), is for a noncontent attribute of information (i.e., information that supplements content in terms of such features as when or where the event in question occurred). Note further that in the everyday world, our source memory is likely to be incidental in form. We surely do not intend to remember where we heard about Smith's retirement, nor are we likely to rehearse the source in an attempt to ensure its memorability. And yet we often do remember sources of information we have acquired, but not always ("Was it on the radio or TV"?). Source memory may have a number of different kinds of information associated with it. For example, was the news reporter on the radio a man or a woman?

Age differences in the proficiency of source memory are studied by giving participants a series of items from different sources and later testing their memories for the source of each item. For example, researchers at the University of Toronto used trivial factual statements as items, with half of the statements delivered by means of an overhead projector and the other half delivered verbally by the investigator. When tested later for the source of each statement (projector or investigator), the proportion of correct source identifications was moderately greater for young adult participants than for older participants. A similar outcome has been found in other laboratory studies with somewhat different content items and somewhat different sources for those items. The implication is that elderly adults generally are somewhat less proficient than younger adults in their everyday applications of source memory. However, in most cases, the accuracy of sources of information is of little consequence, and it is a form of memory that should be of little concern to older people unless it functions very poorly. There is some limited evidence to indicate that source memory involves the brain's frontal lobes, and extremely poor source memory could be a sign of frontal lobe dysfunction. Even benign problems with source memory could result in some mild disagreements between spouses or friends, as is evident by such exchanges as "We saw that on the television news" and "We did not—we read it in the newspaper."

There is a special case of source memory in which accuracy is seemingly very high for adults of all ages. From what source did you hear that President Kennedy had been shot? The majority of people who were adults in 1963 will tell you whether they heard the news on the radio, the television, or from a friend, spouse, or another source—and with great confidence in the accuracy of the source. Memories of dramatic and highly emotional events are often remarkably preserved in their details (memory of the news about the bombing of Pearl Harbor is another example). For this reason, they are called "flashbulb memories." *Flashbulb memories* commonly include the location of where you were when you heard about the dramatic news as well as the source of the news. That is, flashbulb memories consist of both spatial memory (see SPATIAL MEMORY) and source memory.

Span of Apprehension

How much information can you "see" in a brief glance? If several letters of the alphabet were flashed on a screen for 50 milliseconds, how many letters could you recall? The amount of information that can be seen in a glance is called the *span of apprehension,* a characteristic of our iconic memory, a form of sensory memory (see SENSORY MEMORY). For young adults, the span of apprehension averages four or five letters. There is limited evidence that older adults may have a slightly lower span of apprehension.

Some indication of your own span of apprehension may be given by a simple procedure. Have someone throw several beans on a table and then quickly cover them. If asked how many beans there were, you will probably be correct if the number is no more than four or five. If the number is much greater than this, you would need more time than allowed by a glance—enough time to allow you to count the beans before they are removed from view.

Spatial Ability

What would the resulting figure look like if you were to place this segment, ⟨, side by side with this segment, ⟩? The answer, of course, is a diamond-shaped figure. This is a simple example of use of your spatial ability. *Spatial ability* refers to your ability to visualize mentally how objects will appear if they are physically manipulated. This example involves the ability to integrate separated segments to form a whole. Spatial ability also includes the ability to visualize the third dimension of objects from their two-dimensional drawings, and to reproduce three-dimensional designs from two-dimensional drawings. Spatial ability is measured by several components of intelligence tests, including the space test of the Primary Mental Abilities test (see PRIMARY MENTAL ABILITIES [PMA] TEST) and the block design subtest of the Wechsler Adult Intelligence Scale (see WECHSLER INTELLIGENCE TESTS). Both cross-sectional and longitudinal studies have revealed substantial age-related declines in spatial ability as measured by these tests. For example, scores on the block design test show about an 8% decline per decade (relative to scores in early adulthood) in cross-sectional studies. Aging's effects on spatial ability parallels those for the use of imagery in other mental performances (see IMAGERY), and they suggest the possible faster rate of decline with normal aging in the brain's right hemisphere than in the left hemisphere.

The decline in spatial ability with normal aging is unlikely to affect the daily lives of most older people. However, there are professions, such as engineering and architecture, in which proficient spatial ability is very important, and even the decline by middle age may affect job performance and require greater assistance from younger colleagues. Age-related declines in scores on spatial ability tests have been found for engineers with years of experience. However, older engineers and architects still score well above older nonengineers and nonarchitects on such tests, suggesting that they had unusually high spatial abilities when they were young adults (if they did not, they probably would not have become successful engineers or architects).

One minor problem elderly people may encounter is with "you are here" maps found in shopping malls and other large facilities. Canadian researchers have found that older people have much greater difficulty than younger people in navigating through the facility when the map is not upright and is not coordinated with the viewer's position while viewing the map.

Spatial Learning

Do you know where the canned vegetables are in your favorite supermarket? If you start to shop in a new supermarket, how many visits to the store would be required before you knew where they are? Do you know where the Amtrak station is located in your city? Where the bathroom is located in your neighbor's house? You undoubtedly could describe the location in each case. In so doing, you are using mental or cognitive maps of your supermarket, your city, and your neighbor's house. These mental maps are the products of spatial learning that are acquired through frequent exposures to each of these areas.

Are there age differences in the rate at which spatial learning takes place? This is an important question. Adults of all ages do move to different cities, to different neighborhoods within the same city, and to different residences. The acquisition of new mental maps is essential for the adjustment of anyone who has moved from a familiar environment. To simulate spatial learning in the laboratory, researchers recently introduced tasks that are more closely related to everyday spatial learning than the older task of maze learning (see MAZE LEARNING). In effect, participants "take a walk" through a novel environment. Movement through the environment is simulated by having the participants view a series of slides that show various scenes and locations in a strange (to the participants) neighborhood or building. After such a "walk," older participants have consistently been found to acquire less information about components of the novel environment than younger participants. This does not mean that normally aging people are incapable of mastering a novel environment. It simply means that it usually will take them longer and require more exposures to the environment before their spatial learning is complete. It also suggests that it would benefit elderly people to take notes for future reference when they begin their exploration of a new environment.

Spatial learning is especially a problem for elderly residents of a nursing home, even those residents who are mentally alert and ambulatory. Researchers at Oklahoma State University provided a dramatic demonstration of this problem. They showed nursing home residents slides from various areas of both the exterior and interior of their nursing home. The residents were asked to locate on a map of the home where each area in a slide would be found. Even highly distinctive areas, such as the dining room and nursing station, were correctly located by relatively small percentages of the residents. These researchers also found that the older the resident, the lower the accuracy of locations. Surprisingly, they also found that duration of stay in the nursing home was unrelated to accuracy. Spatial learning for residents of nursing homes would surely be greater if the managers of those homes made areas within them more distinctive. Currently most hallways look alike, as do most rooms.

Spatial Memory

"Now where did I leave my keys?" "I don't remember where I parked my car in the mall's lot!" These are examples of the importance of spatial memory in our everyday lives. Unless we always leave our keys in the same place and park our car in the same location every time we go to the mall, we are likely to discover frequently the imperfection of spatial memory. *Spatial memory* is memory for where objects are located in geometric space. At one time memory theorists believed that spatial memory was an automatic form of memory in the sense that spatial information is recorded in memory with little effort of our part and without any effort to rehearse that information. As a form of automatic memory, spatial memory was thought to show little decline in proficiency with normal aging. Laboratory studies, however, have demonstrated that the memory for spatial locations is better when we know our memory will be tested later (intentional memory) than when we are unaware of any future memory test (incidental memory). Some rehearsal that occurs when we are trying to remember spatial locations does seem to help us remember those locations better. In addition, laboratory research has revealed a moderate decline in spatial memory proficiency from early to late adulthood.

A variety of laboratory tasks have been used in spatial memory research. One of the most frequently used tasks is one in which the participants examine a box containing a number of compartments. A different object is placed in each compartment (e.g., a comb in one, a key in another, and so on). After examining the filled box for a period of time, the participants are given the same box now emptied and asked where the comb had been, where the key had been, and so on. Another popular task is one in which participants study a map with different kinds of buildings located at various places on the map. They are then asked the location of the gas station on the map, where the church was, and so on. For both of these tasks older adults remember moderately fewer locations than young adults. Laboratory evidence confirms the frequent complaint that elderly people have difficulty in remember where things are located.

Many of the problems of older people with regard to spatial memory could be remedied if individuals recognized their decline in proficiency and tried to bypass spatial memory as much as possible. For example, individuals should try to place their keys in the same place every time they set them down, and they should try to park in the same general section of the parking lot every time they visit the mall. However, such consistency is not always possible. There are certainly occasions when your favorite section of the parking lot is full, and you have to park your car in a different location. Memory training experts believe your memory for where you are parked will be improved if you do other things besides simply looking where you are and trust that your location will be automatically recorded in your memory. These other things really amount to rehearsing where you are located. One memory aid is forming a mental image of the mall's overall structure and adding to that image a further image of your car in relation to that structure. Hopefully, you will later be able to retrieve the total image and easily find your car. However, older people are not as proficient in imaging as are younger people, and they are unlikely to find this memory trick to be of great value. Another approach may be more helpful. Translate the spatial location to a verbal code. For example, observe where you are and say it to yourself. For example, "I am parked on the west side of the mall, about three-fourths of the distance from the front of the lot." Even the later retrieval of only part of the code should help you find your car.

Speech Perception

"What did you say? Would you mind repeating it?" Such requests are more likely to be made by elderly people than younger people. There is a moderate decline with normal aging in speech perception. When asked to listen to a series of individual words and name each one after hearing it, older adults are likely to misidentify more words than younger adults, with errors being more pronounced among the old-old (people in the 80s and older) than for the young-old (people in their 60s). The misidentification of words occurs for words that have low-pitched sounds as well as for words with higher-pitched sounds. Only high-pitched sounds are likely to be affected by the changes in the ear that accompany normal aging (see HEARING). The difficulty encountered with words of a lower pitch suggests that some of the speech perception impairment in late adulthood is caused by some neural loss in the language centers of the brain that are located in the temporal lobe (usually the temporal lobe of the left cerebral hemisphere).

Most everyday conversations require the comprehension of spoken sentences as a meaningful whole, and not necessarily the complete comprehension of every word in that sentence. Consider, for example, the spoken sentence, "Yesterday I saw several ducks swimming in the lake in the park." Even if you did not fully comprehend the word *swimming*, your mind would probably fill it in. There are few words other than swimming that would make sense with the rest of the sentence. Thus the loss in spoken sentence comprehension with normal aging is not as great as might be expected, given the pronounced hearing loss with aging, thanks to our ability to fill in unheard words when listening to meaningful sentences. When sentences are spoken at a normal conversational rate (about 140 words per minute) and at a loudness well above the listener's threshold value, there is little loss in comprehension until older adults are in their 80s, and even then the loss is only about 10%, in relation to young adults. Nevertheless, it is probably wise to speak a little louder to an older audience than to a younger audience, given the greater thresholds for elderly people. It may also be wise to try to lower the pitch of your voice when you speak to an elderly audience. The extent of hearing impairment for elderly people is much greater for high-pitched sounds than for lower-pitched sounds.

Speech is not always delivered under ideal conditions. For example, there may be a noisy background that must be overcome to hear the spoken sentences. Here an elderly listener is likely to experience a much greater loss of comprehension than a younger listener. This is also likely to be true when the speech is delivered at an excessively fast rate or when there is reverberation in the speech (as may be heard over the loudspeaker at a stadium or at an airport). Fortunately, researchers at the University of Calgary found that much of the difficulty experienced by older listeners with reverberated speech may be eliminated when the speaker pauses before saying important words in the sentences. The lesson should be clear for those who use loudspeakers.

Speed of Behavior

The movements of older adults are slower than those of younger adults. The slowing down of behavior with aging (see SLOWING DOWN PRINCIPLE) has been noted for movements requiring a wide range of tasks, including the writing of words or sentences and digits, the movement of a lever from side to side, sorting cards, and dialing a telephone number. In general, the age-related slowing becomes disproportionately greater as the complexity of the behavior increases. For example, the age difference in speed favoring young adults is much greater for writing unfamiliar sentences than it is for writing familiar sentences. For many tasks, the slower behavior of older adults is of little consequence (after all, the tortoise did win the race). It should matter little how rapidly the cards are shuffled in a card game or how fast they are dealt to the players; the job is completed anyway. Of course, the slower dialing of a telephone number does allow greater time for the number to be forgotten as it is being dialed; however, the number can always be looked up again in the telephone book. A potential serious consequence of the slowing down of behavior with aging occurs when an older adult is required to take some evasive action to avoid being struck by a moving vehicle or a flying object.

Stimulus Persistence

Suppose you see the pattern ⊐⊢⁻ followed a second or so later by the pattern ⊔⊐⎸ . You will undoubtedly see them as two different nonsense figures. Suppose, however, the second pattern follows much less than a second after the first. Now you are likely to see the word 5AT instead of the two distinctive patterns. It takes time for the stimulation within the nervous system produced by an external event (or stimulus) to be "cleared" (i.e., to disappear). That is, the stimulation persists for a time after the event itself has terminated. If the second event occurs after the first event has "cleared" the nervous system, then the two events will be perceived separately and independently of one another. This is the case when a second separates our two patterns. However, if the time separation is much shorter, the two events will fuse and you will see the product of that fusion (in this case, the word). Elderly adults experience the fused event after longer separations of the two patterns than will younger adults. Stimulation in the nervous system seems to persist longer in late adulthood than in earlier adulthood. Evidence supporting the existence of an age difference in duration of persistence is derived from numerous studies employing other kinds of external events. The likely age difference in stimulus persistence seemingly explains the age differences in a number of sensory phenomena, such as visual aftereffects (see AFTEREFFECTS [VISION]).

Strength and Stamina

The typical 170-pound man has about 70 pounds of his weight in muscle at age 30. By late adulthood only about 60 pounds of that muscle is likely to be retained. The lost muscle is gradually replaced by fat, and the remaining muscle slowly declines with aging in strength, flexibility, and tone. Strength declines with aging are generally greater for leg and trunk muscles than for arm muscles. Men, on the average, have greater strength (about 30%) than women at every adult age level.

Physical performances that are dependent on muscular status usually show progressive decline from early to late adulthood. An exceptionally thorough study of age differences in physical performances was conducted in 1981 (the Canada Fitness Survey). Almost 7,000 adults ranging in age from the early 20s to the late 60s were evaluated on such abilities as grip strength, situps, and pushups. Relative to the scores for men in the 21- to 29-year range, men in the 61- to 69-year range showed a loss of about 18% in grip strength, about 60% in situps, and about 72% in pushups. Comparable losses for women in the 61- to 69-year age range (relative to women in the 21- to 29-year age range), were about 12%, 75%, and 62%. Age-related declines are also seen for events such as running a sprint, hurdle racing, and marathon racing, but the degree of decline varies greatly among such events. In general, the age-related decline is greatest for those events that require a massive power output. Running short sprints shows much less decline from the 40s to the 60s than does running a steeplechase or a marathon, even for regular participants in these events. How much of these declines is related to lack of physical fitness and regular exercise rather than the inevitability of massive age-related declines? Muscle atrophy (i.e., loss of some muscle) that occurs with aging probably cannot be reversed. However, muscle strength can be increased despite such loss of muscle, given the maintenance of physical fitness with regular lifelong exercise.

Stress and Coping with Stress

The alarm did not go off this morning, so you overslept and were late for work. You spilled your first cup of morning coffee on the brand-new blouse you were wearing. These are examples of daily stressors experienced by adults of all ages. Usually the stress created by them is mild, and it disappears quickly, regardless of age. Another kind of stress is that created by major negative life events. In such cases one needs to find a way to cope with the stress created by these events. Coping means the use of thoughts and actions to eliminate, or at least diminish, the distress and negative emotions produced by a stressful event.

A popular belief is that late adulthood is an especially stressful period of life, given the negative events likely to be encountered. They include death of a spouse, deaths of friends, retirement (to some elderly people), and similar negative events less likely to occur earlier in life. However, other periods of life have their own stressful events that are less likely to occur later in life. They include a faltering marriage, divorce, new job, loss of job, and so on. Negative life events may be less stressful for many elderly people than younger people believe they would be. Events may be less stressful in that they are not unexpected and therefore are somewhat anticipated. Especially stressful are those unexpected life events, such as the death of a grown child or the loss of one's life savings by bad investments. For this reason, divorce in late adulthood is likely to be more stressful than in earlier adulthood. In fact, divorce has been found to be more stressful for an elderly person than is the death of a spouse. When the latter occurs at older ages, the incidence of subsequent illness and death is lower than it is when widowhood or widowerhood occurs at earlier ages. However, the number of negative life events experienced by older people during a 6-month period is a reasonably good predictor of their physical health status when their initial (before the negative events) health status is considered. Elderly people who are psychologically healthy and well-adjusted experience less stress from negative events than do elderly people who are not as well-adjusted. However, for some older people an accumulation of negative events has been found to be predictive of a decline in mental functioning and the occurrence of depression. In general, the existence of a good social network of friends helps to prevent such mental deterioration.

People play various roles during their lives, those of spouse, parent, grandparent, friend, church member, and so on. For older adults, stressors that occur in roles that are highly important to them have more negative effects on their life satisfaction than do stressors that occur in roles that are less important to them. Researchers at the University of Michigan recently surveyed adults age 65 and older to determine which roles are highly important to them and which are less important. The most important role was found to be that of spouse, with parent and grandparent being second and third, respectively. Less important roles included those of friend, church member, and volunteer worker.

Of interest to researchers of stress is the source to which people attribute their problems and who (or what) is responsible for finding a solution to their problems. Researchers have identified several models that may be followed. The first is the moral model, in which people see themselves as creating their own problems and accept responsibility for solving the problems themselves. The second is the compensatory model, in which people believe they are not responsible for their problems, but they accept the responsibility for solving them. They see themselves as being handicapped in some way by their environments or by forces beyond their own control. The third model is the enlightenment model, in which people accept the responsibility for causing their own problems, but not the responsibility for solving them. For example, they may see their own weakness as being responsible for their excessive drinking, but they turn to Alcoholics Anonymous to solve the problem. The final model is the medical model, in which people neither accept responsibility for their problems nor responsibility for solving them. They need expert help to help to identify their problems and to find solutions to them. Unfortunately, studies in this area have found a greater tendency among older people than for younger people to accept the medical model.

Psychologists have discovered that there are several broad types of coping behaviors when people are confronted by negative life events. One type is called *problem-focused coping*. Here the individual directly tackles the problem causing stress. Thus, if one is experiencing symptoms of illness, problem-focused coping with the stress that the symptoms cause would be to seek medical diagnosis and advice. A second type is called *emotion-focused coping*. Here the person would take an optimistic view and believe that the symptoms are temporary and will soon be gone. A third type of coping is *resignation*, in which the individual experiencing a negative event such as symptoms of illness simply accepts the stressful event and is prepared to take its consequences (e.g., resigned to die after experiencing physical symptoms) and makes no effort to cope with it. Elderly people are more likely to use problem-focused coping than either emotion-focused or resignation coping. In general, if one's resources (health, financial, and social) decline in late adulthood, then his or her ability to cope effectively with stress diminishes. However, if these resources remain intact, the older person should be able to cope with stress as well as younger persons.

The decisions we are often required to make may be stressful. Having to decide when to retire may be such a stressful event for many elderly people, as may having to decide where to live after retirement. Of interest is how elderly people, compared to younger people, cope with difficult decisions. A recent study in Los Angeles compared the coping strategies of middle-aged and elderly men to the conflict created by a difficult decision. Each participant described a major decisional conflict they had recently encountered and how they coped with the problem it created. The researchers identified three different strategies of coping with the conflict: problem solving (direct action to find the best solution), avoidance (trying to escape the problem without making a firm decision), and resignation (accepting the stress without doing anything about it). Both the middle-aged and elderly participants favored the problem-solving strategy for most decisions. The elderly participants made less use of avoidance than did the middle-aged participants, and there was no age difference in the relatively infrequent use of resignation.

An especially harmful way of coping with stress is to engage in excessive drinking of alcoholic beverages. The number of older people with drinking problems is probably fairly low. Those who do have a drinking problem, however, are more likely to be experiencing a chronic source of stress than those who do not have a drinking problem.

Stroke

A stroke occurs when there is a disruption in cerebral blood flow, most often from a blood clot in the brain. A stroke may also be caused (about 30% of strokes) by fat deposits in the carotid artery that block the flow of blood from the heart to the brain. Blockage may be detected by echocardiography (an ultrasound procedure much like that of sonar). If the blockage is severe, surgery may be required in which cuts are made in the carotid artery and fatty deposits are removed. If less severe, medical treatment may be sufficient (e.g., aspirin daily).

It is estimated that more than a half a million Americans have strokes each year; most are elderly people. A stroke is the number three cause of death among Americans, after heart disease and cancer. The risk of death from a stroke is nearly twice as high among black men as it is among white men. The race difference may be genetic in nature.

Recent evidence indicates that the risk of a stroke for elderly people who have thickening of the walls of the heart is three times greater than the average risk for other elderly people. The reason for the connection between such thickening and the risk of stroke is unknown. The thickening of the wall may be detected by echocardiography. The procedure is expensive but is beneficial for those known to be at high risk who may benefit from preventive measures (e.g., smoking cessation and avoidance of alcoholic beverages). High blood pressure and a high level of cholesterol are known to be factors that place elderly people at an especially high risk of stroke.

The parts of the brain that are affected by the loss of blood supply during a stroke are no longer capable of normal functioning. The consequences, contingent on the location of the area of brain in which the stroke occurs, may result in declines in physical, mental, and emotional functioning (see MULTI-INFARCT DEMENTIA). The symptoms of stroke may consist of paralysis in one side of the body, difficulty in speaking (aphasia) or understanding (apraxia) speech, memory impairment, depression, and uncontrollable crying or anger. Recently a medicine has been discovered that may reduce the extent of brain damage caused by stroke if it is given within a few hours of the onset of a stroke. The medicine is tissue plasminogen activator (TPA), a genetically engineered protein. There are, however, risks associated with TPA.

Care of a patient who has had a stroke usually begins with hospitalization during the acute phase of the stroke. The acute phase may last for days and even weeks. Rehabilitation training with one or more therapists (e.g., physical and speech therapists) follows the acute phase. The objectives of rehabilitation are to allow the patient to recover as much of the impaired functions as possible and to teach ways of compensating for those functions that cannot be recovered. The length of the rehabilitation period varies greatly with the severity of the stroke and may last several months to a year or longer.

The welfare of older patients affected by strokes is influenced by the degree to which they are able to find continuity with their life-styles before the stroke. In a survey of a number of older stroke patients, Dr. Gay Becker of the University of California–San Francisco found that many patients do find ways to accomplish this continuity. Those who demonstrated the greatest success in finding some form of continuity were the ones most likely to persevere in their efforts to recover from the stroke. Other researchers have found that the size of the patient's social network is related to the degree of physical limitations after the stroke. Frequent contacts and interactions with friends and family members and participation in group activities are associated with improved physical functioning after the stroke.

Subjective Age

How old do you feel? Younger or older than your actual (chronological) age? Our reference is to your subjective age in contrast to your true age. There is some evidence that subjective age in late adulthood may be more closely related to performance on various tasks than is chronological age. However, this is an area of research that has not received the attention it deserves.

Psychologists measure subjective age by asking participants four questions: What age most clearly corresponds to (1) the way you feel, (2) the way you look, (3) the age of the person who has interests and activities most like yours, and (4) the age you would like to be if you could choose your age right now. Your subjective age is then found by averaging the answers to these four questions. Researchers at Brandeis University recently determined the average subjective age for groups of men and women ranging in age from their teens through their early 80s. What they discovered is that adults of all ages tend to have subjective ages that are lower than their actual ages. Moreover, the discrepancy between subjective age and true age increases progressively from early to late adulthood, and the discrepancy is greater for women than for men. For example, for the true age of 35, men and women averaged subjective ages of about 34 and 28, respectively. For the true age of 65, the average subjective ages were about 55 (men) and 47 (women), and for the true of age of 75, they were about 65 and 50.

Why do older adults maintain younger subjective age identities? A popular theory has been that it is a way of denying their age and thereby avoid the stigma they believe is associated with old age. Moreover, the denial of aging has been regarded by some gerontologists as being important in promoting successful aging and higher life satisfaction. That is, older people with lower subjective ages should have greater life satisfaction than older people with higher subjective ages. In the Brandeis University study, participants were evaluated in terms of their fear of aging and their current life satisfaction. Contrary to the denial theory, the researchers found that fears of aging for their older participants were not strongly related to their subjective ages. The researchers also found no relationship for older men between their subjective ages and their current life satisfaction. They did find a relationship between subjective age and life satisfaction for the older women in their study. However, the relationship was the opposite of that predicted by theory—the older women with the least discrepancy between their subjective age and their true age were found to be the most satisfied with their current lives.

Suicide

Approximately 25,000 people officially commit suicide each year in the United States. This number is probably a gross underestimation because many suicides are ruled as accidental deaths. Depression is the most common reason for suicide. However, the source of the depression typically differs between younger and older individuals who commit suicide. Depression is most likely to be psychological in origin for younger adults, resulting from such factors as perceived rejection. By contrast, depression is more likely to be linked to poor health for older adults who commit suicide. However, psychological depression produced by social isolation may be an important contributing factor for at least some elderly adults who commit suicide.

From 1950 to 1980 there was a drastic increase in the incidence of suicide for young adults, but a pronounced decrease for both middle-aged and elderly adults. However, according to a recent survey conducted by the federal government, the incidence of suicide among people age 65 and older, regardless of sex or race, increased by 21% between the years 1980 and 1986. As a result, the incidence of suicide among people age 65 or older increased from about 18 per 100,000 people in 1980 to about 21.5 per 100,000 people in 1986. The survey further indicated that the incidence increased by 42% for black men and 23% for white men. Since 1986 there has been an additional increase of 4% for people in the 75- to 84-year age range and a 6% increase for those people age 85 and older. However, there was a decrease of 8% for people in the 65- to 74-year age range. In 1988 the suicide rate for adults of all ages was slightly greater than 12 per 100,000. Thus the incidence of suicide is somewhat greater for elderly adults, and especially those in the 75- to 84-year age range, than for younger adults.

The ratio of attempted suicides to actual suicides differs between young and older adults. For young adults the ratio is about seven unsuccessful attempts to one successful attempt. By contrast, the ratio for older adults is about eight successful attempts to one unsuccessful attempt.

The suicide rate for elderly adults is lower among white women and nonwhite men and women than among white men. The high incidence of suicide among older white men is seemingly related to the perceived loss of economic, business, and social power experienced by a number of white men after retirement. The large difference in suicide rates between elderly men and women overall is somewhat misleading in that more elderly women than men attempt suicide. The probable reason for the difference is a sex difference in the choice of method used to attempt suicide. Women are more likely to choose less lethal methods (sleeping pills) than men (a gun).

Syntax

Stored in our permanent memory is our knowledge of the rules of grammar, that is, the *syntax* of our spoken and written language. These rules are automatically and effortlessly employed whenever we speak or write a sentence. You surely realize that people do not become "ungrammatical" as they age. There is no evidence to suggest that normal aging is accompanied by any major changes in the ability to use syntax effectively. However, some more subtle changes in the use of syntax occur as people age. Older adults do tend to have greater difficulty than younger adults in comprehending complex sentences (those containing embedded clauses). Interestingly, a researcher at the University of Kansas has examined diary entries of people who kept a daily diary for many years. She discovered a tendency for sentences entered in the diaries to be syntactically less complex when the diary writers were old than when they were younger.

T

· ·

Taste

If you believe everything you hear from elderly people, you are likely to believe that many of them are "tasteless." Familiar statements by older people are "Everything tastes alike now to me" and "Food just doesn't taste the way it used to taste." Although such statements are probably exaggerated (unless there is a specific biological disease affecting the taste and smell systems), there is some degree of truth behind them. In classic studies by Dr. Susan Schiffman, young adults and adults in their 70s were tested for their ability to identify, while blindfolded a number of blended foods (blending was necessary to prevent identifications by means of the substance's texture). For most of the blended foods, the young adults were considerably more accurate in their identifications than were the elderly adults. For example, the percentages of those identifying apple, strawberry, and fish were 81%, 78%, and 78%, respectively, for the young adults and 55%, 33%, and 59%, respectively, for the elderly adults. However, it is important to note that there were some reversals, specifically for tomato (69% for elderly adults, 52% for the young adults) and potato (38% for the elderly adults, 19% for the young adults).

The problem in assigning the responsibility for the greater difficulty of older people in food identifications to age-related declines in taste sensitivity is the fact that taste plays only a relatively minor role in these identifications. The texture of the food in your mouth provides useful information, and the smell of the food is especially important information. The importance of smell is clearly indicated when young adults are deprived of smell and texture by having them hold their nostrils while attempting to identify blended food substances. When this is done, their accuracy in food identification is no greater than that of older adults. It is apparent that not only is smell important in discriminating among foods regardless of one's age, but also that it is the diminished sense of smell with aging that is largely responsible for the difficulty experienced by many older people in making these discriminations.

What happens to taste itself with aging? We must recognize first that there are only four basic tastes: bitterness, saltiness, sourness, and sweetness. Common foods have varying combinations of these basic tastes, thus accounting in part for their varying tastes (along with their variations in odor and texture). Of interest in aging research is the extent to which sensitivity to each of the four basic tastes decreases with normal aging. As with all of the other senses, sensitivity refers both to threshold sensitivity and suprathreshold (above the threshold) sensitivity.

Threshold sensitivity refers to the ability to detect weak amounts of a taste substance. For example, how much salt must be added to water before you are able to detect the presence of the salt? That amount defines your saltness threshold value. Similarly, how much of a bitter substance, a sour substance, or a sweet substance must be added before you are able to detect bitterness, and so on defines your other sensory thresholds. Studies comparing individuals of various ages indicate that there is only a modest decline in sensitivity for saltiness from early to late adulthood. There is only a modest increase in the absolute threshold for older adults, on the average, relative to young adults. Moreover, the decline in sensitivity may be even less for detecting bitterness, sourness, and sweetness. For all of the four basic tastes, the threshold value for older adults in general may be no more than two to two-and-one-half times that of young adults. The magnitude of the increase in threshold (or decrease in sensitivity) is much less than that found for the other senses. This is especially true for the sense of smell (see SMELL). Part of the moderate decline in taste sensitivity in elderly adults may result from the taking of certain medicines that dull taste sensitivity. These medicines are more likely to be taken by older adults than by younger adults.

Suprathreshold sensitivity refers to the ability to discriminate among varying intensities of a taste substance, all of which are well above threshold intensity. Does a concentration of salt that is twice as high as that of another concentration taste twice as salty? Less than twice as salty—or even more than twice as salty? In general, the evidence indicates that elderly adults have less suprathreshold sensitivity than do young adults, but, as with absolute sensitivity, the age difference is relatively modest. Older subjects do need a greater increase in the concentration of a taste substance than do younger adults before they are able to perceive the fact that the concentration has indeed increased. This seems to be the reason why older adults generally prefer stronger tastes (e.g., more tart) than do younger adults. That is, the greater concentration of the taste substance is actually perceived as being weaker than it is by most elderly adults. The exception, however, is for sweetness. There is evidence to indicate that the preference for less sweet tastes increases from early to late adulthood.

Tear Secretion

Tears are drops of a saline solution that are secreted by the lacrimal glands. The drops are spread between the eye and the eyelid and moisten their parts and aid their motion. One of the problems confronting older people is a reduction in the amount of tear secretion (it may be as much as a 40% reduction). This reduction may produce visual problems for some elderly people. An examination of tear flow should be part of regular eye examinations for elderly people. There are medications to reduce the symptoms of dryness in the eyes.

Teeth, Gums, and Mouth

It is estimated that about 60% of people age 65 and older have some or all of their teeth. However, many of these elderly people make insufficient use of dental services, primarily because most health insurance plans provide no dental coverage and Medicare pays only for the removal of tumors from the mouth. Consequently, many elderly people have considerable discomfort from their teeth and gums. Teeth are likely to be less sensitive to hot or cold substances in late adulthood than in earlier adulthood because nerve and blood supplies to the teeth decrease with age.

About 50% of adults between the ages of 65 and 74 years have some form of periodontal (gum) disease. It develops when plaque accumulates between the teeth and the gums and causes the gums to recede from the teeth. Infection then forms in the resulting open spaces, producing swollen or tender gums, unpleasant breath, and a bad taste in the mouth. Elderly adults with diabetes are at particular risk of infections that result in periodontal problems.

Elderly people who wear dentures also need to visit their dentists at regular intervals. The mouth tends to change its shape somewhat with aging. Consequently, dentures do not fit properly, and they need to be adjusted. Dentists should also check regularly for the possible presence of oral problems other than those of the teeth themselves.

Xerostoma (dry mouth) occurs for some older people because their salivary glands do not function as they should. This is a side effect of many of the medications taken by elderly people. Persons affected by xerostoma feel thirst frequently and have difficulty in speaking. Dry mouth may contribute to tooth decay and periodontal disease. Dentists often recommend that those with dry mouth use sugar-free mints, home air humidifiers, fluoride rinses, and artificial saliva solutions.

Oral cancer often goes undetected in older people because they visit their dentists infrequently and because there is little pain early in the disease. The disease affects more elderly men than elderly women. Those at greatest risk are elderly people who have smoked and have been consumers of alcohol for a number of years.

Television Viewing

In a survey of television viewing conducted several years ago, young adults and older adults were compared in a number of ways. In terms of hours per day spent watching television, less than 13% of the young men and women reported watching more than 3 hours per day. By contrast, 50% of the elderly men and more than 75% of the elderly women watched more than 3 hours per day. The most frequent reason given for watching television was for its entertainment value. This was true for both age levels and for both men and women (over 65% in each sex and age breakdown). Some programs were equally popular among men and women and at each level. Both *The Cosby Show* and *Cheers* were ranked high in popularity for young men, young women, elderly men, and elderly women. Conversely, some programs were much more popular for older people, regardless of sex, than for young adults. Included here were *Murder, She Wrote* and *Golden Girls*. By contrast, other programs, such as *thirtysomething* and *LA Law,* were more popular for young adults than for older adults.

Temperature Sensitivity

What room temperature do you prefer to feel comfortable? There is a modest age difference in this "comfort-point" temperature, with middle-aged and elderly adults averaging only about half a degree higher than young adults. This evidence implies that there is little change with aging in temperature sensitivity. In agreement with this position is the limited evidence indicating the slight age difference in the threshold value for detecting the presence of either cold or heat on the skin. Threshold here refers to the minimal intensity of the source of cold or heat needed to report the experience of cold or heat. Conflicting with this evidence, however, are studies suggesting that older people are less capable than younger people in estimating the temperature of their environments and less capable of detecting a temperature change in their environments.

The diminished capability is probably a contributing factor to the higher incidences of hypothermia (a below normal body temperature—95 degrees Fahrenheit or lower), heatstroke, and frostbite among older adults than among younger adults (see also HEAT STROKE). A survey by researchers at Southwest Texas State University conducted from 1979 to 1985 revealed that there were more than 5,000 deaths of people age 60 and older related to excessive heat or cold. This is less than 1,000 deaths per year, but the incidence is probably underestimated. There are likely to be a number of deaths each year in which the role played by excessive temperatures goes undetected. The researchers found deaths related to excessive cold were responsible for more than three-fourths of the temperature-related deaths. Indicators of low body temperature include irregular heart beat, very slow breathing, and mental confusion. The presence of these indicators calls for immediate emergency treatment.

The researchers in Texas also found that the overall incidence of deaths was about the same for older women and men. However, elderly women were found to die more frequently from excessive heat than from excessive cold, whereas the opposite was true for elderly men. More than 70% of the deaths occurred among elderly adults living in metropolitan areas. Most deaths of elderly people attributable to excessive temperatures could be avoided. Older people forced to live on a meager income often save money for food and rent by reducing their heating and cooling bills. Those who are in danger of death by so doing could readily be discovered by daily visitations to their homes from community volunteers, visiting nurses, or Meals on Wheels volunteers. Financial aid for adjusting the temperature in their rooms could then be provided by various agencies and services. In addition, to avoid hypothermia during cold weather elderly people should be encouraged to wear layers of warm clothing both indoors and outdoors, to wear a hat outdoors, to use extra blankets in bed, and to keep active physically.

Temporal Memory

"Did I go grocery shopping last week on Wednesday or Thursday?" "When did we last play bridge together?" Events are remembered not only for their contents, but also to some degree for the time of their occurrence. *Temporal memory* is memory for the timing of events in one's life. The usual procedure for studying temporal memory in the laboratory is to have participants perceive a series of events and then make temporal judgments about those events. Usually the events are familiar words (e.g., *apple* and *pencil*) presented in a lengthy series. After the series is presented, subjects may be asked such questions as "Which word appeared more recently in the series, *apple* or *pencil*?" Alternatively, the participants may be asked to reconstruct the order in which the words appeared, and their reconstructed order is compared in accuracy with the actual order. Regardless of the task, older adults have been found to be considerably less proficient in temporal memory than are young adults.

The diminished proficiency of temporal memory with normal aging is further demonstrated when words in the series are replaced by actions performed in the laboratory (e.g., touching your nose, shaking your head). After the last action is performed, subjects are asked to reconstruct the order in which the actions were performed. Elderly adults are generally far less accurate than young adults in reconstructing the temporal order of the actions they had just performed. Temporal memory for events does seem to be much more adversely affected by normal aging than is memory for the frequency with which events occur (see FREQUENCY-OF-OCCURRENCE MEMORY). The adverse effect of aging on temporal memory is also probably greater than the adverse effect on spatial memory (see SPATIAL MEMORY).

Terminal Drop Phenomenon

In the early 1960s psychologist Dr. Robert Kleemeier discovered a peculiar phenomenon known as the *terminal drop phenomenon*. He discovered that older people who showed a pronounced decline in intelligence test scores from one time of testing to a later time of testing had an unusually high probability of death within a relatively short period of time after the second testing. Later investigators have generally supported the existence of the terminal drop phenomenon. Declines in scores for several of the subtests of the Wechsler intelligence tests (especially the vocabulary subtest) appear to be particularly associated with impending death. Such declines in test scores are probably an indication of substantial declines in neurological functioning that, in turn, serve as warnings of impending death.

Time-Lag Comparison

Time-lag comparisons are possible when the same task is given at widely separated times to groups of adults who are the same age each time the task is administered. Thus the task may have been given to a group of elderly adults in 1930 and again in 1990. The comparison between the average score on the task in 1930 and the average score in 1990 is a time-lag comparison. If the two averages are approximately equal, then it suggests that performance on the task in question is unaffected either by generational membership or by the time period in which the task was administered. Older adults tested in 1930 obviously came from a much earlier generation than elderly adults tested in 1990. Similarly, the two tests occurred in very different time periods. This is the case, for example, with the digit span task in which it is determined for each participant the longest series of digits that can be remembered in order without an error (see MEMORY SPAN). The average digit span for older adults was about 6.5 in 1930, and it was also about 6.5 for older adults tested in 1990. However, if a time-lag comparison indicates that the average score earned at one time differs greatly from the average score earned at another time, then it is likely that either the variation in generational membership or the variation in time period has affected performance on the task in question.

Tinnitus

Tinnitus is a condition in which the affected individuals "hear" noises, such as a ringing or a buzzing sound, either intermittently or constantly. It may result from various diseases, or it may be the consequence of an allergy, an obstruction in the ear canal, or the buildup of wax in the ear canal. The condition may be accompanied by some hearing loss, and it tends to worsen as hearing sensitivity decreases. Many drugs, including aspirin, may exaggerate tinnitus. Although the percentage of older people with tinnitus is small, the condition is especially stressful. Treatment of the condition in terms of permanent relief is often unsuccessful. If so, elderly people with tinnitus should consult their physician about the use of tranquilizers to reduce the stress they experience or about the acquisition of a "masker" (a device producing noise at frequencies that could cancel the inner ear noise). In some cases a hearing aid may also lessen the annoyance produced by inner ear noise.

Touch

The degree to which touch sensitivity declines with aging varies for different parts of the body. The decline is particularly pronounced for the fingers. This decline is largely the result of the loss of many touch receptors in the skin of the fingers during late adulthood. Some related decline in the ability to locate and identify objects by touch is to be expected as a consequence of normal aging.

Transfer of Learning/Training

After finally learning the names of all of the president's cabinet members, a new president is elected and the process of learning cabinet members' names has to start all over. Now instead of Secretary of State Sanders it is Secretary of State Simpson. This is a situation in which previous learning is likely to have a negative effect on the new learning. The previous name of Sanders keeps intruding while you are trying to learn to relate Simpson to the position of secretary of state, and by so doing interferes with and slows your rate of new learning. A similar slowing down is likely for the other new names to be learned as well. This is an example of what learning psychologists call *transfer of training*—the effect of previous learning (or training) on new learning. In this case, it is an example of specific negative transfer, meaning that the specific content of previous learning interferes to some degree with new learning.

To bring specific transfer into the laboratory, participants are asked to learn successive lists of paired words (paired-associate learning; see VERBAL LEARNING) in which the first word of each pair from the first list is also the first word of each pair in the second list. However, the second word of each pair in the first list is replaced by a new and unrelated word in the second list. For example, *apple* and *king* may be words of a pair in the first list, and *apple* and *pencil* the corresponding words in the second list. Note that *apple* plays the same role as *secretary of state* and *king* and *pencil* the same roles as *Sanders* and *Simpson* in our previous example. Adults of all ages tend to show specific negative transfer in learning the second list. Their rate of new learning is slower than if the pairs in the first list had been completely unrelated to the pairs in the second list. The interference from *king* slows the learning of *pencil* as the new response to be given to *apple,* just as the interference from *Sanders* slows the learning of *Simpson* as the new response to be given to *secretary of state.* Most important, the amount of negative transfer (or slowing down in rate of learning) has generally been found to be no greater for older participants than for younger participants, despite the common belief that elderly people are more susceptible to interference from prior learning (see FORGETTING).

Negative specific transfer is not unusual in learning motor skills. Consider having learned to drive a car with an automatic transmission.

Then, for some reason, you must learn to drive a car with a stick shift. Your previous learning with the automatic shift may make learning the use of the stick shift somewhat more difficult than if you did not have the previous experience with the automatic shift.

Specific transfer may also be positive in its effects. Prior learning may facilitate subsequent learning. Consider a basketball fan in Milwaukee in the 1970s. The city already had a professional basketball team known as the Milwaukee Bucks. A professional women's basketball league was then formed, and Milwaukee was one of the cities involved. The name of the new team? The Milwaukee Does! Having already learned to associate Bucks with Milwaukee should make it easier to now learn to associate Does with Milwaukee. Positive transfer is the expected outcome. It probably is no coincidence that cities with both professional baseball and professional football teams often have team names that lead to positive transfer (e.g., Chicago Cubs and Chicago Bears). To bring specific positive transfer into the laboratory, participants receive successive lists in which the pairs of words are, for example, *apple* and *king* in the first list and *apple* and *queen* in the second. Here the task is like learning *Milwaukee* paired with *Bucks* in the first list and *Milwaukee* paired with *Does* in the second list. Evidence indicates that elderly participants show less positive transfer (facilitation) on such lists than do younger adults, presumably because they are less likely to take advantage of the relatedness of content.

There is another form of transfer known as learning-how-to-learn, or *nonspecific transfer*. The reference is to mastering the skills needed to learn a particular kind of task or needed to perform more proficiently on a task, and then applying these skills to a new version of that task even when the specific content changes with successive tasks. This is the case when participants are given successive lists of paired words in which there is no commonality of the words across the lists. Rate of learning tends to improve from the first list to the second list and perhaps even from the second list to a third list as participants learn skills that make learning faster. Nonspecific transfer is always positive (i.e., it facilitates new learning), and it is likely to be as facilitating for older participants as it is for younger participants. Nonspecific transfer also occurs again, in about equal amounts for both younger and older participants when they are given extensive practice on some reasoning tasks. In such cases participants are acquiring, with practice, more effective skills for solving the kinds of reasoning problems they receive. Older people are not only capable of learning new content, they are also quite competent in learning skills that benefit a wide range of mental performances.

Twins

Identical twins have long played an important part in psychological research. They have identical heredities, making them a critical research asset for determining the relative contributions of inheritance and the environment to individual differences in many kinds of behaviors. Especially important are comparisons between identical twins who were reared together during childhood and identical twins who were separated soon after birth and reared in different environments. If pairs of adult twins are found to be highly similar in a given behavior, regardless of their child-rearing environments, then there is good reason to believe that heredity is a major determinant of proficiency in that behavior. That is, with the same heredity, variation in the environment seems to have little effect on the behavior. This is the case for intelligence. Scores on intelligence tests earned by identical twins, even during late adulthood, tend to be highly similar. Moreover, psychologists at Pennsylvania State University have discovered remarkable similarities in several personality traits between older identical twins (average age 59 years, with many of the twins being much older than 59), again regardless of their togetherness or separation while growing up. The traits are those of emotionality, activity level, and sociability. Identical twins may be expected to be similar in many ways throughout their adult life spans. Their identical heredities ensure their similarities (see also LONGEVITY).

U

. . . .

United States Administration on Aging

The Administration on Aging was established by the Older Americans Act of 1965. The agency's objectives were to administer programs that help elderly people and to distribute information about old age. Accomplishment of these objectives was greatly enhanced by the establishment in 1973 of Area Agencies on Aging, located in many communities across the United States. These community agencies provide a number of services for elderly people, such as counseling, Meals on Wheels, and senior centers (see FOOD AND MEAL SERVICES). For information about the nearest agency call the Administration on Aging's Eldercare Locator at 800-677-1116.

Urinary Incontinence

A rather common health problem in late adulthood is urinary incontinence (involuntary urination). It is estimated to be present in about 38% of community-dwelling elderly women and about 19% of community-dwelling elderly men and in more than half of elderly nursing home residents. However, a substantial percentage of incontinent men and a somewhat smaller percentage of incontinent women report spontaneous remission to continence over a period of months. The gender differences in remission rates is seemingly related to the different types of incontinence present in elderly people. Men are more likely than women to have urge incontinence (uncontrollable urination with no warning) brought about by conditions (e.g., urinary infections, bowel dysfunctions) that may improve even without treatment. Women are more likely to have stress incontinence in which there is a loss of urine at times of exertion (e.g., laughing, sneezing, or bending). Stress incontinence is related to anatomical problems that usually require treatment of some kind. When older people begin to experience incontinence of either type, it is usually mild and may eventually become moderate. Reversals from moderate to mild incontinence are not uncommon. Men whose incontinence progresses from mild to moderate usually experience a change from urge incontinence alone in the mild form to a combination of urge and stress incontinence in the moderate form. Similarly, women whose incontinence progresses from mild to moderate usually have a change from stress incontinence alone in the mild form to a combination of stress and urge incontinence in the moderate form.

A common belief about older people is that incontinence results in social embarrassment and withdrawal from social contacts, and that it is likely to lead to loss of self-esteem, depression, and anxiety. However, the results obtained by researchers at the University of Michigan indicated that incontinence, even in a severe form, is only weakly related to increases in depression and negative emotions and to a lowering of life satisfaction.

Experts recommend a number of steps to manage incontinence. The crucial first step is to avoid denial. The problem cannot be managed without being aware of its presence and the willingness to do something about it. Other steps include avoiding the intake of bladder irritants, such as caffeine and spices, and eating foods high in fiber and carbohydrates. Elderly people who have a problem with incontinence could avoid embarrassment by taking such preventive measurers as alerting the flight attendant on an airplane to the fact that they may have to get up even when the "fasten seat belt" sign is on and asking for directions to the nearest restroom when scheduling an appointment in an unfamiliar building.

Incontinence is especially a problem for nursing home residents who have Alzheimer's disease or some form of dementia. Much of the problem stems from their difficulty in remembering where a facility for urination is located. There is evidence to indicate that some help in solving this problem may be obtained by painting signs on the floors in areas where residents congregate. The intent of the signs is to aid them in finding the facility in each particular area of the nursing home. The most effective signs are those with the word "toilet" printed in large black letters, with arrows pointing in the direction of the facility.

There are organizations dedicated to improving the life-style of people with incontinence. One is called Help for Incontinent People (HIP). It publishes a newsletter and other educational materials with useful information about incontinence. HIP may be contacted by writing to P.O. Box 544, Union, SC 29379 (telephone, 800-BLADDER). A similar organization is the Simon Foundation for Continence, P.O. Box 835, Wilmette, IL 60091 (telephone, 800-23-SIMON).

V

....

Variability of Behavior

Variability on a given task usually refers to the spread or dispersion of scores around the average score earned by individuals. Consider a given task to be playing golf and scores on the task to be the number of strokes needed to play 18 holes. One group of golfers in a charity tournament has an average score of 100 strokes. However, within the group scores vary from 70 to 130, with many scores falling between the two extremes. A second group of golfers in a different tournament also has an average score of 100 strokes, but the scores vary only between 90 and 110. Variability of performance within the group is surely greater for the first group than for the second group. Such within-group variability is quantified by a statistic known as a *standard deviation*. For our golf example, the standard deviation would be considerably greater for the first group than for the second group. In terms of performances on many mental tasks, groups of older participants tend to be more like the first group of golfers and younger participants more like the second group of golfers. That is, within-group variability around an average score is likely to be greater (a larger standard deviation) for older than for younger participants. Why is there greater variability among elderly groups of people? Probably because the effects of aging on performance on a particular mental task vary greatly among elderly people. Some older people show little effect of aging. They may be individuals who have been regular physical exercisers for many years and/or have maintained very active mental lives. By contrast, other individuals, for various reasons, may have shown fairly pronounced declines in the mental ability in question, and many others fall somewhere between the two extremes.

Variability of behavior is also used to refer to variability in performance on the same task on different occasions for the same individual. Consider golf again as an example. One golfer may score 80 on some days, 90 on other days, and 100 or over on still other days, while another golfer always scores between 90 and 100. The first golfer is obviously more variable in his or her performance than is the second golfer. A popular belief is that elderly people are more variable in their performances on the same mental task than are younger people. However, there is evidence to indicate that this is usually not true. Variability in this case is determined by finding the *reliability of scores.* Participants in a group perform a given mental task on at least two different occasions. The correlation between scores earned on that task on the different occasions defines reliability or the consistency of the performances for the members of the group over separate administrations of the task. This correlation has been found to be as high for elderly groups of participants on a number of mental tasks as for groups of younger participants. There is no reason to believe that older adults are any less consistent in their performances on many tasks than are younger adults.

Verbal Ability

Verbal ability refers to one's command of his or her native language. One index of verbal ability is vocabulary level. In general, the extent of vocabulary, as measured by vocabulary tests, grows from early to late adulthood (see INTELLIGENCE; WECHSLER INTELLIGENCE TESTS), strongly suggesting that at least one important component of verbal ability increases with normal aging. On a vocabulary test a participant is given words and asked to define each (e.g., "What does the word *psychology* mean?"). There is another component of verbal ability, however, that seems to show a slight decline from early to late adulthood. It is the ability to find the right word to label a specific idea or thought. Age differences in this ability are tested by giving participants what, in effect, is the opposite of a vocabulary test. For example, you may be asked "What is the name of the mythical animal that is very large and breathes fire?" The use of this kind of test reveals that older participants, generally have more difficulty than younger participants in providing the right word. There is also evidence to indicate that elderly adults experience more tip-of-the-tongue experiences than do younger adults. A *tip-of-the-tongue state* occurs when you know a particular word, but you just can't seem to say it. Often you have an idea of what the missing word sounds like (e.g., *secant* when you are trying to use the word *sextant*). We usually find a way to circumvent the problem by using a synonym of the missing word, and we often discover that the missing word suddenly occurs to you at a later time (when you no longer need it). Age differences in tip-of-the-tongue states are determined by having people of various ages keep a diary for some weeks in which they record each occurrence of such a state. Elderly people, on the average, tend to report about twice as many tip-of-the-tongue experiences per week than young adults. However, there is also evidence to indicate that older adults are about as effective as younger adults in gaining access to the missing word when they exert effort to do so.

Verbal Learning

Elements of language are always involved in verbal learning. They may be words, names, or numbers. In your lifetime you have had many verbal learning experiences. For example, you learned that the name of Chicago's professional football team is the Bears, that the capital of Illinois is Springfield, and that the name belonging with a specific face is Johnson. What you learned in each case is a paired associate that, in turn, is the product of paired-associate learning. Paired-associate learning is one of the two most widely studied forms of verbal learning.

In *paired-associate learning*, you learn to associate two originally unrelated events with each other. Often more than one pair of unrelated events must be learned at essentially the same time. Thus you probably learned the capitals of Illinois, Ohio, and other Midwestern states at the same time. The need for new paired-associate learning continues through late adulthood. Regardless of age, we try to learn the names of new cabinet members each time there is a vacancy (the new secretary of defense is Jones, the new secretary of labor is Smith, and so on). We also try to learn the names of new football teams each time the league expands, and the names to associate with the faces of our new neighbors. Of interest is what happens to paired-associate learning proficiency during late adulthood.

To study paired-associate learning in the laboratory, participants receive a list of initially unrelated elements (usually 10 or 12 pairs). The pairs are composed of either words as both elements or faces as one element and surnames as the other. For example, the words *apple* and *table* may make up one pair, the words *pencil* and *king* another pair, and so on. The pairs are studied together until participants are able to say "table" when *apple* is presented alone, "king" when *pencil* is presented alone, and so on for each of the pairs in the list. Numerous studies have revealed that, with such materials (and with face-name pairs as well), elderly participants do learn paired-associate lists. However, these studies have also revealed a rather substantial age difference in the rate of learning. Learning progresses more slowly for elderly participants than for younger participants. The main reason for this age difference seems to be in the kind of rehearsal favored by older and younger adults. Older adults tend to rehearse the paired elements rotely by simply repeating the elements to themselves (e.g., "apple" "table", "apple" "table"). Rote rehearsal of this kind is not very efficient in promoting rapid learning. By contrast, younger people often short-circuit rote rehearsal by finding some way of relating the seemingly unrelated elements of each pair. This is often through the use of imagery. For example, *apple-table* could be visualized as a large and highly polished red apple located squarely in the middle of a kitchen table. If the image is firmly established, then the word *apple* when presented alone should serve to recover the entire image which, of course, contains the correct word. Older people generally have less capacity for imaginal activity than do younger people (see IMAGERY). Consequently, they are less able to use this form of imaginal rehearsal, and they must therefore rely heavily on rote rehearsal.

The other widely studied form of verbal learning is serial learning. In *serial learning,* you must not only learn a number of verbal elements, but you must also learn the order in which they occur. Examples of past serial learning in your life are learning the names of the months of the year in the correct order, the names of the U.S. presidents in the correct order, your Social Security number, and many telephone numbers. Serial learning is just as much a part of your present life as it was of your past life. You still need to learn new telephone numbers, new zip codes, spellings of new words in your vocabulary, unique names (e.g., Ayatollah Khomeini), and perhaps, even lines of poetry. To study serial learning in the laboratory, participants receive a list of 8 to 12 words and they practice the list until it can be recited in the order given. As with paired-associate learning, there have been numerous studies of age differences in serial learning. Older participants clearly learn serial lists, but, as with paired-associate learning, the rate of learning is much slower than it is for younger participants. It is learning the order of the words that is especially difficult for older participants. Retaining order information is an example of temporal memory, a form of memory known to decline substantially in proficiency from early to late adulthood (see TEMPORAL MEMORY).

Two other aspects of serial learning are of interest. The first is that older participants make many more errors of omission while practicing a serial learning list. An error of omission refers to saying nothing when asked what word comes after another word. By contrast, younger participants make many more errors of commission than do older participants. An error of commission refers to saying a word but at the wrong place in the serial order. The high omission rate of elderly participants is often cited as evidence for their greater cautiousness (see CAUTIOUSNESS). The other aspect of interest is the pronounced difference found for rate of learning of words at different positions in a serial list. The words in the middle of the list are much more difficult to learn in their correct order than are the words near the beginning and the end of the list. These differences in learning among positions are known as *serial position effects*. They are as ubiquitous for elderly participants as they are for younger participants. A familiar everyday example of serial position effects is the fact that spelling errors occur much more frequently for letters in the middle of a word than for letters at either end.

Verbosity

Elderly adults are commonly believed to be excessively talkative or verbose in the sense that their conversations seem to wander aimlessly away from the topic at hand and therefore prolong their conversations unnecessarily. Are elderly adults truly verbose? Probably more so than younger adults, but only for a minority of older adults. Researchers at Concordia University in Canada conducted interviews with a number of adults of all ages. They analyzed the contents of the answers of the participants to the questions they were asked in terms of the information given that was irrelevant to those questions (e.g., information about themselves, comments about the interviewer, and so on). They discovered that the percentage of elderly adults who were verbose was relatively small, but it was nevertheless higher than the percentage of younger adults. Those older adults identified as being verbose were generally socially outgoing people who were having some difficulty in functioning well in their daily lives. The more verbose elderly participants were also found to be more socially active, more extroverted, and experiencing greater stress than the less verbose elderly participants. The researchers also found no difference in memory between their verbose and nonverbose older participants, but they did find that verbose participants scored lower on a test of nonverbal intelligence than the nonverbose participants and also showed more signs of difficulty in inhibiting irrelevant thoughts.

Very Long-Term Memory

Try to remember—what was your third grade teacher's name? How many names of your grade school teachers can you recall? High school teachers? How is your memory for the foreign language words you acquired in your high school language class? The names of television programs from 10 years ago? These are all examples of *very long-term memory* (also called *remote* or *tertiary memory* by memory researchers) for impersonal events experienced years ago that you shared with other people. You certainly were not the only person who had Miss Johnson for a third grade teacher, the only one in the language class, or the only one watching television years ago. Very long-term memory refers to the retention of such past information, in contrast to long-term or secondary memory, which refers to the retention of newly acquired information (see EPISODIC MEMORY). Very long-term memory also consists of memory for your own personally experienced events, that is, autobiographical memory (see AUTOBIOGRAPHICAL MEMORY). Our present interest is only for those remote events of a more impersonal nature, such as teachers' names.

There is convincing evidence that many of these events are rapidly forgotten, with most of the forgetting taking place within 6 or so years after the events were encountered. Usually, only 20% to 40% of the information seems to be retained and held in what is called a "permastore" state (i.e., permanently available and highly resistant to forgetting from interference created by similar events occurring both before and after the events to be remembered, e.g., names of other people, including names of your children's teachers, names of other television programs before and after those of 10 years ago). Those events that remain in permastore are likely to be those that were especially well learned or overlearned. Thus memory for those events is likely, on the average, about what it was some years ago, and probably as good as the memory for comparable events for people age 30, 40, or 50 who are beyond the "6-year barrier." Elderly people frequently remark that their memories for remote events (tertiary memory) are very good; it is their memories for recent events that are not as good (secondary memory). Many of them are probably correct in their assessments of their own memories.

Vigilance

Vigilance refers to one's ability to maintain alertness to detect a change in otherwise constant conditions. For example, the parent of a sleeping infant stays vigilant until the infant begins to stir and cry. Here the constant condition is silence from the infant's crib, and the change is the occurrence of sounds from that crib. Similarly, a quality control inspector observes a steady stream of objects. The inspector maintains a state of vigilance while looking for an occasional object that fails to meet some standard established by the industry and must therefore be withdrawn.

The possibility of a decline with aging in the ability to detect occasional "odd" events in a series of otherwise of like events has been investigated in a number of studies. Research has been directed at two different kinds of vigilance. The first kind is *simple vigilance*. In tests of simple vigilance the demand placed on the observer is slight in that the "odd" event is clearly distinguishable from the like events. Laboratory research has concentrated on age differences in the accuracy of detecting the occurrences of the odd events. This research has made use of a clocklike device with a single moving hand and a large number of markers that resemble those indicating seconds on a true clock. Participants in research with this device watch the hand move from marker to marker for an hour. During that time the hand moves 3,600 times, of which only 23 are odd events. An odd event consists of a double jump of the hand. Participants are asked to signal when each double jump occurs. These double jumps occur at random times during the hour. As might be expected, accuracy in detecting a double jump decreases during the course of the hour. Fatigue does set in, and it makes its presence felt by failures to detect the double jumps that occur late in the series of jumps. However, there is convincing evidence to indicate that the decline in accuracy over time is no greater for older adults than for younger adults. In fact, accuracy throughout the tedious hour-long session is as high for elderly adults as for young adults.

The second kind of vigilance is *complex vigilance*. Here conditions are such that it is more difficult for the observer to detect the difference between the odd event and the like events. Consider, for example, the greater difficulty of a parent in detecting an infant's crying when the parent is busy vacuuming a rug rather than sitting in silence. Researchers at Catholic University created a laboratory situation in which complex vigilance had to be maintained. Their participants watched a series of numbers displayed on the screen. They were to signal whenever a zero appeared. Complexity was varied by the amount of visual degrading (blurring) of the numbers projected on the screen. Regardless of a participant's age, accuracy in detecting the zeros decreased as the degree of blurring increased. In addition, they found their older participants to be less accurate than their young participants even when the degree of blurring was relatively low. Other researchers have investigated age differences with various other ways of increasing the complexity of maintaining vigilance. They also found older adults to be less accurate than younger adults.

Unlike simple vigilance, complex vigilance does seem to decline moderately in proficiency with aging.

Vision

Visual impairment is one of the most prevalent physical impairments confronting elderly people. It is estimated that 13% of the overall elderly population of the United States has some form of visual impairment. For those age 85 and older it is estimated that 27% are visually impaired. Visual impairment accompanying normal aging brings with it a number of problems in daily living. Older people with considerable visual decline report greater difficulty in performing the normal functions of daily living (e.g., preparing meals) and in maintaining social interactions than elderly people who have relatively little visual decline. They are also likely to report lower morale and greater depression, again compared with older people with relatively little decline.

Visual decline is usually thought of in terms of static acuity (the ability to discriminate the fine details of a spatial pattern). Static acuity is measured by the familiar Snellen chart (rows of letters of different sizes that are read during an eye examination) and expressed by such scores as 20/20. Static acuity begins to decline at about age 40. By age 70 it has decreased by about 30% relative to the static acuity of people in their 20s. However, even with this decline it is estimated that only 1% of the elderly population meets the criterion for legal blindness (20/200 or worse vision in the better eye or a field of vision constricted to 20 degrees or less). The decline in static acuity is by no means the only form of visual impairment with normal aging. An even more dramatic decline occurs for dynamic acuity. Dynamic acuity is basically defined in terms of the smallest movement of an object that can be detected as movement by an observer. The decline in dynamic acuity begins at an earlier age than the decline in static acuity, and it progresses to the point where the loss is, on the average, nearly 60% for people in their 70s, relative to people in their 20s. However, evidence indicates that the impairment in dynamic acuity experienced by many older people may be greatly reduced when the moving target is exposed at a high level of illumination. The implication is that at least part of the decline in dynamic acuity is the result of the reduction of illumination that reaches the retina through the lens.

A number of other visual impairments accompany normal aging. Elderly people are more susceptible to the disrupting effects of glare than are younger people, and their peripheral vision is less extensive than that of younger people. The ability to locate the past position of objects in the visual field is less accurate among elderly people than younger people. This may be demonstrated by projecting on a computer screen a visual object at a certain position and then terminating the exposure. Participants are then asked to locate by a cursor where the target had been located on the screen. Recent research with this procedure has indicated that elderly participants are about 40% less accurate than young adult participants in correctly identifying the locations. Older adults are also less sensitive in detecting weak-intensity lights than younger adults. Elderly adults have a much higher absolute threshold for brightness than young adults. The absolute threshold is measured by presenting initially very dim lights and then increasing the brightness of the light until an intensity is reached where the light is detected half of the time it occurs. This intensity is the absolute threshold. The age difference in brightness sensitivity is also apparent for brightnesses that are well above the absolute threshold value. For example, if a light doubles in its brightness intensity, older adults will perceive it as increasing less than will younger adults. (For other changes in vision with aging, see COLOR PERCEPTION; CONSTANCIES OF PERCEPTION; DARK ADAPTATION; DEPTH PERCEPTION; FORM PERCEPTION; VISUAL DISORDERS.)

Visual Disorders

The visual impairment that occurs with normal aging (see VISION) is often compounded by abnormalities of the eye that are more common in late adulthood than in earlier adulthood. Foremost among these abnormalities are cataracts and glaucoma. A cataract is a clouding of the lens that lessens the sharpness of the image transmitted to the retina, resulting in blurred vision and an increased susceptibility to glare. Cataracts may be removed surgically by a procedure that is performed thousands of times annually in the United States. Glaucoma, a disease that rarely occurs before age 40, consists of an elevation of pressure within the eyeball that may, if not treated, damage the visual receptors in the retina. Often the symptoms of glaucoma are not noticed by individuals until the disease has progressed considerably. Consequently, regular eye examinations are important for early detection, especially for individuals age 40 and older. Treatment requires normalizing pressure within the eye, and it may be done by drugs such as beta-blockers or by laser surgery.

Other visual disorders that are less prevalent in late adulthood than cataracts or glaucoma, but more prevalent than in earlier adulthood, are macular degeneration and diabetic retinopathy. Macular degeneration consists of degeneration of visual receptor cells (cones) in the macular section of the retina (at its center is the fovea, the area most densely packed with cones and the most sensitive part of the retina), where most of our perception of finer details takes place. Elderly whites are more susceptible to degeneration than are elderly blacks. Loss of these cells results in the inability to resolve finer visual details. Consequently, reading and driving become very difficult tasks. The receptors in the periphery of the retina are rarely involved; thus, affected individuals are usually able to see sufficiently to move about and to care for themselves. There are two kinds of macular degeneration, dry and wet. In dry degeneration there is no leaking of fluid into or below the retina. In wet degeneration a pool of fluid and blood accumulates beneath the retina. Wet degeneration is sometimes (5% or less) reduced by means of laser coagulation. Diabetic retinopathy, or damage to the retina from vascular hemorrhages, may occur after years of diabetes. In some cases it may be treated by laser therapy or by surgery.

Visual disorders are much more likely to be present in nursing home residents than in others of the same ages living in the community. A survey of about 500 nursing home residents in Baltimore found them over 10 times more likely to be blind than were community dwellers. Many of the visual problems nursing home residents have could be corrected simply by having them obtain new glasses. The need for new, updated glasses is often overlooked by caregivers in nursing homes. Their attention is likely to be concentrated on more life-threatening illnesses of their patients. Relatives of patients in nursing homes should make sure that the patients receive eye examinations at regular intervals. Improving the vision of residents should greatly increase the quality of their lives.

Voice

In late adulthood the voices of many people tend to increase slightly in pitch as the vocal cords stiffen and vibrate at a higher frequency than earlier in life. For some elderly people the volume of their voices may decrease somewhat, and there may also be a quaver in the voice through some loss of control over the vocal cords. However, it remains uncertain whether these voice changes are a normal consequence of aging for many people or whether they are the consequence of poor health and the presence of a disease.

W

. . . .

Wechsler Intelligence Tests

For a number of years the Stanford-Binet test was the only individually administered intelligence test. This test was developed by Lewis Terman to measure the mental ages and intelligence quotients (IQs) of children and adolescents, and its use with adults was generally viewed as inappropriate. The void in individually administered intelligence tests was finally filled in 1939 by the appearance of the Wechsler-Bellevue Intelligence Test. The test was developed and standardized by Dr. David Wechsler, a psychologist at New York City's Bellevue Hospital. Several revisions of the test have appeared over the years, including the Wechsler Adult Intelligence Scale (WAIS) and the Wechsler Adult Intelligence Scale-Revised (WAIS-R; the version currently in use). The Wechsler tests have had wide use in both academic and clinical settings as a reliable measure of adult intelligence.

From the beginning, the Wechsler tests have had several distinguishing features. First, the tests yield a global or overall IQ score, but also separate IQ scores for two major components of intelligence that Wechsler called Verbal Intelligence and Performance Intelligence. Second, an individual's scores (overall, verbal, and performance) on the tests are evaluated relative to people of the same age who were included in Wechsler's standardization sample. That is, there are age norms for different age ranges from early to late adulthood (see NORMS). Thus older adults' scores on any of the test versions are interpreted relative to people their own age rather than to scores obtained by younger adults. An adult in his or her early 60s who has an IQ of 100 on any of the versions is therefore considered to be average with respect to people of that age. Third, each version of the Wechsler tests consists of 11 subtests, each considered to be a component of either verbal intelligence or performance intelligence. Scores on these subtests do correlate moderately highly with each other. These correlations (i.e., people who score high on one subtest have a greater than chance probability of scoring high on the other subtests as well) suggest that each subtest is measuring an ability determined in part by some general factor of intelligence that influences to some degree each specific ability. There are six verbal subtests and five performance tests. The six verbal subtests are information, comprehension, vocabulary, memory span, similarities, and arithmetic. The five performance subtests are picture arrangement, picture completion, block design, object assembly, and digit symbol.

Various subtests of the Wechsler tests have been widely used apart from their contributions to overall IQ scores and separate verbal and performance IQ scores. For example, the vocabulary subtest is a popular test for measuring verbal ability and for comparing adults of different ages (see VERBAL ABILITY). Similarly, the block design subtest is often used to compare adults of different ages in their spatial abilities (see SPATIAL ABILITY), and the digit symbol subtest to compare adults of different ages in their response speed (see SPEED OF BEHAVIOR).

Adult age differences in test scores (points earned on the test before they are converted into IQ scores) have been frequently found for total scores, verbal component only scores, and performance component only scores. Regardless of whether age differences are determined cross-sectionally or longitudinally, the scores tend to peak for people in their early 20s and then show a progressive decline from this age on. The rate of decline, however, is far more pronounced for performance scores than for verbal scores. In fact, when age groups are equated for educational level (there is moderately high correlation between years of education and test scores), scores on the verbal component have often been found to show an increase from early to late adulthood. The rate of decline in scores on the performance component has also been found to be reduced considerably when age groups are matched for educational level.

The various subtests show greatly different age effects. Some subtests are considered to be "hold" tests that show little decline in scores with advancing age (e.g., vocabulary, information), whereas other subtests are considered to be "don't hold" tests that show pronounced decline with advancing age (e.g., digit symbol, block design). Still other subtests, such as object assembly and picture completion, fall between the hold and don't hold subtests. That is, they show age-related declines in scores, but to a lesser degree than found for the don't hold subtests.

Most current researchers on intelligence make a distinction between crystallized intelligence and fluid intelligence as the two basic forms of intelligence in preference to Wechsler's distinction between verbal and performance intelligence (see INTELLIGENCE). However, the verbal component of the Wechsler test may be considered to approximate a measure of crystallized intelligence, and the performance component to approximate a measure of fluid intelligence. It is only an approximation, however. To many experts in intelligence testing, several subtests of the verbal component (e.g., memory span) are considered to be tests of fluid intelligence rather than crystallized intelligence.

Wechsler Memory Scale

The Wechsler Memory Scale is a widely used clinical test for diagnosing memory impairment, including moderate impairment shown with normal aging and more severe impairment with organic amnesia, Alzheimer's disease, and other forms of dementia. Included in the scale are subtests that evaluate proficiency in paired-associate learning (see VERBAL LEARNING) and story memory (see DISCOURSE MEMORY). The popularity of the scale is based largely on the availability of age norms that provide some indication of the deviation of a client from the average score for people of the client's age. However, the adequacy of these norms in determining whether an older client is experiencing a benign age-related decline in memory proficiency or is experiencing a more serious pathological decline is questionable.

Well-Being (Psychological)

Well-being is a broad concept that refers to an individual's current level of happiness or distress and his or her current satisfaction with life. Much of the research on age differences in well-being has been on the life satisfaction component of well-being (see LIFE SATISFACTION). However, other research has centered on the negative and positive affective (emotional) states of people of various ages. One of the tests used for this purpose is the General Well-Being Schedule. Participants taking this test are asked such questions as "Have you been anxious, worried, or upset during the past month?" to measure negative affect and such questions as "How happy, satisfied, or pleased have you been with your personal life during the past month?" to measure positive affect. Research with this test and similar tests has revealed that psychological well-being as defined by emotional states is remarkably stable from early adulthood through late adulthood. That is, the subjective experience of well-being of elderly adults seems to differ little from that of younger adults. Research on life satisfaction has generally yielded the same outcome. Satisfaction with one's present life does not seem to differ greatly among adults of different ages.

Most of the research on well-being has focused on what psychologists and sociologists believe to be the major determinants of the degree of well-being. Of further interest is what older individuals themselves believe to be the important determinants. This information was provided by Dr. Carol D. Ryff of the University of Wisconsin–Madison. She interviewed a number of middle-aged and elderly adults. Positive well-being was found to be associated with being an individual who is "others oriented," that is, being caring and having sound relationships with other people. In addition, middle-age individuals generally viewed a positive attitude toward one's self as being an important determinant of positive well-being. This was deemed less important by older adults. They instead viewed the ability to accept change as an important determinant of positive well-being; change was defined both in the sense of the respondents' own biological aging and in the world in which they live. They also believed personal growth to be a positive contributor to well-being. Personal growth refers to having a sense of continued development and self-realization. Dr. Ryff's evidence indicated that personal growth declines from young adulthood to middle age and declines even more to late adulthood. She also found that women of all ages report higher levels of personal growth than do men of all ages. For the very old (age 85 and older), positive well-being has been found to be associated with their independence in performing the activities of daily living (e.g., doing their own shopping, managing their own finances) and with their ability to control the events of their lives.

Other researchers have found well-being and life satisfaction to be greater for older adults who have a number of roles in their lives (e.g., employee, volunteer worker, spouse, parent, grandparent, and so on) than it is for older adults who have fewer roles to play. The positive effect of multiple roles tends to be greater for men than for women and greater for black men than for black women, white men, or white women.

Werner Syndrome

Werner syndrome is a rare inherited disease characterized by premature aging. Affected individuals have a normal childhood, but growth ordinarily ceases in the early teens. Signs of aging, such as cataracts and old-looking skin, appear when they are in their 20s. Heart disease is common, and death often occurs when the individuals are in their 40s.

White House Conferences on Aging

There is a White House Conference on Aging in each decade. For each conference several thousand delegates from the community and from professional organizations gather to discuss issues relevant to the welfare of elderly people and to conclude with recommendations directed at improving that welfare. The first conference was held in 1961. Recommendations from that conference eventually led to the creation of the Medicare and Medicaid programs. The second conference, held in 1971, resulted in the creation of the Meals on Wheels program. The most recent conference, held in May, 1995, was the first to address issues relevant to younger adults as well as elderly adults. Rather than proposing new legislation and new programs, the theme of this conference was to "hold the line"—that is, to maintain Social Security, Medicare, and other programs relevant to elderly people at their present levels, rather than reducing benefits.

Why Aging? (Biological Theories of Aging)

Biological aging is as inevitable as death and taxes; yet why the human organism ages is not fully understood. Many theories have been proposed, but no single theory has become universally accepted as *the* most valid theory. Conceivably, aging is the result of a number of changes in the human body as we grow older, and each theory may have some element of truth.

Some biological theories of aging are based on the principle of a biological clock that is genetically present in all of us. Generally, the "clock" is assumed to be in some area of the brain, and a signal of some kind from the brain triggers a number of the biological changes associated with aging. One theory based on the principle of a biological clock has the pacemaker for regulating the clock located in the neurons of higher brain centers. Stimulation from these neurons causes changes in the body's endocrine system and/or changes in the metabolic activity of various organs. Alternatively, only prematurity stages of development are programmed genetically, and genetic regulation of development ends at maturity. From this point on, the body is susceptible to the ravages of "wear and tear," in which the parts of the body accumulate defects from use and misuse, and from intruders to the body from disease, pollution, and so on. The analogy here is that of a machine whose parts eventually wear out at different rates from constant use. The analogy is not a perfect one, however. Biological systems, unlike machines, have the capability of self-repair. For some systems (e.g., the skin), new cells form to replace old ones; for other systems (e.g., muscles), new cells are not formed, but other self-repair mechanisms occur.

Biological theories of aging also differ in the particular location of where the changes responsible for aging take place. One class of theories places the location at the level of the body's cells. Theories in this class may then be further divided into genetic and nongenetic theories. Genetic theories typically view damage by radiation or mutation to cellular deoxyribonucleic acid (DNA) as the cause of aging. DNA controls the formation of the proteins that are needed by cells to sustain life. However, there is little support for this theory. Another possibility is an increase in errors of transferring information from DNA cellular molecules to ribonucleic acid (RNA) cellular molecules. Such errors are believed to produce one or more proteins that are not exact copies of the original protein in the cell. The inexact copy cannot execute its mission of maintaining cellular life, and cells age and die as a result. This theory is a promising one, but one that has been difficult to prove. Another genetic theory is that cells are programmed to reproduce themselves only so many times, and without reproduction they die.

Nongenetic theories stress that the aging and death of cells is the result of their accumulation of metabolic wastes and harmful substances (such as lipofuscin, a fibrous protein known to increase in cellular amount with aging), which interfere with cellular functioning. This theory has not received much support. Yet another cellular theory is the free radical theory. Unstable chemical compounds are believed to accumulate in the cells and interact with other normal cellular molecules to alter proteins essential for life. The evidence in support of the theory has not been great (see also ANTIOXIDANTS).

The other major class of theories places the location at the level of a particular organ or system of organs. One such theory, and probably the most viable one, is the immunological theory of aging. The body's immune system protects the body against invading microorganisms and atypical cell mutants (e.g., cancer). Through the immune system the body generates antibodies that react with the proteins of foreign organisms and form defensive cells that digest the foreign bodies. Aging is known to affect the immune system. The production of antibodies declines with aging, as does the ability of antibodies that are formed to recognize mutated cells (thus accounting for the increased incidence of cancer in late adulthood). The net effect is to produce those biological decrements associated with normal aging.

Why Aging? (Psychological Theories of Aging)

Most psychological theories of aging stress that both decline and growth occur for mental functioning and behaviors throughout adult development. Decline is brought about by biological changes that alter the brain and other parts of the body (see WHY AGING? [BIOLOGICAL THEORIES OF AGING]) and result in slower mental processes, diminished working memory capacity, slower reaction times, and so on. At the same time, growth occurs through increases in knowledge and experience over the entire course of adult development. Growth is manifested in the ability to alter our behaviors in response to changes in the physical and social context (or environment) in which people live as they grow older. This theoretical position is known as *contextualism.* Dr. Paul Baltes, a prominent gerontologist at the Max Planck Institute for Human Development and Education in Berlin, argues effectively that people play an active role in changing themselves through accumulated wisdom and experience to meet new challenges and new life crises brought about by their changing context. Further growth in the form of reversing declines that often appear in late adulthood may take place through interventions of various kinds (see PLASTICITY THEORY).

Another strong advocate of positive growth in late adulthood is Dr. Gisele Labouvie-Vief of Wayne State University. She has observed that many of the age differences seen in mental performance are the result of qualitative rather than quantitative changes in late adulthood (see CONTINUITY VS. DISCONTINUITY IN ADULT DEVELOPMENT). Consider, for example, a likely age difference in response to information given that a wife has threatened to leave her husband if he comes home drunk one more time—and eventually he does. Young adults typically respond with the seemingly logical conclusion that she will certainly leave her husband. Many elderly adults, however, will go beyond the information given and consider situational factors (i.e., the context) that may be involved. For example, the husband may have heard that day of the death of a close friend, and he had a few drinks to help relieve his sorrow.

A theoretical approach that has been followed by a number of gerontologists is the dialecticism introduced by the late Dr. Klaus Riegel. From a dialectical perspective, internal factors, such as physiological states and personality traits, are viewed as interacting with external factors in the physical, social, occupational, and familial environments. Crises in a person's life occur when internal and external factors are out of synchrony. The types of asynchrony and resulting crises people encounter differ at different stages of their lives. However, the ability to resolve crises is as true of elderly adults as it is of younger adults (see PERSONALITY STAGES).

Widowhood and Widowerhood

Widowhood and widowerhood refer to the state of a woman or man, respectively, who has not remarried after the death of a spouse. There are more widows than widowers in the United States, partly because longevity is greater for women and partly because men aged 65 and older are less likely than women of the same age range to survive long after the death of a spouse. Another contributing factor is the greater probability of remarriage by widowers (often with younger women) than by widows. Widows who either remarry or consider remarrying tend to be younger than those widows who do not.

The first stage of widowhood or widowerhood is usually that of grief. Evidence indicates that grief persists at least 30 months (and probably longer) after the death of a spouse for most widows and many widowers. However, elderly men are more likely than elderly women to repress their emotional distress after the death of a spouse. Such repression may contribute to the earlier death after widowerhood for men than after widowhood for women. Researchers at the University of Southern California found that men who survive the initial 18 months of widowerhood are likely to live the same life span as they would without the death of their spouse.

The resolution of grief or bereavement is generally viewed as depending on the coping strengths of the individual experiencing the bereavement as well as the nature of the social network available to that individual. Gerontologists continue to debate whether grief is experienced more intensely by widows or by widowers. After 6 or so months, grief, and the loneliness that accompanies it, is typically followed by a reorganization of the widow's or widower's life. The reorganization requires a role transition from being a member of a husband-wife team to being on one's own. Most of the research by gerontologists has focused on the social networks of the widow or widower that may either aid or hinder the role transition. This research has revealed that a network of friends is of greater aid than is a network of family members. Research at Portland State University has provided information as to why this difference probably exists. Widows and widowers perceive friends to be more flexible in their relations with them than family members. Family members are perceived as frequently placing unwanted commitments on the widow or widower (e.g., frequent babysitting of grandchildren).

Bereaved widows and widowers are also likely to view their late spouses more positively and their marriage as having been more satisfying than do nonbereaved elderly married people. The results of a recent survey of bereaved and nonbereaved older people in California indicated further that the more positive widows and widowers viewed their marriage retrospectively, the more likely they were to feel depressed. By contrast, the opposite was true for elderly people who were still married. That is, they were more likely to feel depressed when they viewed their ongoing marriage as being less satisfactory.

Widows who have remarried tend to express fewer concerns about financial matters, home maintenance, and so on than either widows who did not remarry or widows who considered remarriage but did not. Moreover, widows who remarry tend to report fewer concerns about these matters than they recall having during the period after their first husband's death. By contrast, widows who consider remarriage (but do not remarry) tend to report, on the average, more concerns than they experienced after their husband's death.

Of further interest is the possible difference between the bereavement experienced by elderly widows and widowers whose spouses died suddenly and unexpectedly and the bereavement experienced by elderly widows and widowers whose spouses died from natural causes and whose death was therefore largely expected. Recent surveys have indicated that the survivors of suicide and other forms of sudden, unexpected death (e.g., from an automobile accident) differed from survivors of natural death in the greater intensity of emotional distress. Widows and widowers of spouses who suffered from a lingering terminal illness tend to experience anticipatory grieving that accompanies the illness. Such anticipation of grief seems to ease their emotional strain after the spouse's death. Anticipatory grieving probably accounts for the fact that the depression and anxiety experienced 6 or so months after a spouse's death is less for elderly survivors than it is for young survivors.

Wisdom

The definition of *wisdom* in a dictionary is likely to read something like "the ability to judge soundly and deal well with facts, especially as they relate to life and conduct." Wisdom does seem to be related to intelligence, especially to that form of intelligence known as crystallized intelligence (see INTELLIGENCE) in which life's experiences add to our accumulated knowledge. However, intelligence is usually used in reference to knowledge of words (vocabulary), knowledge about famous people ("Who wrote *Hamlet?*"), knowledge about famous events ("When did the Civil War begin?"), knowledge about geography ("What's the largest city in Ethiopia?"), and so on—the kind of knowledge we find being tested daily on such television shows as *Jeopardy.*

Wisdom means a different kind of knowledge, but one, nevertheless, likely to accumulate with years of living. Researchers at the Max Planck Institute in Berlin have been vigorously conducting research on wisdom. As they define it, *wisdom* consists of an expert knowledge system dealing with the pragmatics of life, such as life planning and life management. They believe that not all elderly people excel in wisdom, relative to younger people, but they also believe that the percentage of older people who excel in wisdom is significantly greater than the percentage of younger people. Their research studies lend considerable support to their belief. Participants of various ages are given problems that deal with such topics as life planning and asked how the problem might be resolved. For example, in one of the problems the dilemma facing a 60-year-old widow is described. She had recently received a business degree and had opened her own business, an activity very important to her. However, she heard that her son had been left with two small children in his care. What should she do—close her business and move in with her son to care for the children, or should she arrange for financial aid for her son to cover the cost of child care? The quality of the solutions proposed has been found to be higher for older adults than for younger adults. However, the quality of solutions was also found to be slightly higher for young adults when the problem concerned one facing a young adult. Wisdom does seem to be a mental ability that increases with age, rather than declines (as is also true for the kinds of knowledge considered to be part of crystallized intelligence).

Word Associations

For each of the following words, give the first word that comes to mind: *table, king, bread.*

A fairly safe prediction is that the words you gave were "chair," "queen," and "butter." These are examples of word associations. When *table, king,* and *bread* are given to a group of people, most of the members of the group will respond with "chair," "queen," and "butter." The most popular, or frequently given, association to a given word is called the *primary associate*. Table, king, and bread are examples of words that have strong (highly probable) primary associates. This is true regardless of the adult age level of the group members giving the associates. It is also true that most word associates are of a particular form known as a paradigmatic associate. This is again true for both younger and normally aging older adults. A *paradigmatic associate* is one that is of the same grammatical group or form as the word to which it is given (e.g., both nouns, as in the case of "queen" to *king*). Paradigmatic associates may also usually replace each other in a sentence without a major change in the meaning of that sentence. For example, "The _____ sat on the throne"—either king or queen may fill the blank meaningfully.

Not all words have strong primary associates. Consider the word *deep*. Associates are likely to include "shallow," "dark," and "water." "Shallow" is the primary associate, but it is given by fewer than 20% of a group of adults, again regardless of the members' age level. Incidentally, "water" as an associate to *deep* is an example of what is called a syntagmatic associate. A *syntagmatic associate* is of a different grammatical class than the word to which it is associated (e.g., noun and adjective for water and deep), and they do not replace each other in a sentence. Normally aging adults and younger adults give relatively few syntagmatic associates. By contrast, children and patients with Alzheimer's disease give frequent syntagmatic associates.

The pronounced similarity of word associations among adults of different ages strongly suggests that there is little change in the organization or structure of our mental dictionaries or lexicons (see LEXICON). Another type of word association adds to our conviction that aging has little, if any, effect on the structure of the lexicon. Here, participants are given taxonomic categories, such as "a metal" and "a four-footed animal," and they are asked to name several instances or exemplars of each category. Categorical names are an important part of the organization of related words in our lexicons. Most people will respond with "iron," "copper," and "gold" when asked to name metals and with "dog," "cat," and "horse" when asked to name four-footed animals. This is as true for normally aging elderly adults as it is for younger adults.

Work

According to the U.S. Department of Labor, the percentage of men older than age of 65 who participated in the labor force decreased from nearly 50% in 1950 to about 17% in 1991. Moreover, the percentage of men between the ages of 55 and 64 decreased from about 90% to nearly 50% during the same period. The decline is especially pronounced for blue-collar workers. Various surveys conducted in the 1980s indicated that blue-collar workers retire at a younger age than do white-collar workers, with the average age of retirement for service workers between the two. Although the decline in participation has been less pronounced for women, a similar trend of decreasing work involvement is apparent. The declining participation of older people in the labor force, combined with increases in longevity for many older people, means that the ratio of retired elderly people to employed younger people has been steadily increasing. The net effect has been to increase the tax burden on those in the labor force to finance programs directly relevant to elderly people (e.g., Social Security, Medicare).

A recent survey of men age 69 to 84 revealed that about 1 in 6 was currently employed and about 1 in 5 had worked at some time in the prior year. About a third of those employed worked full time. The reasons given for working were good health and a strong dislike for retirement. Of those surveyed who were not working, very few indicated a desire to be working. The probability of employment was found to be positively related to educational level (the higher the level, the greater the likelihood of employment), negatively related to amount of income (the higher the income, the lower the likelihood of employment), and negatively related to age (the higher the age, the lower the likelihood of employment).

The trend toward fewer working older people has taken place even though the legal minimum mandatory age increased from 65 to 70 in 1978 and has since been eliminated for many workers. Why are so many older people withdrawing from the labor force? One of the more frequent reasons people give for withdrawal is their health status. Men who report their health to be poor do retire an average of more than a year earlier than men who report their health to be at least good. However, it seems unlikely that poor health is the major reason for the decline of older people in the labor force. In general, the health status of older people has been increasing, not decreasing, over the past 40 years. Many older people may cite declining health as the reason for their retirement because they believe it to be a more socially acceptable reason than the real reason (e.g., wanting more leisure time), or they may be seeking disability benefits. A more important reason for retiring at age 65 (and often earlier) is the financial benefit often received by so doing. About 90% of retired people have at least some of their retirement income from Social Security. People who retire beyond age 65 are penalized in terms of their Social

Security benefits relative to what they would have received if they had retired at age 65 or earlier. The same is true for people receiving private pensions on retirement (about 35% of retirees do). That is, it is financially to their benefit to retire earlier rather than later.

Another important issue regarding aging and work is the relationship between the ages of workers and their satisfaction with their jobs. In general, the evidence indicates that job satisfaction increases with age. Older workers tend to express greater satisfaction with their jobs than do younger workers. A recent study of city and county managers in Florida revealed the probable reason for this increase in job satisfaction with increasing age. Older workers tend to perceive their jobs as having characteristics that more closely match their own needs than do younger workers. This is a likely reason that absenteeism from the job, both voluntary and involuntary, has been found to be inversely related to age. Older workers are absent less frequently than are younger workers. This seems to be true at least until workers approach some fixed retirement age. A study by researchers at the University of Kansas Medical Center revealed that the closer male workers came to that age, the more burdensome their jobs became in terms of tension and fatigue experienced at work.

Our society needs to recognize that future generations of elderly people will be healthier and better educated than the present generation. Future elderly people are therefore more likely than current elderly people to want to work in what are considered to be the retirement years. Means of finding ways of enabling them to do so need to be found, such as increasing the opportunity for training on new jobs or retraining on old jobs that have had new technological advances.

Working Memory

Memory researchers believe that a very important part of the human memory system is a component they call *working memory*. Working memory functions like a "mental box" that is divided into two parts. The first part is a store for holding prior information briefly (see SHORT-TERM MEMORY); the second part is a place for performing various mental operations. Consider what you are doing when you add the numbers 9, 5, and 7. The first two numbers are summed to give 14. This information is held in the store component of working memory while you identify the next number and add it to 14 to give 21 (this is accomplished within the operations component). The operations component is especially important for long-term memory. It is here that new information is encoded and placed in the long-term store, and it is also here where a memory search is conducted to recall or recognize information previously placed in the long-term store.

Working memory is believed to have a limited capacity both for the storage of prior information and for conducting such mental operations as encoding new information for memorization. Most researchers of memory aging believe that the capacity of working memory diminishes during the course of the adult life span, becoming moderately less in late adulthood than in early adulthood. Whether capacity diminishes with aging only for storage or only for conducting mental operations, or for both, is not fully understood. However, the evidence to date suggests that storage capacity decreases only slightly, and the operations capacity decreases somewhat more, on the average.

Working memory's overall capacity is usually determined by measuring a participant's reading span. The participant is first given a sentence that must be answered true or false while at the same time remembering the last word in the sentence. For example, consider "Beaches are often found by an ocean" as the sentence. "True" is the correct answer, and "ocean" is the word to be remembered. If the last word is remembered correctly, the participant is then given two consecutive sentences, each to be answered true or false and each to have its last word remembered. For example, the participant may read the sentences "Cats are members of the canine family" and "A rose is a flower found in many gardens." The sentences are answered "false" and "true," respectively, and "family" and "gardens" are the words to be remembered. If both last words are remembered correctly, then the participant receives three consecutive sentences, with three last words to be remembered. This procedure continues until the number of sentences in the series is too large to permit memory of all of the last words. The largest number of sentences that can be spanned without a memory error defines the participant's reading span. The reading span of elderly participants has been found to average about one sentence less than that of young adult participants, presumably reflecting the decrease in working memory's capacity with aging.

Individual differences among elderly participants in their reading spans have been found to be related to their scores on various memory tasks, such as the recall of a story's content. Older participants with greater span scores (and presumably greater working memory capacity) are more proficient memorizers than elderly participants with smaller span scores (and presumably smaller working memory capacities).

A decline in working memory's capacity is not necessarily an inevitable consequence of normal aging. There is evidence to indicate that working memory is one of the abilities that are positively affected by long-term regular physical exercise (see EXERCISE AND PHYSI-CAL/MENTAL PERFORMANCE). Elderly people who have been regular exercisers for years tend to have larger reading span scores than elderly people who have had less active physical lives. The extent to which highly active mental lives may slow any age-related decline in working memory's capacity is unknown.

Index of
Entries and Cross-References

. . . .

Index of
Entries by Broad Topics

· ·